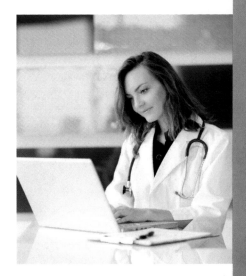

Oral and Maxillofacial Radiology

Editor

DANIA TAMIMI

RADIOLOGIC CLINICS OF NORTH AMERICA

www.radiologic.theclinics.com

Consulting Editor
FRANK H. MILLER

January 2018 • Volume 56 • Number 1

ELSEVIER

1600 John F. Kennedy Boulevard • Suite 1800 • Philadelphia, Pennsylvania, 19103-2899

http://www.theclinics.com

RADIOLOGIC CLINICS OF NORTH AMERICA Volume 56, Number 1
January 2018 ISSN 0033-8389, ISBN 13: 978-0-323-56655-1

Editor: John Vassallo (j.vassallo@elsevier.com)
Developmental Editor: Donald Mumford

Radiologic Clinics of North America (ISSN 0033-8389) is published bimonthly by Elsevier Inc., 360 Park Avenue South, New York, NY 10010-1710. Months of issue are January, March, May, July, September, and November. Periodicals postage paid at New York, NY and additional mailing offices. Subscription prices are USD 493 per year for US individuals, USD 889 per year for US institutions, USD 100 per year for US students and residents, USD 573 per year for Canadian individuals, USD 1136 per year for Canadian institutions, USD 680 per year for international individuals, USD 1136 per year for international institutions, and USD 315 per year for Canadian and international students/residents. To receive student and resident rate, orders must be accompanied by name of affiliated institution, date of term and the signature of program/residency coordinatior on institution letterhead. Orders will be billed at individual rate until proof of status is received. Foreign air speed delivery is included in all *Clinics* subscription prices. All prices are subject to change without notice. **POSTMASTER:** Send address changes to *Radiologic Clinics of North America*, Elsevier Health Sciences Division, Subscription Customer Service, 3251 Riverport Lane, Maryland Heights, MO63043. **Customer Service: Telephone: 1-800-654-2452** (U.S. and Canada); **1-314-447-8871** (outside U.S. and Canada). **Fax: 1-314-447-8029. E-mail: journalscustomerservice-usa@ elsevier.com (for print support); journalsonlinesupport-usa@elsevier.com (for online support)**.

Reprints. For copies of 100 or more of articles in this publication, please contact the Commercial Reprints Department, Elsevier Inc., 360 Park Avenue South, New York, New York 10010-1710. Tel.: +1-212-633-3874; Fax: +1-212-633-3820; E-mail: reprints@elsevier.com.

Radiologic Clinics of North America also published in Greek Paschalidis Medical Publications, Athens, Greece.

Radiologic Clinics of North America is covered in *MEDLINE/PubMed (Index Medicus), EMBASE/Excerpta Medica, Current Contents/Life Sciences, Current Contents/Clinical Medicine, RSNA Index to Imaging Literature, BIOSIS, Science Citation Index,* and *ISI/BIOMED.*

Printed in the United States of America.

Contributors

CONSULTING EDITOR

FRANK H. MILLER, MD
Chief, Body Imaging Section and Fellowship
Program, Medical Director of MRI, Professor,
Department of Radiology, Northwestern
University Feinberg School of Medicine,
Chicago, Illinois, USA

EDITOR

DANIA TAMIMI, BDS, DMSc
Consultant, Oral and Maxillofacial Radiology,
Private Practice, Orlando, Florida, USA

AUTHORS

MANSUR AHMAD, BDS, PhD
Associate Professor, Department of Diagnostic
and Biological Sciences, University of
Minnesota School of Dentistry, Minneapolis,
Minnesota, USA

**ASMA'A ABDURRAHMAN AL-EKRISH,
MDS, Cert Diag Sci (OMFR)**
Associate Professor, Department of Oral
Medicine and Diagnostic Sciences, Division of
Oral and Maxillofacial Radiology, College of
Dentistry, King Saud University, Riyadh, Saudi
Arabia

REYHANEH ALIMOHAMMADI, DDS
Oral and Maxillofacial Radiology, The
University of Texas Health Science Center at
San Antonio, School of Dentistry, San Antonio,
Texas, USA

BRUNO AZEVEDO, DDS, MS
Assistant Professor, Radiology and Imaging
Sciences, Department of Surgical & Hospital
Dentistry, University of Louisville, Louisville,
Kentucky, USA

ERIKA BENAVIDES, DDS, PhD
Diplomate, American Board of Oral and
Maxillofacial Radiology, Clinical Associate
Professor, Department of Periodontics and
Oral Medicine, University of Michigan, School
of Dentistry, Ann Arbor, Michigan, USA

LAURENCE GAALAAS, DDS, MS
Assistant Professor, Department of Diagnostic
and Biological Sciences, University of
Minnesota School of Dentistry, Minneapolis,
Minnesota, USA

ANITA GOHEL, BDS, PhD
Clinical Professor and Program Director, Oral
and Maxillofacial Radiology, Division of Oral
and Maxillofacial Pathology and Radiology,
The Ohio State University College of Dentistry,
Columbus, Ohio, USA

DAVID HATCHER, DDS, MSc
Private Practice, Diagnostic Digital Imaging,
Sacramento, California, USA

MOHAMMED ABBAS HUSAIN, DDS
Assistant Clinical Professor, Section of Oral
and Maxillofacial Radiology, UCLA School of
Dentistry, Los Angeles, California, USA

ELNAZ JALALI, DDS, MDSc
Private Practice, Miami, Florida, USA

SANJAY M. MALLYA, BDS, MDS, PhD
Associate Professor and Chair, Section of
Oral and Maxillofacial Radiology, UCLA
School of Dentistry, Los Angeles, California,
USA

SHAZA MARDINI, DDS, MS
Oral Maxillofacial Radiologist, BeamReaders
Inc, Knoxville, Tennessee, USA

FARAH MASOOD, BDS, DDS, MS
Diplomate, American Board of Oral
and Maxillofacial Radiology, Professor,
Department Oral Diagnosis and
Radiology, The University of Oklahoma
College of Dentistry, Oklahoma City,
Oklahoma, USA

MEL MUPPARAPU, DMD, MDS
Professor of Oral Medicine, Director of
Radiology, University of Pennsylvania School
of Dental Medicine, Philadelphia,
Pennsylvania, USA

MITRA SADRAMELI, DMD, MS
Clinical Assistant Professor, The University of
British Columbia, Private Practice, Vancouver,
British Columbia, Canada

WILLIAM C. SCARFE, BDS, FRACDS, MS
Professor and Director, Radiology and Imaging
Sciences, Department of Surgical & Hospital
Dentistry, University of Louisville, Louisville,
Kentucky, USA

DOUGLAS D. STEFFY, DDS, MS
Oral and Maxillofacial Radiologist, United
States Navy, Captain James A. Lovell Federal
Health Care Center, North Chicago, Illinois,
USA

DANIA TAMIMI, BDS, DMSc
Consultant, Oral and Maxillofacial Radiology,
Private Practice, Orlando, Florida, USA

CLARENCE S. TANG, DDS, MD
Oral and Maxillofacial Surgeon, United States
Navy, Captain James A. Lovell Federal Health
Care Center, North Chicago, Illinois, USA

SOTIRIOS TETRADIS, DDS, PhD
Senior Associate Dean and Professor, Section of
Oral and Maxillofacial Radiology, UCLA School
of Dentistry, Los Angeles, California, USA

SHIVA TOGHYANI, DDS, MS
Assistant Professor, Radiology and Imaging
Sciences, Department of Surgical & Hospital
Dentistry, University of Louisville, Louisville,
Kentucky, USA

SUSAN M. WHITE, DDS
Private Practice, Merrimack, New Hampshire,
USA

Contents

Head and neck imaging studies frequently encompass the oral cavity and human dentition. Given the relatively wide prevalence of dental disease, the likelihood of detecting incidental dental pathology is high. This article provides an overview of dental terminology, anatomy, restorations, and associated computed tomography imaging artifacts necessary to more effectively interpret and communicate findings related to teeth.

This article deals with identification and descriptions of intraoral and extraoral anatomy of the dental and maxillofacial structures. The anatomic landmarks are highlighted and described based on their radiographic appearance and their clinical significance is provided. Cone-beam computed tomography–based images are described in detail using the multiplanar reconstructions. The skull views are depicted via line diagrams in addition to their normal radiographic appearance to make identification of anatomic structures easier for clinicians. The authors cover most of the anatomic structures commonly noted via radiographs and their descriptions. This article serves as a clinician's guide to oral and maxillofacial radiographic anatomy.

Odontogenic infections represent a common clinical problem in patients of all ages. The presence of teeth enables the direct spread of inflammatory products from dental caries, trauma, and/or periodontal disease into the maxilla and mandible. The radiographic changes seen depend on the type and duration of the inflammatory process and host body response. Imaging plays a central role in identifying the source of infection and the extent of the disease spread and in detecting any complications. Many different imaging modalities can be used. The radiographic features associated with acute and chronic inflammatory processes are discussed.

Numerous benign cysts or solid tumors may present in the jaws. These arise from tooth-forming tissues in the dental alveolus or from nonodontogenic tissues in the basal bone of the mandible and maxilla. Radiologists provide 2 deliverables to assist in diagnosis and management: (1) appropriately formatted images demonstrating the location and extent of the lesion and (2) interpretive reports highlighting specific radiologic findings and an impression providing a radiologic differential diagnosis.

This article provides guidance on essential image protocols for planning treatments, a radiologic differential diagnostic algorithm based on location and pattern recognition, and a summary of the main features of benign odontogenic lesions.

Malignant Lesions in the Dentomaxillofacial Complex

Susan M. White

Malignancies in the maxillofacial region are rare but comprise a broad spectrum of lesions. Given the potential for malignancies to mimic dental/sinus/temporomandibular joint pathology or remain asymptomatic, the judicious radiologist will be familiar with the initial and unique malignant changes affecting the dentition, periodontium, and supporting osseous structures on conventional film, dental, and sinus imaging. This article is meant to serve as a complement to the many excellent texts dedicated to advanced imaging techniques for the staging of known malignancies. The lesions discussed are a representative sample of malignancies involving hard tissues of the maxillofacial complex but are far from complete.

Imaging of Radiation- and Medication-Related Osteonecrosis

Sanjay M. Mallya and Sotirios Tetradis

Osteonecrosis is the devitalization of bone and consequent lytic changes. In the jaws, osteonecrosis is a pathologic consequence of prior radiation therapy (osteoradionecrosis) or certain antiresorptive medications. Herein, we review the pathogenesis and clinical manifestations of these lesions, and describe the spectrum of radiologic findings in these conditions, and highlight the similarities and differences between the imaging appearances of these 2 entities.

Fibro-osseous and Other Lesions of Bone in the Jaws

Mansur Ahmad and Laurence Gaalaas

Fibro-osseous lesions in the jaws have similar histologic and radiographic features. Despite their similarity, management varies significantly. In this article, common fibro-osseous lesions and key radiographic features are described. Many of the fibro-osseous lesions are diagnosed radiographically, without performing histologic examinations. For some of the fibro-osseous lesions, for example, periapical osseous dysplasia, histologic examination is contraindicated. Cherubism and fibrous dysplasia have specific radiographic findings; these conditions can be diagnosed radiographically. Accurate diagnosis of conditions is essential; some conditions do not require any intervention, whereas others require surgical resection. Patient demographics, for example, age, gender, and race, play important roles in diagnosis.

Imaging of Dentoalveolar and Jaw Trauma

Reyhaneh Alimohammadi

Before the invention of cone-beam computed tomography (CT), use of 2-dimensional plain film imaging for trauma involving the mandible was common practice, with CT imaging opted for in cases of more complex situations, especially in the maxilla and related structures. Cone-beam CT has emerged as a reasonable and reliable alternative considering radiation dosage, image quality, and comfort for the patient. This article presents an overview of the patterns of dental and maxillofacial fractures using conventional and advanced imaging techniques illustrated with multiple clinical examples selected from the author's oral and maxillofacial radiology practice database.

A variety of factors can affect the normal development of tissues and may lead to variation in the normal compliment of teeth and development of alterations in the shape and size of teeth. These anomalies can be congenital, developmental, or acquired. Dental anomalies can present as isolated traits or be associated with systemic conditions and syndromes for which early diagnosis and genetic testing may result in better treatment outcomes and quality of life. Dentists play an essential role in the multidisciplinary management of these abnormalities. This article discusses some of these tooth alterations and associated systemic and genetic conditions.

The article presents an overview of the goal of imaging at each stage of implant therapy and the usefulness and limitations of multidetector computed tomography (MDCT) in achieving those goals. Various MDCT protocols of use in implant imaging also are presented, with an emphasis on dose reduction and the use of iterative reconstruction techniques. Also discussed are options for viewing and analysis of CT images, issues related to appropriate image reformatting and interpretation, interactive treatment planning, and transfer of information from the images to the surgical field during implant surgery using surgical guides and CT-guided navigation systems.

The temporomandibular joint (TMJ) is an anatomically and biomechanically complex structure. Understanding how this structure grows and functions is essential to accurate radiographic evaluation. This article discusses the anatomy, function, and growth and development of the TMJ and how growth changes can affect the morphology of the craniofacial structures. Accordingly, the radiographic appearance of the entities that may alter the TMJ are discussed, including developmental, degenerative, inflammatory, and traumatic changes. Both osseous imaging and soft tissue imaging are shown.

Sleep-disordered breathing and obstructive sleep apnea are becoming more prevalent in today's population. Management of these conditions can be difficult, and this diagnosis is often overlooked by clinicians. An increased awareness and understanding of craniofacial structures and anatomic relationships can aid the clinician in identifying at-risk patients, and improve treatment outcomes. An airway review of 3-dimensional computed tomography imaging can identify (1) anatomic variations that contribute to obstructive airway complications, and (2) measurable dimensions to identify at-risk patients. This article provides instruction on the key anatomic landmarks and imaging protocols for radiographic airway evaluation.

PROGRAM OBJECTIVE

The objective of the *Radiologic Clinics of North America* is to keep practicing radiologists and radiology residents up to date with current clinical practice in radiology by providing timely articles reviewing the state of the art in patient care.

TARGET AUDIENCE

Practicing radiologists, radiology residents, and other healthcare professionals who provide patient care utilizing radiologic findings.

LEARNING OBJECTIVES

Upon completion of this activity, participants will be able to:
1. Review oral and maxillofacial anatomy and terminology for the radiologist.
2. Discuss imaging of benign and malignant odontogenic and dento-maxillofacial lesions.
3. Recognize imaging of systemic issues, jaw trauma, and other oral and maxillofacial concerns.

ACCREDITATION

The Elsevier Office of Continuing Medical Education (EOCME) is accredited by the Accreditation Council for Continuing Medical Education (ACCME) to provide continuing medical education for physicians.

The EOCME designates this enduring material for a maximum of 15 *AMA PRA Category 1 Credit*(s)™. Physicians should claim only the credit commensurate with the extent of their participation in the activity.

All other healthcare professionals requesting continuing education credit for this enduring material will be issued a certificate of participation.

DISCLOSURE OF CONFLICTS OF INTEREST

The EOCME assesses conflict of interest with its instructors, faculty, planners, and other individuals who are in a position to control the content of CME activities. All relevant conflicts of interest that are identified are thoroughly vetted by EOCME for fair balance, scientific objectivity, and patient care recommendations. EOCME is committed to providing its learners with CME activities that promote improvements or quality in healthcare and not a specific proprietary business or a commercial interest.

The planning committee, staff, authors and editors listed below have identified no financial relationships or relationships to products or devices they or their spouse/life partner have with commercial interest related to the content of this CME activity:

Mansur Ahmad, BDS, PhD; Asma'a Abdurrahman Al-Ekrish, MDS, Cert Diag Sci (OMFR); Reyhaneh Alimohammadi, DDS; Bruno Azevedo, DDS, MS; Erika Benavides, DDS, PhD; Anjali Fortna; Laurence Gaalaas, DDS, MS; Anita Gohel, BDS, PhD; David Hatcher, DDS, MSc; Mohammed Abbas Husain, DDS; Elnaz Jalali, DDS, MDSc; Leah Logan; Sanjay M. Mallya, BDS, MDS, PhD; Shaza Mardini, DDS, MS; Farah Masood, BDS, DDS, MS; Mel Mupparapu, DMD, MDS; Mitra Sadrameli, DMD, MS; William C. Scarfe, BDS, FRACDS, MS; Douglas D. Steffy, DDS, MS; Karthik Subramaniam; Dania Tamimi, BDS, DMSc; Clarence S. Tang, DDS, MD; Shiva Toghyani, DDS, MS; John Vassallo; Susan M. White, DDS.

The planning committee, staff, authors and editors listed below have identified financial relationships or relationships to products or devices they or their spouse/life partner have with commercial interest related to the content of this CME activity:

Sotirios Tetradis, DDS, PhD is a consultant/advisor, with research support from, Amgen Inc.

UNAPPROVED/OFF-LABEL USE DISCLOSURE

The EOCME requires CME faculty to disclose to the participants:
1. When products or procedures being discussed are off-label, unlabelled, experimental, and/or investigational (not US Food and Drug Administration [FDA] approved); and
2. Any limitations on the information presented, such as data that are preliminary or that represent ongoing research, interim analyses, and/or unsupported opinions. Faculty may discuss information about pharmaceutical agents that is outside of FDA-approved labelling. This information is intended solely for CME and is not intended to promote off-label use of these medications. If you have any questions, contact the medical affairs department of the manufacturer for the most recent prescribing information.

TO ENROLL

To enroll in the PET Clinics Continuing Medical Education program, call customer service at 1-800-654-2452 or sign up online at http://www.theclinics.com/home/cme. The CME program is available to subscribers for an additional annual fee of USD 315.

METHOD OF PARTICIPATION

In order to claim credit, participants must complete the following:
1. Complete enrolment as indicated above.
2. Read the activity.

3. Complete the CME Test and Evaluation. Participants must achieve a score of 70% on the test. All CME Tests and Evaluations must be completed online.

CME INQUIRIES/SPECIAL NEEDS

For all CME inquiries or special needs, please contact elsevierCME@elsevier.com.

RADIOLOGIC CLINICS OF NORTH AMERICA

THE CLINICS ARE AVAILABLE ONLINE!
Access your subscription at:
www.theclinics.com

Preface
Oral and Maxillofacial Radiology

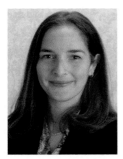

Dania Tamimi, BDS, DMSc
Editor

The oral and maxillofacial area is a very complex anatomic location that is of interest to multiple medical and dental specialists. Dentists are often called upon to treat conditions of the teeth and supporting structures as well as disorders of the temporomandibular joint (TMJ). Otolaryngologists, oncologists, head and neck surgeons, and neuro-radiologists need to be aware of some of the conditions affecting the oral and maxillofacial complex in order to render a complete and accurate diagnosis as symptoms may be referred from this area to others in the head and neck. There are also dental manifestations of systemic disease, such as the dental signs of metastasis, syndromes, and metabolic disorders that medical observers should know in order to complete the assessment of the patient.

This issue of *Radiologic Clinics of North America* is written by dentists, mostly specializing in the field of oral and maxillofacial radiology. The articles reflect their insight into the conditions of the jaws and teeth and aim to bridge the gap between the knowledge of the dental observer and the medical observer. Although not all conditions of this region were covered in this issue, most of the key diagnoses and specialized analyses were included. For more information of the imaging of this region, reviewing specialized imaging textbook on the subject of oral and maxillofacial radiology is recommended.

As the imaging primarily seen by oral and maxillofacial radiologists is plain films and cone beam computed tomography (CBCT) imaging, as well as MR imaging of the TMJs, the majority of the imaging in this issue will reflect the cases that we see in our practices.

The issue starts with a review of dental anatomy and nomenclature, which come naturally to dentists but may not be familiar to our medical colleagues. This review aims at helping the general radiologist speak the language of their referring dental clinicians.

The article on oral and maxillofacial anatomy aims primarily at aiding in the identification of normal anatomy as seen on head films, specifically, specialized dental views, such as the panoramic, lateral cephalometric, and frontal cephalometric. Cross-sectional imaging as seen on CBCT is also reviewed. As head and neck surgeons and neuroradiologists are familiar with the cross-sectional imaging anatomy on CT and MR imaging, this information is readily available in their literature and is not covered in this issue.

The pathology articles review infection, benign and malignant neoplasia, bone dysplasia, osteonecrosis, and trauma. Even though these processes can have soft tissue manifestations, the focus of these articles is to describe the osseous and dental clues that the oral and maxillofacial radiologist looks for on the osseous imaging provided in their practices. Some of the developmental and acquired changes in the dentition that can occur with systemic disease are also reviewed.

The final three articles present some of the specialized analyses that oral and maxillofacial radiologists are often called upon to perform for their

Radiol Clin N Am 56 (2018) xi–xii
https://doi.org/10.1016/j.rcl.2017.10.001
0033-8389/18/© 2017 Published by Elsevier Inc.

radiologic.theclinics.com

fellow dentists. These include analysis of the TMJ, upper respiratory tract for Sleep Dentistry purposes, and dental implant planning and show the dental thought process from a radiologist's standpoint.

I would like to thank my colleagues, Phillip Chapman, MD, Joel Curé, MD and Marcel Noujeim, DDS for their generous case contributions to this issue.

I hope that the information contained in this issue will be useful to our medical colleagues and will open up paths for future collaboration. I believe that, in the end, we are all working toward a common goal: To ensure that our patients receive the very best care that they possibly can get, and that the appropriate treatment can only be rendered with an accurate diagnosis.

Dania Tamimi, BDS, DMSc
Oral and Maxillofacial Radiology
Private Practice
Orlando, FL, USA

E-mail address:
daniatamimi2005@gmail.com

Dental Anatomy and Nomenclature for the Radiologist

Mohammed Abbas Husain, DDS

KEYWORDS

- Tooth naming • Dental anatomy • Dental restorations • CT imaging

KEY POINTS

- The Universal and Federation Dentaire International systems are the major systems for numbering teeth.
- In the United States, the universal system assigns a number 1 to 32 to each of the permanent teeth, and letters A to T to each of the primary teeth.
- Teeth consist of a crown and one or more roots. The crown is visible within the oral cavity; the root is embedded in the alveolar bone.
- Teeth are made up of 4 dental tissues (enamel, dentin, pulp and cementum), most of which have distinct radiographic densities on computed tomography (CT) imaging.
- Dental restorations are common and include fillings, crowns, root canal obturation materials, and dental implants. On CT imaging, most of these materials create substantial metallic artifacts.

INTRODUCTION

The dentition is frequently encompassed in imaging studies of the head and neck. As a result, incidental abnormalities of the dentition are frequently visualized by interpreting radiologists. The abnormalities encountered can potentially alter the course of patient treatment and may require referral to dental practitioners. To effectively identify and communicate the abnormalities that are observed, a good understanding of dental development, morphology, and terminology is required. This article provides an overview of dental anatomy and nomenclature, allowing the radiologist to communicate confidently and accurately with regard to the dentition.

TOOTH NOMENCLATURE, NAMING, AND NUMBERING

Humans develop 2 sets of dentitions, often referred to as the primary (deciduous) and permanent (succedaneous) dentition. Whether primary or permanent, the dentitions are further subdivided based on the location of a tooth in the upper or lower jaw, or within a specific quadrant of the oral cavity. The teeth in the upper jaw are referred to as the maxillary teeth and in the lower jaw as the mandibular teeth. The 4 quadrants of the oral cavity are designated the maxillary right, maxillary left, mandibular left, and mandibular right quadrants (**Fig. 1**). The division into quadrants serves as a convenient basis for 1 type of tooth classification system described elsewhere in this article, because the types of teeth in each quadrant are repeated. For example, the permanent dentition consists of 8 teeth in each quadrant: 2 incisors (central and lateral), a canine, 2 premolars, and 3 molars, yielding a total of 32 teeth (**Fig. 2**A). In the primary dentition, each quadrant contains 5 teeth: 2 incisors (central and lateral), a canine, and 2 molars (**Fig. 2**B). These teeth are repeated in each of the 4 quadrants of the oral cavity giving a total of 20 teeth.

Disclosures: None.
Section of Oral and Maxillofacial Radiology, UCLA School of Dentistry, 10833 Le Conte Avenue, 53-067A CHS, Box 951668, Los Angeles, CA 90095-1668, USA
E-mail address: mhusain@dentistry.ucla.edu

Radiol Clin N Am 56 (2018) 1–11
http://dx.doi.org/10.1016/j.rcl.2017.08.001

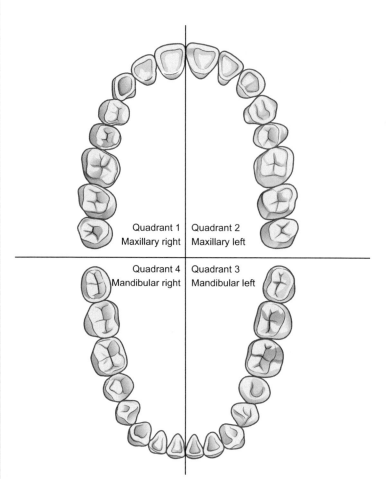

Quadrant 1 | Quadrant 2
Maxillary right | Maxillary left

Quadrant 4 | Quadrant 3
Mandibular right | Mandibular left

Fig. 1. Graphic drawing demonstrates division of the oral cavity into 4 quadrants. (*Courtesy of* dentalcare.com.)

Teeth can be referred to by name or by number. Naming teeth is generally more cumbersome owing to the multiple qualifiers necessary to specify a given tooth. Nonetheless, the nomenclature of tooth naming is universally accepted and so is useful when there is doubt about the appropriate number assigned for a tooth. This may arise if there is uncertainty about the classification system being used (such as when interpreting international studies), or when teeth may have moved position secondary to extractions or orthodontic tooth movement. This is a common scenario after orthodontic extraction of the first premolars. The second premolars frequently have moved into the position of the first premolars, and this may create confusion about its appropriate tooth number. The convention for naming teeth should follow this sequence: dentition (primary or permanent), jaw (maxillary or mandibular), side (right or left), tooth name (incisor, canine, premolar, or molar).[1] An example of a tooth name following this convention would

be as follows: permanent maxillary right central incisor. The qualifier specifying the type of dentition, permanent or primary, is unnecessary once all the primary teeth have been exfoliated. Additionally, it is unnecessary when referring to permanent teeth that have no primary analog, such as the first and second premolars and third molars.

Two main classification systems exist for the numbering of teeth: the universal system and the Federation Dentaire International system. Despite its name, the universal system is actually quite country specific; it is the system adopted in the United States by the American Dental Association.[2] In this system, only teeth are numbered. The numbering begins in the upper right quadrant with #1 referring to the maxillary right third molar (**Fig. 3**A). The numbering continues along the maxillary arch from the right side to the left ending with the maxillary left third molar, which is assigned #16. The numbering then drops to the lower left quadrant beginning with the mandibular

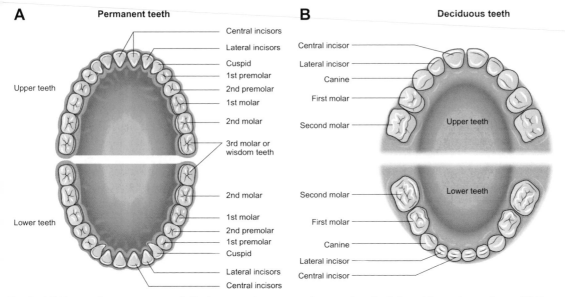

Fig. 2. (*A*) Types of permanent teeth (incisors, canines, premolars, and molars) found in each quadrant. (*B*) Types of primary teeth (incisors, canines, and molars) found in each quadrant. Note the repetition in types of teeth found across the quadrants.

left third molar, assigned #17, and continues around the mandibular arch. The last tooth in this system is the mandibular right third molar, which is assigned #32. The universal system classifies the primary dentition in an analogous fashion, but using letters of the alphabet A through T rather than #1 to #32 (**Fig. 3**B). The primary maxillary right

second molar is the first tooth in the series assigned letter A, and the primary mandibular right second molar is the last tooth in the series and assigned the letter T.

The Federation Dentaire International system is more widely used globally and adopted by the World Health Organization and the

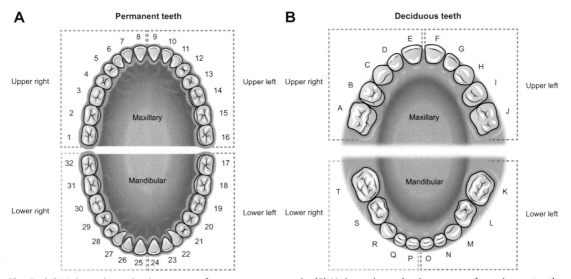

Fig. 3. (*A*) Universal numbering system for permanent teeth. (*B*) Universal numbering system for primary teeth. The universal numbering system is the most widely accepted system in the United States. Note that numbering always begins in the maxillary right quadrant and ends in the mandibular right quadrant.

International Association For Dental Research.[2] It is a system in which both dental quadrants as well as the teeth are numbered. Each quadrant is assigned a number, 1 to 4, starting with the upper right, assigned number 1, and continuing clockwise to the lower right quadrant, assigned number 4. Individual teeth are also numbered, but only within a specific quadrant. This numbering begins from the midline with the central incisor, assigned number 1, and continues posteriorly to the third molar, which is assigned number 8. The total number assigned to any given tooth is a combination of the quadrant number and tooth number. For example, the permanent maxillary left canine is assigned the number 23 (spoken as "two–three" rather than "twenty-three"). The "2" in "23" reflects the position of the tooth in the upper left quadrant, and the "3" reflects the position of the tooth within the quadrant relative to the midline (**Fig. 4**A). Primary teeth are numbered in a similar way, except that the quadrants are assigned the numbers 5 to 8, rather than 1 to 4. The individual teeth in each quadrant are numbered 1 to 5, reflecting the fewer number of primary teeth (**Fig. 4**B).

One of the most common anatomic variants involving the dentition with implications for tooth numbering is hyperdontia, or the presence of supernumerary teeth. When such teeth are present

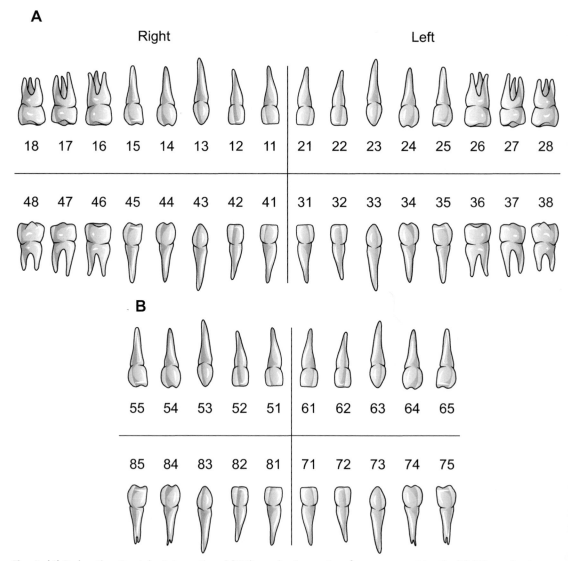

Fig. 4. (*A*) Federation Dentaire International (FDI) numbering system for permanent teeth. (*B*) FDI numbering system for primary teeth.

they are named in the universal system using a combination of numbers and letters, referencing the closest erupted permanent tooth. For example, a supernumerary tooth located buccal to tooth number #20 would be referred to as tooth #20A (**Fig. 5**). Hyperdontia commonly occurs as a phenomenon in isolation. However, in cases of multiple, unerupted supernumerary teeth the possibility of a hereditary syndrome such as Gardner syndrome or cleidocranial dysplasia should be considered.[3] Hypodontia, or the lack of development of 1 or more teeth, is also a common anatomic variant that mostly occurs in isolation, but can also be associated with a hereditary syndrome.[4] However, it usually has no implications for tooth naming.

ANATOMIC RELATIONSHIPS IN THE DENTOALVEOLAR ARCH

Terminology used to describe the relationship of teeth, or objects in relation to teeth, differ from conventional anatomic nomenclature. Although still generally understood, terminology such as inferior, posterior, medial, lateral, anterior, and posterior are less commonly used when speaking about objects in the dentoalveolar arch. More common are the terms mesial, distal, facial, lingual, coronal, and apical. The use of the terms mesial and distal are somewhat analogous to

anterior and posterior, but refer specifically to the proximity of objects or surfaces to the dental arch midline (**Fig. 6**). Objects closer to the dental midline are mesial, whereas those further away are distal. The terms facial and lingual are similar to the terms medial and lateral, although the point of reference is the alveolar arch. More specific terms are sometimes used in lieu of the terms facial and lingual. The term palatal is sometimes used to describe objects lingual to the maxillary teeth. Additionally, the terms labial or buccal can be used for objects facial to the dental arch based on proximity to the lips (anterior teeth) or cheeks (posterior teeth). Finally, coronal and apical are terms used in a similar way to the terms superior and inferior, but describe the relationship of objects in specific relationship to the crown and apices of a tooth. Objects that are closer to the crown or superior to it are coronal, whereas those that are closer to the apices or inferior to them are apical.

TOOTH ANATOMY

Teeth are made up of 2 basic components: a crown and 1 or more roots. The crown of a tooth is generally that which is seen clinically within the mouth in a patient without periodontal bone loss. To be precise, the exact boundary of the crown and root(s) of a tooth is the cementoenamel junction. This is a junction, clearly evident on tooth specimens, where 2 distinct dental tissues (described in more detail later) meet on a given tooth. That which is above the cementoenamel

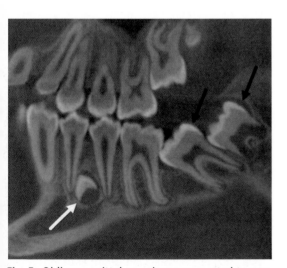

Fig. 5. Oblique sagittal cone-beam computed tomography demonstrates a supernumerary tooth follicle between the roots of the mandibular left premolars (*white arrow*). The tooth would conventionally be referred to as #20A or #21A given its proximity to these teeth. Note also the orientation of the mandibular molars, #17 and #18, which are mesioangularly impacted (*black arrow*).

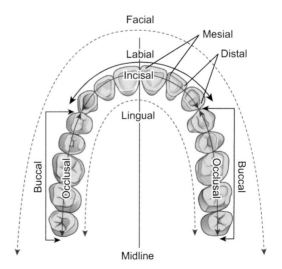

Fig. 6. Common terminology used to specify tooth surfaces: mesial/distal, facial/lingual, and occlusal/incisal.

junction is covered by enamel and makes up the crown, and that which is below is covered by cementum and makes up the roots. The crowns of different teeth vary greatly in their morphology, depending on where they are in the mouth. Anterior teeth, which include the central and lateral incisors and canines, have prominent incisal edges, whereas the posterior teeth (premolars and molars) have multiple cusps and large occlusal tables. Differences in the morphology of the anterior and posterior teeth reflect their varied functions. The incisal edges of anterior teeth function in cutting, whereas the broad occlusal tables of posterior teeth facilitate chewing.

The roots of teeth differ in their morphology, depending on the type of tooth in question. Teeth can either be single rooted or multirooted. The incisors, canines, and premolars other than the maxillary first premolars are generally single rooted. Molar teeth and the maxillary first premolars are multirooted. However, exceptions to these general trends are not uncommon and should be expected. In particular, third molars tend to have the most variable root morphology. When naming individual roots in a multirooted teeth, the point of reference is the furcational area, or the area between the roots of the tooth. Common terms used to describe the roots in 2 rooted teeth are mesial/distal or buccal/lingual and in 3 rooted (maxillary) teeth are mesiobuccal, distobuccal, and palatal (or lingual). Additionally, for the purposes of description, tooth roots are divided into thirds: the cervical, middle, and apical. The cervical third is that which is closest to the crown, whereas the apical is that which includes the root terminus.

The terminology used to designate different surfaces of teeth is similar to that which is used to specify anatomic relationships in the dentoalveolar area. Teeth either have 4 or 5 surfaces depending on whether they are anterior or posterior teeth. All teeth have a buccal/facial, lingual/palatal, mesial, and distal surfaces. Posterior teeth have an additional occlusal surface that forms the occlusal table. The contacting surfaces of adjacent teeth may also be referred to as the proximal surfaces.

As for the physical makeup of teeth, they are made up of 4 basic dental tissues: enamel, dentin, cementum, and pulp (**Fig. 7**). The first 3 dental tissues are mineralized hard tissues, whereas the pulp is a nonmineralized soft tissue. The outer aspect of the crown of teeth is made of enamel. Enamel is the most mineralized substance in the human body and is distinctly radiopaque on radiographs. Deep to the enamel is dentin, which makes up the bulk of the crown and roots, and is

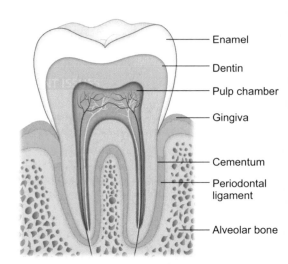

Fig. 7. A molar tooth shows the various dental tissues that compose the tooth (enamel, dentin, cementum, and pulp) as well as the distinction between crown and roots. The components of the periodontium (gingiva, alveolar bone, and periodontal ligament) are identified.

somewhat less calcified than the enamel. The dentin surrounds both the pulpal tissues within the tooth. Where the enamel and dentin meet is what is called the dentinoenamel junction. Within the roots of teeth, cementum is the outermost tissue and surrounds the underlying dentin. The mineral content of cementum is similar to that of dentin and is, therefore, isoattenuating on radiographs (**Fig. 8**) and difficult to differentiate radiographically. Where the enamel and cementum meet makes up the cementoenamel junction. As described, this junction marks the boundary between the crown and roots of a tooth.

The pulp tissues fill the internal cavities of a tooth, both the pulpal chamber and root canal. The pulp tissues are made of nerves and vessels that enter through the apical foramen of a tooth. The pulp tissue has a number of functions, including a nutritive and sensory function. Through the pulp, sensations of pain are mediated and blood flow is controlled. Given the soft tissue nature of the pulp, it demonstrates the most radiolucent appearance relative to other dental tissues. The pulpal tissues are subdivided into 2 distinct areas. The pulpal tissues at the center of the crown of a tooth are referred to as the pulpal chamber and can make up a significant portion of the crown, particularly in the posterior teeth of young adults. The pulp tissue within the roots of teeth are referred to as the pulpal canals and are usually centered within the roots. The pulpal canals extend from the apical foramen to the pulpal

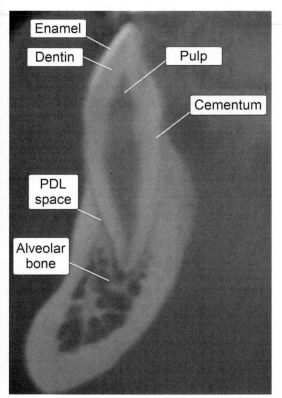

Fig. 8. Sagittal cone-beam computed tomography cross-section of the mandibular right canine (tooth #27) shows the various components of the tooth (enamel, dentin, pulp, and cementum) and periodontal tissues. PDL, periodontal ligament.

chamber. When the pulpal tissues necrose, the tooth is said to have "died" or lost vitality. Pulpal necrosis and infection are indications for root canal treatment.

Thus far, descriptions of tooth anatomy have taken as their point of reference the permanent dentition. However, some general anatomic differences should be noted between primary and permanent teeth. Primary teeth differ from permanent teeth in general by having more bulbous crowns, thinner layers of enamel, relatively larger pulpal chambers, and roots that are more slender and splayed.

PERIODONTIUM

The term periodontium, originates from Greek and literally means that which is "around the tooth." It collectively refers to the alveolar bone, periodontal ligament (PDL) and gingival tissues (gums; see **Fig. 7**). The periodontium is a group of dynamic tissues that support the teeth by adapting to increased occlusal forces and variations in function. Evidence for this is seen when teeth are

lost. The occlusal stimulus to the periodontium is absent and the periodontal bone is resorbed. The periodontium refers specifically to that portion of the maxilla and mandible that surrounds the roots of teeth. The superior most portion of the periodontal bone demonstrates a cortication and is referred to as the alveolar crest. Additionally, a thin area of corticated bone is noted surrounding the roots of teeth and is called the lamina dura. When the cortications of the alveolar crest or lamina dura are lost, this is a sign of pathology. Between the lamina dura and the root of tooth is a thin radiolucent zone that contains the PDL (see **Fig. 8**). The PDL contains fibers that attach the roots of teeth to the alveolar socket and serve a proprioceptive role. Normally, the PDL should have uniform thickness around the root of the tooth. Localized widening of the PDL space is a common sign of pathology, usually inflammatory in nature.

The soft tissue, which covers the periodontal bone, is the gingiva, also known colloquially as the "gums." The gingiva also attached directly to the roots of teeth, creating a small gingival sulcus. Inflammation of the gingival tissues can lead to apical migration of the gingival attachments and periodontal bone loss.

TOOTH DEVELOPMENT AND ERUPTION

The development of teeth can be seen as having 2 distinct components: tooth formation and tooth eruption. The process of tooth formation is a complex process beginning early in utero. Primary teeth begin development at approximately 6 to 8 weeks in utero, whereas permanent teeth begin at approximately 20 weeks in utero.[5] Tooth development is initiated by embryonic cells, which differentiate into cells that produce dental tissues. These embryonic cells are referred to as the tooth germ, derived from the ectoderm of the first pharyngeal arch and the ectomesenchyme of the neural crest.[6] The tooth germ has 3 main components, the enamel organ, the dental papilla, and the dental follicle, each of which give rise to the different dental tissues that compose a tooth. The enamel organ contains precursors of cells that produce enamel and the dental papilla contains cells, which eventually produce dentin and pulpal tissues. The dental follicle gives rise to the cementoblasts, osteoblasts, and fibroblasts that form cementum, alveolar bone and the PDL, respectively.[7] For a more detailed description of stages of odontogenesis and regulatory signaling pathways, the reader is referred to more comprehensive descriptions found elsewhere.[5–7]

The process of odontogenesis as previously summarized is relatively resilient to environmental factors, whereas the mechanism of eruption of teeth is more easily altered by external factors, such as tooth obstructions, early tooth loss, or infection. The mechanism of tooth eruption is not fully understood, although the most widely held theory holds that although multiple factors might be involved, the PDL plays the main role in promoting the eruption of a tooth.[8] Tooth eruption occurs concurrently with the root resorption of the deciduous teeth and root formation of the erupting tooth. When the tooth has fully erupted, the root is often not fully formed, but forms sometime after its emergence.

The tooth eruption process is often divided into 3 broad stages: the primary, transitional (mixed), and permanent stage. The primary stage begins with the eruption of primary central incisors into the oral at about 6 to 12 months postnatal. By approximately 3 years of age, all the deciduous teeth have erupted and root development is complete.[2] Some variability in the exact chronology of tooth development is common, and mirrors the variability seen in other similar growth indicators.

The mixed dentition stage refers to the phase of development when both primary and permanent teeth are present within the dental arches (**Fig. 9**). This begins at approximately 6 years of age with the eruption of the first mandibular molars and lasts until approximately 11 to 12 years of age, with the exfoliation of the last deciduous teeth (usually the primary second molars or canines).

The final stage of eruption is that of the permanent dentition and begins after all the deciduous teeth have been exfoliated. With the exception of the third molars, the permanent teeth fully erupt by approximately the age of 13 to 14. The third molars erupt significantly later at approximately the ages of 18 to 25.

Frequently, teeth do not erupt within their expected developmental timeframe. This delay may occur for a variety of reasons, including malpositioning of the tooth, inadequate arch space, genetic abnormalities affecting the eruption mechanism, or the presence of pathology or dense bone along the eruption pathway. Inadequate arch space is the most frequent cause of tooth impaction. The most frequently impacted teeth are the third molars and maxillary canines.[9] Generally, impacted third molars are considered for surgical removal. Other teeth, such as the canines, may be surgically exposed and brought into the dental arch using orthodontic techniques. Terminology describing an impacted tooth describes its angulation and the extent to which it is covered by bone. Teeth that are mostly submerged within the alveolar process are described as full bony impacted. Those that are partially covered by alveolar bone are partial bony impacted.[10] Depending on the angulation of the long axis of the impacted tooth, the impaction is classified as mesioangular, distoangular, buccoangular, linguoangular, horizontal, vertical, or inverted (see **Fig. 5**). These descriptive terms communicate to some degree the difficulty that might be expected in the surgical removal of the tooth.[11] Teeth that are impacted are predisposed to a number of complications, including local infection of the periodontium (periodontal disease) or overlying soft tissue (pericoronitis). Dentigerous cyst formation may also occur within the follicle of an impacted tooth.[11]

DENTAL RESTORATIONS

A variety of materials and dental prostheses are used to restore the form and function of teeth within the oral cavity. Depending on the type of restoration, a different set of materials may be used. For example, direct partial coverage restorations, commonly known as "fillings," typically use 1 of 2 different filling materials: amalgam or composite. Dental amalgam is probably the more widespread material and is actually a combination of different metals including silver, mercury, and tin. Fillings of this material are commonly referred to as "silver fillings." This dental material is highly radiopaque and thus distinct from other dental tissues (**Fig. 10**). On CT imaging, the material creates a metallic artifact that can interfere with the assessment of dental disease. Composite material is a resin material and the main alternative to amalgam. Its use has gained increasing popularity, largely for aesthetic reasons. Most patients find the tooth-colored nature of the material aesthetically preferable to the silver color of dental amalgam. Composite material bonds with the underlying tooth structure. Radiographically, it appears less opaque than dental amalgam but more opaque than enamel. Earlier versions of composite material, however, appeared radiolucent radiographically. This feature should not be mistaken on radiographs for dental caries.

Full coverage coronal restorations are also known as dental crowns. These restorations are usually made of full metal, full porcelain, or a combination as in the case of porcelain fused to metal crowns. The restorations require tooth preparation before placement. The tooth

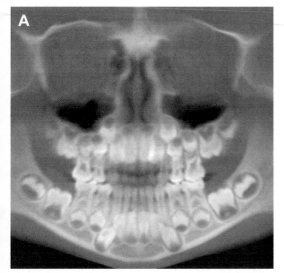

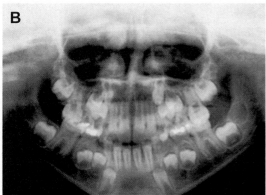

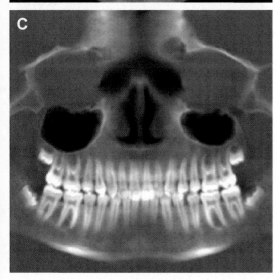

structure around the periphery of the crown of a tooth must be removed to make space for the dental prosthesis. The dental crown is placed over the prepared tooth to restore the form and function of the tooth. On CT imaging, the crown appears opaque, regardless of which of the 3 materials is used (**Fig. 11**). Moreover, full metal crowns tend to have the most opaque appearance and create the most metallic artifact.

A fixed partial denture, or bridge, is a dental prosthesis designed to replace one or a small number of missing teeth. A bridge can be thought of as a series of fused dental crowns, one or more of which fill an edentulous space. The most common type of bridge is a 3-unit bridge, which consists of 2 dental crowns placed on teeth adjacent to an edentulous area. These crowns are fused to a third crown, or pontic, that replaces a missing tooth (**Fig. 12**). The restorative materials available to make a bridge are identical to those available to make a dental crown, and have a similar radiographic appearance.

Root canal therapy is a type of endodontic treatment used to treat infected or necrotic pulp. The procedure involves accessing, cleaning, and disinfecting the pulpal chamber and canals. Once this is completed, the pulpal canals are instrumented and filled with gutta-percha and sealer cement. Gutta-percha is a cone-shaped, nontoxic, latex material that is flexible and highly radiopaque. The material should fill the entire length of the pulpal canal. On CT imaging, the material has a radiodensity of metal and creates an analogous artifact (**Fig. 13**). It is used in conjunction with sealer cement that fills any gaps left by the gutta-percha within the pulpal canal. The gutta-percha or sealer may, on occasion, extend beyond the radiographic apex of a tooth. In most cases, however, this is of no consequence owing to the biocompatibility of the materials used.

Dental implants are, at present, the preferred method of replacing missing teeth and are seen more frequently in older patients who are more likely to be edentulous. Although different types of implants exist, the most common and contemporary type is the root form implant. This type of implant demonstrates a cylindrical shape

Fig. 9. Cone-beam computed tomography panoramic reformats of patients in the 3 stages of tooth eruption. (*A*) Primary dentition: only primary teeth are erupted and permanent teeth follicles are visualized but unerupted. (*B*) Mixed dentition stage: a mixture of primary and permanent teeth are erupted into the oral cavity; some permanent tooth follicles are unerupted. (*C*) Permanent dentition: complete exfoliation of all primary teeth, only permanent teeth remain in the oral cavity. (*From* Koenig JL, Tamimi DF, Petrikowski CG, et al. Diagnostic imaging: oral and maxillofacial. 2nd edition. Philadelphia: Elsevier, 2017; with permission.)

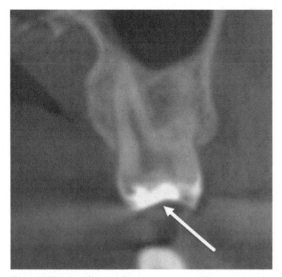

Fig. 10. Coronal cone-beam computed tomography through the area of the first molar tooth shows an amalgam restoration (white *arrow*) on the occlusal surface. Note the increased attenuation of the material relative to the dental tissues.

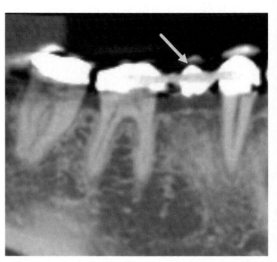

Fig. 12. Oblique sagittal cone-beam computed tomography of the posterior left mandible demonstrates a fixed partial denture (bridge) extending from teeth #19 to #21. Note the pontic (*yellow arrow*) in the edentulous space of tooth #20 that is attached to the adjacent crowns.

mimicking that of a tooth root. Dental implants are usually made of titanium and are surgically placed into the alveolar bone. After a period of integration with the surrounding alveolar bone, a crown is placed onto the implant to restore tooth function. On CT imaging, the implant appears highly radiopaque, with significant metallic artifact (**Fig. 14**). This artifact can obscure evaluation of periimplant bone, an important factor in assessing the prognosis of an implant. In these cases, clinical evaluation and intraoral imaging are helpful supplements for more comprehensive evaluation.

DENTAL APPLIANCES

Dental appliances used for orthodontic treatment are common findings, particularly in young

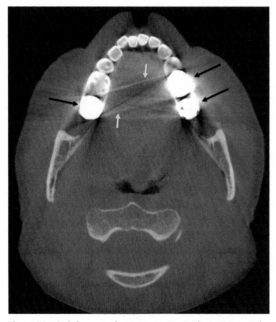

Fig. 11. Axial cone-beam computed tomography through the crowns of the mandibular teeth shows full coverage coronal restorations, commonly referred to as dental crowns, on most of the mandibular molars (*black arrows*). Extensive metallic streaking artifact is noted emanating from the crowns (*yellow arrows*).

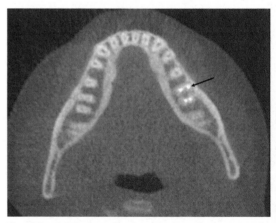

Fig. 13. Axial cone-beam computed tomography through the roots of the mandibular teeth shows a root canal treated mandibular left first molar (*black arrow*).

molars and serve as a way of anchoring the orthodontic appliance. All the features of a standard orthodontic appliance are metallic in nature and create significant metallic artifact on CT imaging.

SUMMARY

Incidental abnormalities involving the dentition are likely to be encountered by the radiologist interpreting studies of the head and neck region, particularly on CT imaging. Proper identification and communication of the abnormalities involving the dentition first require an understanding of normal dental anatomy, dental development, and a familiarity with the radiographic appearance of common dental restorations. This article has introduced the basic language of dental anatomy, the 3 stages of tooth eruption, and specific features of dental restorations to assist radiologists in communicating effectively with their dental colleagues.

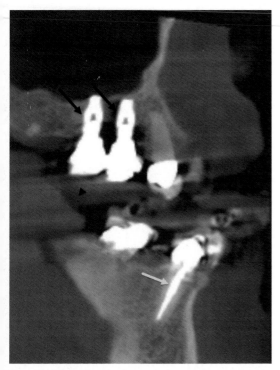

Fig. 14. Sagittal cone-beam computed tomography demonstrates 2 osseointegrated implants within the maxillary alveolar ridge at the sites of the missing maxillary right first and second molars (*black arrows*). The right mandibular first premolar is endodontically treated and demonstrates gutta-percha within its root canal (*yellow arrow*).

patients. They present as brackets and wires fixed to the facial aspect of most maxillary and mandibular teeth (**Fig. 15**). Metallic bands may also be seen on the maxillary and mandibular

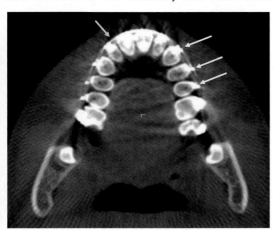

Fig. 15. Axial cone-beam computed tomography shows a conventional fixed orthodontic appliance that consists of brackets bonded to the facial surfaces of teeth (*white arrows*) and an arch wire (*yellow arrow*) that runs through the brackets and is held in place by elastic bands.

REFERENCES

1. Koenig, LJ. Diagnostic imaging: oral and maxillofacial. Salt Lake City: Amirsys Pub; 2012.
2. Nelson SJ. Wheeler's dental anatomy, physiology and occlusion. St Louis (MO): Elsevier Health Sciences; 2014.
3. Primosch RE. Anterior supernumerary teeth-assessment and surgical intervention in children. Pediatr Dent 1981;3(2):204–15.
4. Larmour CJ, Mossey PA, Thind BS, et al. Hypodontia—a retrospective review of prevalence and etiology. Part I. Quintessence Int 2005;36(4):263–70.
5. Yildirim S. Dental pulp stem cells. Springer Science & Business Media; 2012.
6. Nanci A. Ten cate's oral histology-pageburst on vitalsource: development, structure, and function. Elsevier Health Sciences; 2007.
7. Thesleff I, Sharpe P. Signalling networks regulating dental development. Mech Dev 1997;67(2):111–23.
8. Wise G, King G. Mechanisms of tooth eruption and orthodontic tooth movement. J Dent Res 2008; 87(5):414–34.
9. Dachi SF, Howell FV. A survey of 3,874 routine full-mouth radiographs: II. A study of impacted teeth. Oral Surg Oral Med Oral Pathol 1961;14(10): 1165–9.
10. Haug RH, Perrott DH, Gonzalez ML, et al. The American Association of Oral and Maxillofacial Surgeons age-related third molar study. J Oral Maxillofac Surg 2005;63(8):1106–14.
11. Miloro M, Ghali GE, Larsen P, et al. Peterson's principles of oral and maxillofacial surgery, vol. 1. PMPH-USA; 2004.

Oral and Maxillofacial Anatomy

Mitra Sadrameli, DMD, MS[a], Mel Mupparapu, DMD, MDS[b],*

KEYWORDS

- Intraoral radiography • Extraoral radiography • Panoramic imaging • Cone beam CT imaging
- Multiplanar reconstructions • Dental anatomy • Maxillofacial anatomy • Radiographic anatomy

KEY POINTS

- Oral and maxillofacial anatomy is intricate and best evaluated via multiple forms of radiographs and techniques. This article outlines the various anatomic structures and their common radiographic appearances using intraoral, extraoral, and cone beam CT images
- Intraoral radiographs have a superior anatomic resolution, hence can be used to evaluate dental and periodontal structures. The limitation of such a radiographic method is often the amount of anatomic area covered; hence, there is a need for extraoral imaging to evaluate larger dental and maxillofacial structures.
- Extraoral imaging includes skull views; using a variety of images and line drawings, the anatomic areas are highlighted and the descriptions are concise yet useful for a medical or dental practitioner.
- Cone beam CT–based anatomic descriptions are complementary to the extraoral anatomy noted via skull views and are more objective due to the 3-D aspect of the images. Multiplanar reconstructions ie, axial, coronal and sagittal views are used to describe the anatomy.

INTRAORAL IMAGING

Proper radiographic interpretation requires a thorough knowledge of normal anatomy, variations of anatomic structures, and changes caused by pathology. Anatomic landmarks are not fully visible in intraoral radiographs; however, small areas of anatomy may be seen depending on the angulation used to acquire the radiograph. Intraoral images demonstrate the teeth and the supporting structures in detail. The 2 most commonly used intraoral radiographs, the periapical (PA) and bitewing radiographic examination types, provide clinicians with specific and different information concerning the health of the teeth.

Interproximal examination or bitewing examination is used to investigate to identify caries in the interproximal surfaces of the teeth on cross-sectional mediolateral views, showing the crown and root portion of the teeth in both arches (**Fig. 1**).

PA examination provides information on the cross-sectional mesiodistal view of the tooth and the surrounding structures. It presents the entire length of the tooth and the surrounding structures. Enamel, dentin, periodontal ligament space, and the lamina dura are clearly noted in each and every tooth due to their inherent differences in the densities. PAs typically show a 3-teeth to 4-teeth span in 1 arch only (**Fig. 2**).

Maxillary Anterior Anatomy

The median maxillary suture (median palatal suture) is a located between the 2 palatal (palatine) processes of the maxillae, extending from between the maxillary central incisors posteriorly.[1] A funnel-shaped widening at the

[a] The University of British Columbia, 2194 Health Sciences Mall, Vancouver, British Columbia V6T 1Z3, Canada;
[b] University of Pennsylvania School of Dental Medicine, 240 South 40th Street, Philadelphia, PA 19104, USA
* Corresponding author.
E-mail address: mmd@upenn.edu

Radiol Clin N Am 56 (2018) 13–29
http://dx.doi.org/10.1016/j.rcl.2017.08.002

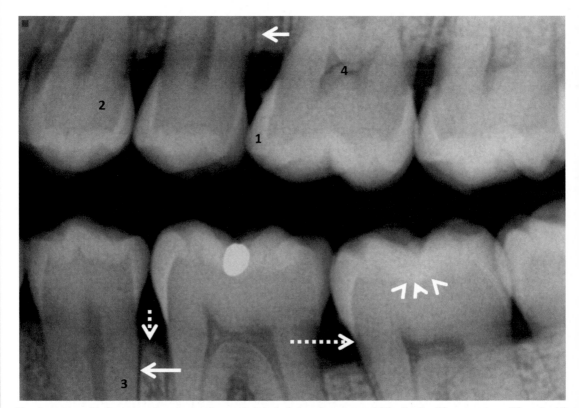

Fig. 1. Intraoral left molar bitewing radiograph labeled showing enamel (1), dentin (2), cementum (3), pulp (4), lamina dura (*short white arrow*), periodontal ligament space (*long white arrow*), crest of the alveolar bone (*short dotted arrow*), dentinoenamel junction (*arrowheads*), and cementoenamel junction (*long dotted arrow*).

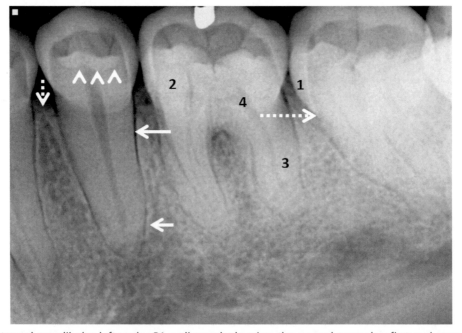

Fig. 2. Intraoral mandibular left molar PA radiograph showing the second premolar, first and second molars along with their periodontal structures. As shown in the bitewing radiograph, enamel (1), dentin (2), cementum (3), pulp (4), lamina dura (*short white arrow*), periodontal ligament space (*long white arrow*), crest of the alveolar bone (*short dotted arrow*), dentinoenamel junction (*arrow heads*), and cementoenamel junction (*long dotted arrow*) are shown in this radiograph as well.

anterior aspect is known as the anterior median maxillary cleft.[1]

The maxillary nasopalatine (incisive) canal is an osseous channel through which the nasopalatine nerves and the anterior branches of the descending palatine vessels traverse. The nasopalatine nerve is a branch from the sphenopalatine ganglion innervating the nasal roof and septum, extending downward and forward in a groove in the vomer bone and the cartilaginous septum.[1] The incisive canal varies greatly in length and width.[2] At the anterior portion of the nasal floor, the nasopalatine nerve enters and travels through the canal of Stensen to finally emerge on the hard palate through the incisive foramen. The foramen is a radiolucent area located posterior to the maxillary central incisors and is formed by the 2 palatal processes of the maxilla.[1] Although the canal itself may not be seen in its entirety on intraoral imaging, the lateral borders of the incisive foramen are best visible in the anterior PA radiograph of the maxillary central incisors (**Fig. 3**). Its location, size, and shape vary depending on the angulation during image acquisition, resulting in its imaged anterior border to assume close proximity to the alveolar crest or some distance superior to it. The foramen's visual presentation in the PA radiographs as a result varies in relationship to the roots of the central maxillary incisor teeth. On a maxillary central incisor PA, the foramen may be a symmetrically oval, round, or heart-shaped radiolucency without cortical borders, sometimes superimposed on the apical thirds of the roots[1] (**Fig. 4**). Presence of a cortical border may indicate transformation into a nasopalatine (incisive) cyst.[1] On a maxillary incisor PA, it may be a symmetrically oval, round, or heart-shaped radiolucency sometimes superimposed on the apical thirds of the roots.[1] Superior foramina of the nasopalatine canal are ovoid radiolucencies, which are noted superior to the maxillary central incisor apices and lateral to the nasal septum. A review of the tooth in question in other neighboring images clears it of any associated pathology. When in doubt, examination of the integrity of the lamina dura and PDL space should be considered. Intact PDL spaces and lamina dura are radiographic indications of absence of disease. The superior foramina of the nasopalatine canal are also known as foramina of Scarpa and only occasionally noted on radiographs depending on the angulation of the x-ray beam.

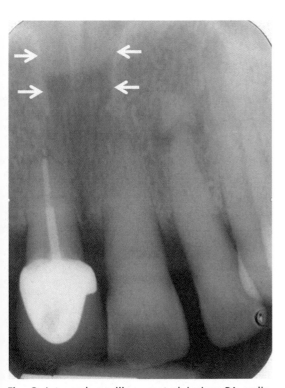

Fig. 3. Intraoral maxillary central incisor PA radiograph showing the 2 nasopalatine canals (*arrows*) before their confluence to the incisive canal and foramen. Note the radiopaque area attached to the apex of maxillary left lateral incisor radiographically consistent with apical cemental dysplasia.

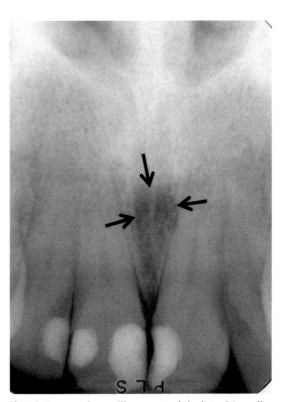

Fig. 4. Intraoral maxillary central incisor PA radiograph showing the incisive foramen (*arrows*).

Pathologies such as nasopalatine canal cyst mostly presents as a round lesion with well-defined border.[2] Superimposition of the incisive foramen on the apices of the maxillary lateral or central incisors may mimic a PA pathosis. The clinician should keep an eye on the developmental anomalies (**Fig. 5**) that can be seen in this region, notably the mesiodens (a small supernumerary tooth located in the vicinity of central or lateral incisors). The floor of the nasal fossa is generally depicted as a linear radiopacity in the maxillary anterior radiographs and meets the floor of the maxillary sinus as it ascends to form the lateral wall of the nasal cavity. This forms an inverted Y line (**Fig. 6**) known as the Y line of Ennis[3]

Maxillary Posterior Anatomy

The floor of the maxillary sinuses (see **Fig. 6**) appears as a thin radiopaque partially curved line in the superior aspect of the PA radiograph in the maxillary molar teeth regions. In radiographs acquired with nonideal angulation, the corticated sinus floor may superimpose on the apical third of

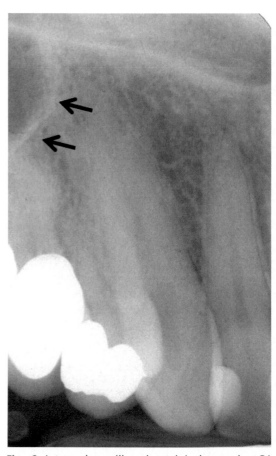

Fig. 6. Intraoral maxillary lateral incisor-canine PA radiograph showing the Y line of Ennis. The cured linear radiopacity (*arrows*) is the floor of the right maxillary sinus. The straight radiopaque line noted in the radiograph is the floor of the nasal fossa.

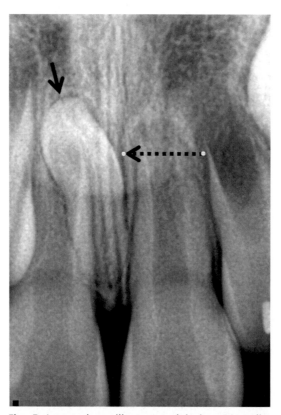

Fig. 5. Intraoral maxillary central incisor PA radiograph showing a mesiodens (*short black arrow*) and the midmaxillary suture (*long dotted arrow*). Note that the root apices are still open suggesting that the roots are still developing.

the roots of the maxillary molar teeth. The maxillary sinus appears as an air density cavity superior to the maxillary sinus floors.

The maxillary tuberosities are elevated, rounded, posterior regions of the terminal aspects of the maxillary alveolar processes (**Fig. 7**).[1] Complete pneumatization of the tuberosities by the maxillary sinuses is considered variations of normal anatomy.

The zygomatic process appears as a radiopaque structure and is almost always present in maxillary posterior teeth radiographs (see **Fig. 7**).[2] It is generally positioned superiolateral to the maxillary first molar tooth. It is a structure of varying dimensions and extends superiorly.[2] In intraoral radiographs, it usually appears as an inverted radiopaque loop, which represents the cortex of the inferior aspect of the process.[2] The malar bone is continuous with the zygomatic process and extends posteriorly, appearing as a

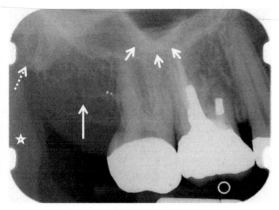

Fig. 7. Intraoral maxillary molar PA radiograph showing the zygomatic process (*short white arrows*), maxillary tuberosity (*long white arrow*), coronoid process of the mandible (*star*), pterygoid process (*dotted arrow*).

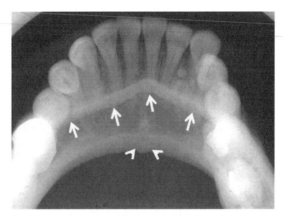

Fig. 8. Intraoral mandibular symphysis occlusal radiograph showing the mental ridge (*short arrows*) and the genial tubercles (*arrowheads*).

shadow of lesser and more uniform radiopacity.[2] Incorrect vertical angulation results in superimposition of these structures.

As the mouth is opened to its fullest extent, the coronoid process moves anteroinferiorly and may be seen superimposed on or inferior to the maxillary molar teeth (see **Fig. 7**). When present, it is important to identify this mandibular anatomic landmark on a maxillary molar radiograph.

The hamular process is a bony projection that arises from the sphenoid bone inferioposteriorly and seen in the proximity of the tuberosity of the maxilla. Great degree of anatomic variation in length, width, and shape is noted; however, the usual appearance is a bulbous or tapered point.

Mandibular Anterior Anatomy

The genial tubercles are located parasymphyseal in the lingual surface of the midmandible, between the superior and inferior borders (**Fig. 8**). They appear as dense opacities on all intraoral images.

The mental ridge (**Fig. 9**) is located on the anterior aspect and near the inferior border of the mandible and extends from the premolar to the symphysis.[2] On an anterior mandibular PA radiograph, it is seen as an inverse V-shaped radiopaque line of varying prominence inferior to the apices of the anterior teeth. Superimposition of the ridge may partially obscure the roots of mandibular anterior teeth.[2]

The nutrient canals (**Fig. 10**) contain blood vessels and nerves that supply the teeth, interdental spaces, and gingivae.[2] These canals appear as radiolucent lines of uniform width and they sometimes exhibit radiopaque borders.[2] Compared with the maxilla, nutrient canals of the mandible

are often better visualized.[2] Nutrient canals arising from the mandibular canal extend superiorly to the apices of the existing teeth or to the interdental space. The canals may appear prominently in areas of significant periodontal bone loss. In other words, the appearance of these preexisting canals is enhanced due to the loss of mineralized tissues around.

The lingual foramen is located on the lingual surface of the mandible at the symphysis, through which a branch of the lingual artery enters the mandible.[2] In PA images of the anterior mandibular teeth, it appears as a small, corticated radiolucent circle. The corticated appearance is caused by the superimposition of the cortices of the genial tubercles.[2]

Mandibular Posterior Anatomy

The external oblique ridge (see **Fig. 9**) is the forward and downward continuation of the anterior border of the ramus toward the mandibular alveolar housing and extending to the mental ridge.[2]

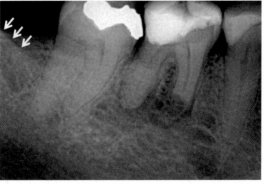

Fig. 9. Intraoral mandibular right molar PA radiograph showing the external oblique ridge (*arrows*).

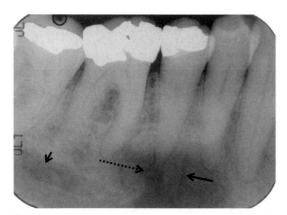

Fig. 10. Intraoral mandibular right premolar PA radiograph showing the mandibular canal (*short black arrow*), the mental foramen (*long dotted arrow*), and a nutrient canal (*long black arrow*).

It presents as a radiopaque line with varying width and density passing anteriorly and across the molar region.[2] With generalized crestal atrophy of the edentulous posterior mandible in which the alveolar ridge has undergone extensive to complete resorption, the external oblique ridge may be seen at the level of the superior border of the body of the mandible.[2]

The mylohyoid (internal oblique) ridge appears as a radiopaque area of varying size, which begins on the anterior and medial aspect of the ramus and extends downward and forward diagonally on the lingual surface of the mandible extending toward the symphysis area and often best visualized at the junction of the retromolar and molar regions.[2] The ridge's posterior portion is the most prominent, ranging from a very faint, narrow to broad, and/or dense radiopaque line. Mylohyoid ridge runs inferior to the external oblique ridge with its image sometimes superimposed on the roots of the molar teeth.[2] In the presence of a deep depression of the mandibular fossa, the radiographic region inferior to the ridge may appear prominently radiolucent mimicking pathology, such as a cystic condition.[2]

The mandibular canal is most often seen in mandibular posterior PAs carrying neurovascular tissues through the mandible, starting at the mandibular foramen and generally ending at the mental foramen (see **Fig. 10**). The mandibular canal varies in size, location, and proximity to the apices of the premolar and molar teeth. Medial to the mental foramen, the mandibular canal is called the incisive canal and it becomes progressively smaller, either extending partway to the midline or disappearing from the radiographic view. The mental foramen, usually located inferior to the mandibular premolars, is an oval or round foramen through which the mental nerve and blood vessels exit.[2] Its location varies in relation to the apices of the premolars and occasionally those of the first molar teeth. In intraoral PA radiographs, the superimposition of the mental foramina on the apices of the mandibular teeth may mimic PA pathosis. An intact lamina dura when visible is confirmation of superimposition of the mental foramina on the apices rather than presence of pathosis.

EXTRAORAL IMAGING

Knowledge of extraoral maxillofacial radiography is essential for a thorough understanding of the complex disease processes that influence the way anatomy is displayed for interpretation. Extraoral radiography, which was entirely film based in the past, is currently a digital modality. Extraoral digital imaging can be performed via either storage phosphor system (a vast majority of medical facilities and hospitals) or using solid state technologies (using positioning devices called cephalostats that are attached to the panoramic units, individual skull units, or CBCT units). No matter which technique is used for imaging, the skull in a dental setting, the patient is almost always in a vertical position. Hospital skull units are typically designed for supine position skull view acquisitions. Extraoral imaging techniques used in dentistry vary from skull views to panoramic radiography and to more advanced imaging like tomography and CT. In addition, MR imaging and ultrasound are used when indicated for imaging of the maxillofacial structures but are not discussed in the scope of this article.

Extraoral Anatomy of Maxillofacial Region as Seen on Radiographs

Table 1 lists the structures that can be readily identified on plain film or digital extraoral imaging.[4] Any alterations of anatomy or absence of any of these landmarks alert the clinician of the possibility of an anomaly or an impending pathology. Most the structures identified here are bony that are sometimes pneumatized. The presence of soft tissue in relation to these bony or air-filled structures can be identified by intermediate attenuation and occasionally need some additional views or techniques. For identification of complex anatomic structures and trauma, the preferred extraoral imaging is either CT or MRI.

Skull Radiographs

The use of skull radiography has declined and rarely used since the advent CT and more recently the introduction of CBCT. Mastering the anatomy of maxillofacial structures is an essential and

Table 1
Commonly evaluated bony landmarks using extraoral radiographic (2-D) techniques

Anatomic Area	Technique Commonly Viewed with	Description
Frontal sinus	PA skull	Bilateral pneumatized structures noted in between orbits superior to ethmoid air cells
Crista galli	PA skull	Linear radiopacity noted in the middle of the frontal sinuses
Cribriform plate of ethmoid	PA skull	Noted between the orbits in PA views
Petrous ridge	PA skull	Superimposed over the lower third of the orbital cavities. It is seen inferior to orbits in PA cephalogram.
Maxillary sinus	Waters view	Bilateral pneumatized structure. Largest of the paranasal sinuses
Nasal septum	PA skull	Linear opacity within nasal cavity extending vertically from the region of anterior nasal spine to nasion
Mastoid air cells	PA skull	Bilateral pneumatized air cells within the mastoid processes
Inferior orbital rim	PA skull, Waters view	Lower border of the orbit
Ethmoid sinuses	PA skull	Pneumatized ethmoid air cells
Sagittal suture, lambdoid suture, frontal suture	PA skull	Cranial sutures superimposed over frontal and temporal bones Frontal suture is usually noted clearly on PA cephalogram.
Zygomatic bone, zygomatic arch, coronoid process of the mandible, odontoid process	Waters view	These structures are seen clearly on the Waters view due to their position within the skull and the angulation of the x-ray beam.
Sphenoid air cells	SMV view	Seen within the sphenoid bone
Mandibular condyles, coronoid processes	SMV	Bilaterally noted in the temporomandibular joint area
Mandible, maxilla, sella turcica	Lateral skull and lateral cephalogram	Mandible and maxilla are superimposed. Sella turcica (pituitary fossa) is noted within the sphenoid.

necessary skill especially when CT scans are not readily available. The most common skull radiographs that are still in use are lateral cephalogram, Waters view, PA view, submentovertex (SMV), and reverse Towne view. The lateral oblique views that were widely used at one time have become outdated since the introduction of panoramic radiography. Lateral cephalograms demonstrate the nasal bone, frontal sinus, and sphenoid sinus (**Figs. 11** and **12**). A PA view of the skull is a useful view that shows numerous useful anatomic landmarks. These include the structures of the face and skull (**Fig. 13**). Waters view is used to evaluate maxillary sinus, frontal sinus, nasal septum,

mastoid air cells, zygomatic bone, and odontoid process of second cervical vertebra (C2) (**Figs. 14** and **15**). The SMV radiograph is used for evaluation of zygomatic arch and sphenoid sinus. A modified SMV view with reduced exposure is used for viewing the zygomatic arches by intentionally underexposing the skull. Only thin bones like the zygomatic arches get appropriate exposures and the rest of the skull is underexposed. This is called a jug handle view (**Fig. 16**). Reverse Towne radiographs are used for evaluation of mandibular condyles. Although somewhat dated now, the lateral oblique radiographs were used for evaluation of both the body of the mandible

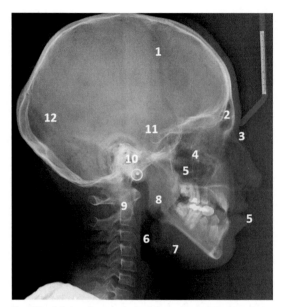

Fig. 11. A lateral cephalometric radiograph showing a properly positioned patient within a cephalostat. The round opaque area noted posterior to the mandibular condyles and superior to the first cervical vertebra (C1) is the ear rod that is designed to show the proximity of the external auditory meatus. Note the following structures on this radiograph—coronal suture (1), frontal sinus (2), nasal bone (3), zygomatic process (4), lower lip (5), common pharynx (6), hyoid bone (7), ramus of the mandible (8), odontoid process (9), external auditory meatus (10), sella turcica (11), and lambdoid suture (12).

and the ramus, including the coronoid and condyloid processes. These were replaced by panoramic radiographs.

A panoramic radiograph is used for evaluation of mandibular body, ramus, maxilla, upper and lower teeth, glenoid fossa, and zygomatic bone.

Panoramic Imaging

Panoramic radiographs are widely used as part of the dental and medical imaging arsenal. The American Dental Association recommendation of 2 bitewing radiographs in conjunction with a panoramic radiograph for assessment of patients with no clinically visible oral cavity lesions and caries is widely known and well-practiced and falls within the scope of the Food and Drug Administration/American Dental Association dental radiographic guidelines.[5]

Panoramic radiographs allow a larger coverage of the oral maxillofacial region, with relatively undistorted anatomic images and minimal superimposition of anatomic structures.[1]

Dental panoramic radiographs allow isolation and study of a particular plane or layer of an individual's maxillofacial anatomy. The images are created with the sensor and x-ray tube turning in opposite directions around a patient's head. The synchronized movement during image acquisition allows blurring out of structures above and below the plane housing the teeth and the jaws,

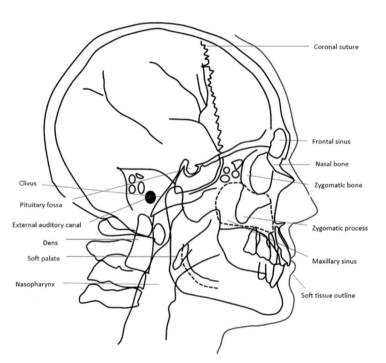

Fig. 12. Labeled, diagrammatic lateral cephalometric radiograph.

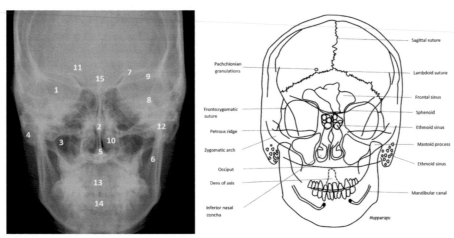

Fig. 13. Labeled PA radiograph on the left and its diagrammatic version on the right. Note the radiographic landmarks noted on this skull view—orbit (1), nasal septum (2), maxillary sinus (3), mastoid process (4), anterior nasal spine (5), ramus (6), supraorbital margin (7), greater wing of sphenoid (8), lesser wing of sphenoid (9), inferior nasal concha (10), frontal sinus (11), mandibular condyle (12), maxillary teeth (13), mandibular teeth (14), and crista galli (15).

highlighting the desired layer (teeth and jaws) referred to as the image layer.[6]

Panoramic radiographs are useful in assessment of jaws for abnormalities and midmaxillofacial assessment not visible by the intraoral radiographs (Fig. 17). Compared with the intraoral radiographs, they exhibit significantly greater amount of information.[6,7] The technology allowing acquisition of panoramic images introduces unique peculiarities, which have to be well understood and familiarized with.[6,7] These peculiarities may be explained by 1 or more of the following 7 concepts[1]:

- Maxillofacial structures are flattened and spread out.
- Midline structures may project as single images and double images.
- Ghost images are formed and are located on the opposite side of the image, higher and more blurry (Fig. 18).

Fig. 14. Labeled, diagrammatic Waters view radiograph.

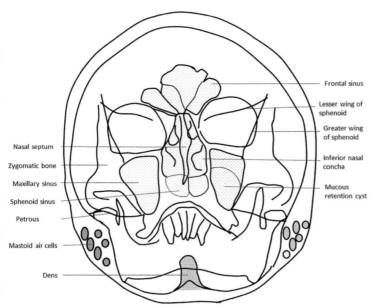

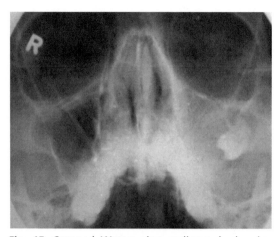

Fig. 15. Cropped Waters view radiograph showing normal right maxillary sinus and an opacified left maxillary sinus. Note the presence of a tooth within the left sinus that appears to have been displaced from the dental arch. The radiographic appearance is consistent with a dentigerous cyst within the left maxillary sinus.

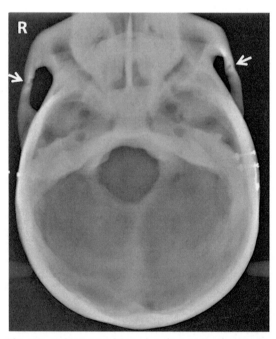

Fig. 16. An SMV positioned radiograph of a plastic skull to show the appearance of jug handle when the radiograph is intentionally underexposed to enhance the visualization of the 2 zygomatic arches. This was a common radiograph to rule out depressed fractures of the zygomatic arch if a CT scan was not available. In a typical underexposed jug handle view, none of the structures other than the zygomatic arches is discernible. The *arrows* point to the zygomatic arches bilaterally.

- Soft tissue outlines may be seen.
- Air spaces, such as the hypopharynx, oropharynx and nasopharynx, maxillary sinuses, and nasal fossa, are noted.
- Relative radiolucencies and radiopacities are visible.
  - Hard tissue (teeth and bone), soft tissue (eg, cartilage and fluid), and air are the components noted on the panoramic radiographs.
  - Hard tissue intersected by air space appear more radiolucent.
  - Hard tissue intersected by soft tissue appear less radiolucent.
- Angular interrelationships of structures are anatomically accurate.

The anatomic structures in a panoramic image is larger than the object that was imaged, mainly as a result of a nonuniform magnification of up to 20%.[6] It is also vital to remember to that only the structures within the desired image layer are in focus.[6] This image layer is narrower in the anterior and wider in the posterior regions.[1,6]

Interpretation of panoramic radiographs requires a systematic approach. To start, the radiograph may be divided into zones that allow comparison of bilateral structures seen superior to the maxillary teeth (zone 1), inferior to the lower border of the mandible that covers the entire neck bilaterally (zone 2), and on the right and left side of the radiograph lateral to the pterygomaxillary and retromolar regions (zones 3 and 4) as well as the maxillary and mandibular teeth, mandibular canal, mental foramen, and so forth (zone 5) (see **Fig. 17**). Bilateral structures in these areas should be compared with one another. In an ideally placed head position, these bilateral structures present with similar dimensions and shape. Variations from bilateral similarities may require further evaluation, assuming the head positioning is ideal.

Objects in the center of a patient's head, such as the cervical spine and the hyoid bone, are depicted on the sides of the panoramic radiograph, a peculiarity that is caused by the flattening and spreading out of the image. Although there is but 1 cervical spine and hyoid bone in the center of the head and neck region, the images are seen on both sides of the radiograph.[1,7]

The last area to be evaluated should be the dentition. The anatomic structures, discussed later, are reviewed with ease on a panoramic radiograph (**Fig. 19**). There are other structures that can also be reviewed but not marked on this radiographic image. These can be found in any standard oral and maxillofacial radiology text book.

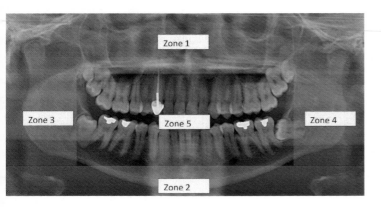

Cone Beam CT imaging

Advanced imaging modality like cone beam CT (CBCT) has become a useful tool for depicting the 3-D anatomy of the skull[7–9] and the maxillofacial structures, including teeth and the alveolar bone. The need for higher resolution is dictated by the demands of the area being investigated. Generally, the smaller the field of view, the higher the resolution because the pixel size gets smaller.

Typically, the CBCT skull anatomy can be reviewed using sagittal, coronal, or axial slices and using 3-D reconstructions; the volumes can be used for reviewing anatomy before and after orthognathic surgery, preoperative mock surgery using models, and implant treatment planning.

In CBCT anatomy of the mandible and maxilla, the anatomic slices observed are from a large volume CBCT at an isotropic voxel resolution of 400 μm × 400 μm × 400 μm (native resolution). If structures are examined at thicker slices, some of the fine anatomic details are lost but can be recaptured with the native resolution. The resolutions that are common in CBCT capture are 400 μm, 300 μm, 250 μm, 200 μm, 100 μm, and several resolutions less than 100 μm for volumetric

examination of smaller areas (limited volume CBCT).

Axial views

Radiographic anatomy of skull is viewed systematically. One common approach is to read the slices caudal to cephalic (inferior to superior), and the anatomy of the neck is viewed from cephalic to caudal. Bony maxillofacial anatomy starts from the identification of hyoid bone, the epiglottis, and the pharyngeal airway along with the symphysis of the mandible (**Fig. 20**) and also noted at that level is the fourth cervical vertebra. More superiorly, mandible is depicted in more detail (**Fig. 21**). Third cervical vertebra is noted at this level. Even more superiorly, the odontoid process of C2 (dens) is noted surrounded by the anterior and posterior arches of the atlas. At this level, mandibular foramen can be viewed. More cephalically, maxillary sinuses are noted along with bilateral rami; mastoid air cells and foramen magnum are seen at this level (**Fig. 22**). More superiorly, the maxillary sinuses can be viewed clearly along with zygomatic arches. The condyles can be viewed clearly at this level. Nasal anatomy can be visualized in all of the slices starting from the floor of the nasal fossa. Jugular bulb

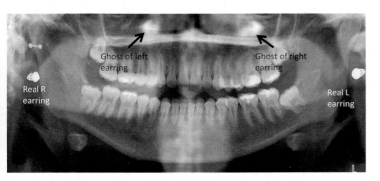

Fig. 18. A panoramic radiograph showing the ghosting of the ear rings. The real ear ring images as well as the ghosted ear ring artifacts (*arrows*) are as shown. In addition to the ear rings bilaterally, there is another piercing noted corresponding to the tragus of the ear on the right side. The ghost shadow of this ear rod would be even superior to the current ear ring ghosts and hence not seen on the image. L, left; R, right.

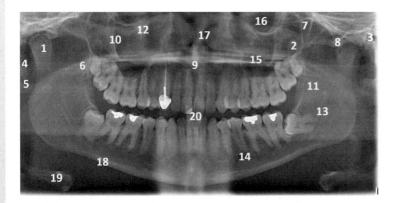

Fig. 19. A labeled panoramic radiograph showing the right mandibular condyle (1), coronoid processes (2), external auditory meatus (3), mastoid process (4), styloid process (5), pterygoid plates (6), pterygomaxillary fissure (7), articular eminence (8) anterior nasal spine (9), zygomatic process (10), mandibular ramus (11), infraorbital foramen (12), mandibular canal (13), mental foramen (14), maxillary sinus (15), orbit (16), nasal septum (17). Inferior border of the mandible (18), hyoid bone (19), and plastic bite block (20).

as well as the vertical portion of carotid canal can be viewed at this level. A bit superior, the slices show nasolacrimal ducts, horizontal portion of the carotid canals, the vidian canal, and the floor of the sphenoid sinus (**Fig. 23**). More cephalic slices from this point show the superior-most portions of the maxillary sinus, central sphenoid sinus, inferior orbital fissure, middle cranial fossa, and also posterior cranial fossa. Even more cephalically, the ethmoid air cells are depicted well and the superior orbital fissure can be seen clearly (**Fig. 24**). Both Optic canal and the clinoid processes can be seen at this level. The slice superior to this shows frontal sinus and the crista galli and as well as the parietal bones.

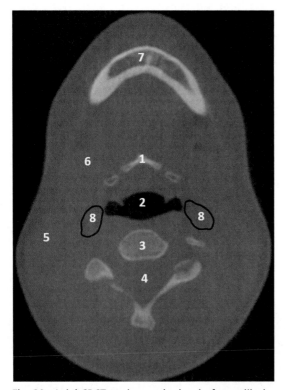

Fig. 20. Axial CBCT section at the level of mandibular symphysis demonstrating the hyoid bone (1), pharyngeal airway (2), body of C4 vertebra (3), vertebral foramen (4), sternocleidomastoid muscle (5), submandibular gland (6), mandibular symphysis (7), and the carotid sheath (8).

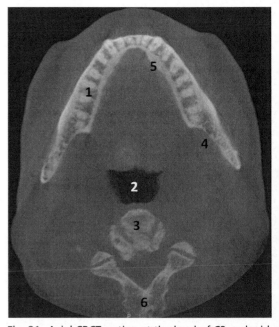

Fig. 21. Axial CBCT section at the level of C3 and midmandibular region demonstrating the body of the mandible (1), pharyngeal airway (2), body of C3 (3), submandibular fossa of the mandible (4), mandibular torus (5), transverse process of C3 (6).

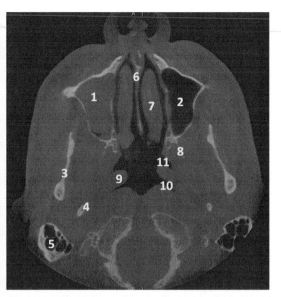

Fig. 22. Axial CBCT section at the level of pterygoid plates and inferior conchae demonstrating the mucous thickening in the right maxillary sinus (1), a normal left maxillary sinus (2), ramus of the mandible (3), styloid process (4), mastoid air cells (5), nasal septum (6), inferior nasal concha (7), lateral pterygoid plate (8), torus tubarius (9), fossa of Rosenmüller (10), and the eustachian tube (11).

Coronal views
Similar to axial view CBCT anatomy, the sectional anatomy is best viewed from anterior to posterior (**Fig. 25**). The anatomic areas of

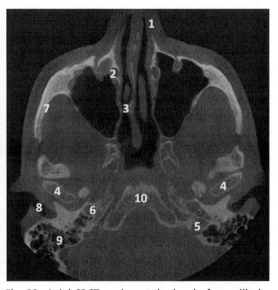

Fig. 23. Axial CBCT section at the level of mandibular condyles showing the ala of the nose (1), nasolacrimal duct (2), nasal spine (3), mandibular condyle (4), jugular bulb (5), vertical portion of the carotid canal (6), zygomatic arch (7), external auditory meatus (8), mastoid air cells (9) and clivus (10).

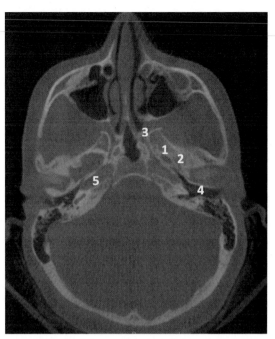

Fig. 24. Axial CBCT section at the level of base of the skull showing the foramen ovale (1), foramen spinosum (2), vidian canal (3), external auditory meatus (4), and the horizontal portion of the carotid canal (5).

interest start from the anterior aspects of mandible, maxilla, orbits, and the frontal bone. Symphysis menti can be viewed along with some anterior teeth and in this vertical plane, the anterior portion of the maxillary sinuses, nasal anatomy, ethmoid air cells, orbits, and frontal sinus can be seen. Moving posteriorly, the shadow of the tongue and bony anatomy of the mandible (now bilateral) along with either mental foramen or inferior alveolar nerve canal on either side, maxillary sinuses in full view along with nasal septum, bilateral nasal conchae (mostly inferior and middle), the uncinated process, ethmoid air cells, lamina paparacea, the cribriform plate of ethmoid, crista galli, and the frontal bone can be identified. More posteriorly, the zygomaticofrontal suture, zygomaticofacial foramen, and, within the mandible, the submandibular gland fossa along with all other anatomic landmarks discussed previously can be appreciated. Continuation of the anatomy more posteriorly is the visualization of sphenoid air cells, the pterygoid plates (both medial and lateral), the vomerine bone, the mandibular rami bilaterally. As the pharyngeal air space is entered, the fossa of Rosenmüller can be visualized. Incidentally, this is the plane where foramen rotundum can be noted. Foramen rotundum transmits the

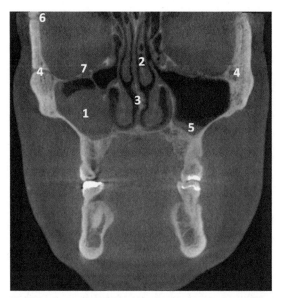

Fig. 25. Coronal CBCT section at the level of maxillary sinuses showing a mucous retention cyst in the right maxillary sinus (1), concha bullosa of the middle concha (2), deviated nasal septum (3), zygomaticofacial foramen and canal (4), mild mucous thickening on the floor of the left maxillary sinus (5), zygomaticofrontal suture (6), and infraorbital foramen (7).

the anterior arch of C1, the clivus, and condylar heads bilaterally along with the glenoid fossa and the clear visualization of the part of middle cranial fossa in this region. Once in the vicinity of the sphenoid bone, the sphenoid sinuses, fading foramen rotundum, optic canal, fading pterygoid fossa, and the fading hyoid bone are noted. The most posterior slice that can be visualized are the slice through the cervical vertebrae and the foramen magnum. Noted anatomy is the cervical vertebrae, the dens, the occipital bone, the external auditory meatus bilaterally, and the contents of the middle ear.

Sagittal views

Because anatomy is identical on both sides of the face (not necessarily symmetric), the sagittal anatomy can be visualized and a replica on the other side expected and, when the anatomy changes on one side, the more normal side acts as a control for comparison purposes. Starting with the midsagittal plane, structures, including both soft tissue and bony, can be identified readily via this slicing. The mandible, genial tubercles, hard palate, soft palate, epiglottis, anterior nasal spine, posterior nasal spine, nasal bone, frontal sinus, sphenoid sinus, dorsum sellae and planum sphenoidale, clivus, anterior and posterior arches of atlas, and the dens are some of the structures that can be identified on this section (**Fig. 26**). In the midline, the uvula, the incisive foramen in the maxilla, the lingual foramen in the mandible, frontal sinus, and the clivus can be noted more clearly. Posterior pharyngeal wall can be noted on this view more clearly. More

maxillary branch of the trigeminal nerve. Even more posteriorly, the greater palatine foramina can be identified within the posterior part of the hard palate. The ethmoid air cells are vividly noted along with fading anatomy of the zygoma. Toward the posterior wall of the pharyngeal air space, the bony landmarks are the hyoid bone,

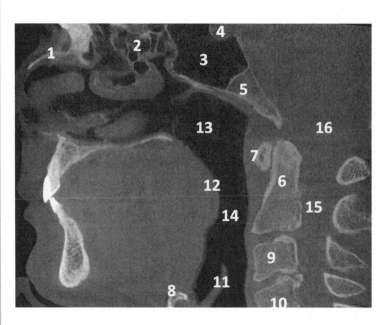

Fig. 26. Midsagittal CBCT section showing the nasal bone (1), posterior ethmoid sinuses (2), sphenoid sinus (3), sella turcica (4), clivus (5), dens (6), anterior arch of atlas (7), hyoid bone (8), C3 (9), C4 (10), epiglottis (11), uvula (12), nasopharynx (13), oropharynx (14), vertebral foramen (15), and foramen magnum (16).

laterally, the conchae can be identified along with the rest of the palate, the ethmoid sinuses, and lateral part of the pharyngeal airway. Only parts of the cervical vertebrae can be noted. A more lateral view from this point is the appearance of the condyle, glenoid fossa, external auditory meatus, and articular eminence and the mastoid process.

Cross-sectional views (orthogonal views)

Along with the anatomic depiction in the multiplanar reconstructions, a series of sequential anatomy via the display mechanism using the CBCT software can be noted. These are serial slices of orthogonal views at any preferred anatomy within the maxilla and mandible. An example of such an anatomic view is seen in **Fig. 27**. The Cross-sectional slices are reconstructed for the purposes of evaluation and measurement of alveolar bone for variety of reasons, the most common being root form dental implant placement. Preimplant assessment of alveolar bone is done this way. Other indications for this form of imaging are evaluating eruption sequence or impaction of the unerupted teeth and evaluating their follicular space, path of eruption, extent of root resorption of permanent teeth, and so forth.

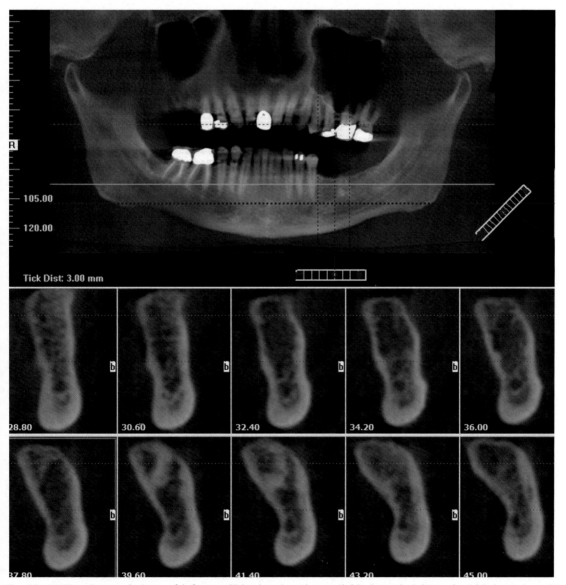

Fig. 27. CBCT orthogonal views of left mandible showing the available bone height and width in regions 17 (slice 28.80) through 19 (slice 45.00). Note the excellent visualization of the mandibular canal and presence of idiopathic osteosclerosis in the region corresponding to 18. These are also called cross-sectional views.

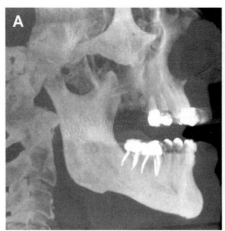
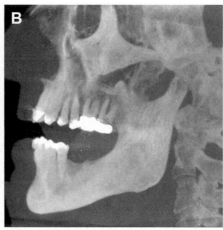

Fig. 28. MIPs of a CBCT volume that was referred for a preimplant assessment of the partially edentulous left mandible (*B*) and dentate right mandible (*A*).

Maximum intensity projections and 3-D reconstructions

Maximum intensity projections (MIPs) are image reconstructions using a volume rendering method for 3-D data that projects in the visual plane the maximum intensity voxels. This technique was invented by Wallis and colleagues[10] in 1989 for use in nuclear medicine and was originally called maximum activity projection. In maxillofacial imaging, this technique has value in detecting calcifications within head and neck that are new and represent soft tissue calcifications (**Fig. 28**) as well as calcifications within vessels[10] (for instance neck carotid calcifications [**Fig. 29**]). MIP images are used routinely in medicine for interpreting PET or magnetic resonance angiography studies.

3-D reconstructions (**Fig. 30**) are part of the display in most software applications and Digital imaging and Communication in Medicine (DICOM) viewers. The reconstruction algorithms allow for accurate depiction of bony anatomy.[11] These can be used for certain diagnostic tasks, 3-D image printing for patient education, and preoperative and postoperative orthognathic surgery.

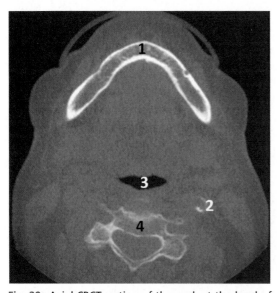

Fig. 29. Axial CBCT section of the neck at the level of the mandibular symphysis demonstrating calcification within common carotid artery. Mandibular symphysis (1), common carotid calcification (2), common pharynx (3), and body of fourth cervical vertebra (4) are as noted.

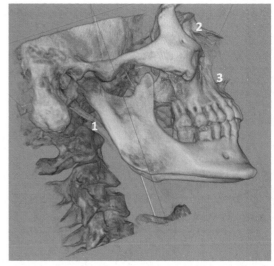

Fig. 30. A 3-D reconstruction of the skull showing detail of the bony components and the teeth in occlusion. Note the slightly elongated styloid processes bilaterally (1) and the appearance of the nasal bone (2) as well as the anterior nasal spine (3).

Clinical applications of CBCT imaging span from detection of bony pathoses to 3-D evaluation of the proposed implant site.[12]

SUMMARY

Oral and maxillofacial imaging includes imaging of teeth and surrounding dental structures, a thorough anatomic depiction of the jaws that house the teeth, and also the skull anatomy as contiguous structures. Digital 2-D as well as 3-D imaging can be successfully used to evaluate the bony anatomy of this area. This anatomy article complements other articles in this issue to understand the oral and maxillofacial pathophysiology.

REFERENCES

1. Langland O, Langlais R, Preece J. Principles of dental imaging. 2nd edition. Philadelphia: Lippincott Williams & Wilkins; 2002.

2. Stafne EC, Bibilisco JA. Oral roentgenographic diagnosis. 4th edition. Philadelphia: W. B. Saunders Company; 1975.

3. Worth HM. Principles and practice of oral radiographic interpretation. Chicago: Year Book Medical Publishers; 1963. p. 15–54, 55–72.

4. White SC, Pharoah MJ. Oral radiology principles and interpretation. St Louis (MO): Elsevier Mosby; 2014. p. 153–65.

5. Available at: http://www.ada.org/en/publications/ada-news/2012-archive/november/ada-updates-dental-radiograph-recommendations. Accessed February 13, 2017.

6. Farman AG. Panoramic radiology seminars on maxillofacial imaging and interpretation. New York: Springer-Verlag; 2007.

7. Mupparapu M, Nadeau C. Oral and maxillofacial imaging. Dent Clin North Am 2016;60:1–37.

8. Angelopoulos C. Anatomy of the maxillofacial region in the three planes of section. Dent Clin North Am 2014;58:497–521.

9. Angelopoulos C. Cone beam tomographic imaging anatomy of the maxillofacial region. Dent Clin North Am 2008;52:731–52.

10. Wallis JW, Miller TR, Lerner CA, et al. Three-dimensional display in nuclear medicine. IEEE Trans Med Imaging 1989;8:297–303.

11. Miracle AC, Mukherji SK. Cone beam CT of the head and neck. Part : physical principles. AJNR Am J Neuroradiol 2009;30:1088–95.

12. Miracle AC, Mukherji SK. Cone beam CT of the head and neck. Part 2: clinical applications. AJNR Am J Neuroradiol 2009;30:1285–92.

Imaging of Odontogenic Infections

Shaza Mardini, DDS, MS[a],*, Anita Gohel, BDS, PhD[b]

KEYWORDS

- Odontogenic infection • Osteomyelitis • Head and neck spaces • Cross-sectional imaging
- Panoramic radiography

KEY POINTS

- Odontogenic infections represent a common clinical problem in patients of all ages.
- The presence of teeth enables the direct spread of inflammatory products from dental caries, trauma, and/or periodontal disease into the maxilla and mandible.
- The radiographic changes seen depend on the type and duration of the inflammatory process and host body response.
- Imaging plays a central role in identifying the source of infection and the extent of the disease spread, and in detecting any complications.
- The imaging modalities used can range from conventional radiography, cone-beam computed tomography, contrast-enhanced computed tomography, MR imaging, and nuclear medicine studies.

INTRODUCTION

Infections in the jaws have diverse clinical courses and outcomes, as the origin and the spread of these infections involve various tissues and anatomic spaces. Infection in the jaws and surrounding structures may be odontogenic or nonodontogenic in origin. Odontogenic infection is that which arises from the tooth or structures closely surrounding the tooth. Inflammatory lesions are the most common pathology condition of the jaws.[1] Infections from the teeth can directly spread into adjacent osseous and soft tissues. Imaging plays a key role in identifying the source of infections, the extent of the disease process, and detecting any complications.[2] This article explores the various odontogenic infections, including dental caries, periodontal disease, pulpal disease, pericoronitis, osteomyelitis, and the appropriate imaging for their diagnoses, as well as the

extension of these infections into the surrounding maxillofacial spaces.

The role of diagnostic imaging is to define the location of the infection and to explore for possible spread of the disease beyond the site of origin.[3] Plain radiography still is an important component of diagnosing dental caries and periodontal disease. Computed tomography (CT), including cone-beam CT (CBCT) plays an important role in detecting bony changes and periosteal reactions. However, CT is superior to CBCT in the assessment of soft tissue spread of infections. Magnetic resonance (MR) imaging is the ideal imaging protocol to diagnose soft tissue infections due to the high spatial and contrast resolution provided in these images. T1-weighted images are ideal for evaluating anatomy and short-T inversion recovery (STIR) or T2-weighted images provide information about soft tissue edema.[4]

There are no commercial or financial conflicts of interest for either author.
[a] BeamReaders, Inc, 7117 West Hood Place, Suite 110, Kennewick, WA 99336, USA; [b] Oral and Maxillofacial Radiology, Division of Oral and Maxillofacial Pathology and Radiology, The Ohio State University College of Dentistry, 3165 Postle Hall, 305 West 12th Avenue, Columbus, OH 43210-1267, USA
* Corresponding author.
E-mail address: shaza@beamreaders.com

Radiol Clin N Am 56 (2018) 31–44
http://dx.doi.org/10.1016/j.rcl.2017.08.003

radiologic.theclinics.com

CARIES

Definition

Dental caries occurs when there is loss of mineral in the tooth structure caused by bacterial by-products. Dental caries is a highly prevalent disease affecting up to 92% of adults.[5]

Etiology

The cariogenic bacteria that initially are at the tooth surface create a demineralization of the outer tooth structure and through that damaged surface can enter the tooth. Caries is a dynamic process with alternative phases of demineralization and remineralization.[6] The surface lesion may then progress to a larger lesion below the surface. Root caries that do not occur as a spread from coronal tooth caries may be the result of an oral environment lacking saliva to wash away the plaque and organisms; that is, drug-induced or radiation-induced xerostomia. Caries affecting the pulp chamber of the tooth will compromise the pulpal tissues and will progress to an inflammatory process within the root canal system and eventually lead to the death of the pulpal tissues. Caries may also recur after dental restorations have been placed where the margins are maladapted to the tooth surface and bacteria have a path to enter.

Radiographic Findings

Initial demineralization of the tooth surface occurs within the enamel as a cavitation or lucent zone commonly on the interproximal surfaces of the teeth. Caries that progresses below the surface appears as a triangle shape showing the spread from a larger base near the enamel surface and narrowing to a point toward the tooth center. The dentinoenamel junction (DEJ) is an important radiographic landmark, as it marks where the caries enters the dentin and then changes radiographic shape. If caries is limited to the enamel and has not reached the DEJ, it is called "incipient caries." As the caries encroaches on the dentin, it spreads along the DEJ to create another wide base that tapers to a point at the pulp. Larger carious lesions may then spread in multiple directions, into the pulp and further into the root, and are called "severe caries." **Fig. 1** shows the stages of caries from simple demineralization of the enamel surface to the larger caries extending into the pulp. The pattern for root caries is an isolated radiographic lucency on the root of the tooth superior to the crestal bone (**Fig. 2**). Recurrent dental caries is common and will appear as a lucent area at the edge of the dental restoration (**Fig. 3**).

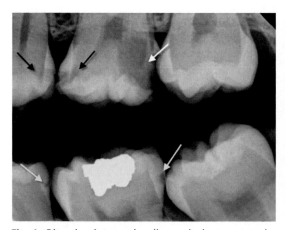

Fig. 1. Bitewing intraoral radiograph shows examples of carious lesions. The yellow arrows indicate incipient lesions that are limited to the enamel. The black arrows indicate caries into the DEJ and the white arrow indicates severe caries that has reached the pulp.

Intraoral dental radiography is the most appropriate imaging modality for diagnosis of caries. This includes periapical and bitewing radiographs. The resolution of these radiographs allows for detailed analysis of caries progression as well as analysis of the bone surrounding the tooth. One of the drawbacks of bitewing radiography is that it cannot differentiate between the clinical state of the surface; whether it is intact or cavitated.[7]

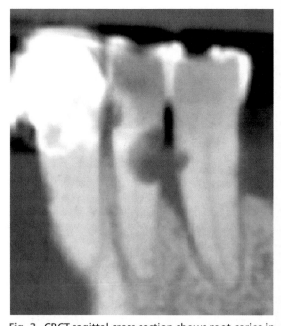

Fig. 2. CBCT sagittal cross section shows root caries in the mandibular left premolars. These lesions appear scooped out and are located at or below the CEJ and are usually associated with periodontal bone loss.

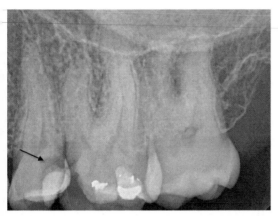

Fig. 3. Periapical radiograph shows recurrent caries (*black arrow*) under a previous restoration.

Panoramic dental imaging may provide an overall screening of any large carious lesions; however, smaller lesions will not be seen, as they have a lower resolution compared with intraoral radiographs. Caries can be seen on 3-dimensional (3D) imaging of the jaws, such as CBCT; however, due to factors such as metal artifacts, recurrent caries is very difficult to diagnosis on CT (**Fig. 4**). CBCT images may be more accurate in detecting occlusal and deep dentinal lesions but the increase in sensitivity correlates to a simultaneous decrease in specificity.[8]

Treatment

Small cavitations that are confined to the enamel may be remineralized with a variety of products, including fluoride and calcium phosphate treatments among many.[9] Deeper dental caries reaching the DEJ require removal and restoration with the preservation of the surrounding healthy tooth

structure. A variety of dental restorative materials are available, including materials that range from radiolucent to radiopaque. If the pulp is compromised, then root canal therapy is indicated even if there are no radiographic signs of apical pathology.

PERIODONTAL DISEASE
Definition

Periodontitis is a complex disease characterized by infection and inflammation of the supporting structures of the teeth.[10] There may be localized disease of the periodontium of a single tooth or may be widespread and generalized throughout the dentition. It is characterized by the loss of bone that supports the teeth.

Etiology

Periodontitis is preceded by gingivitis, which is the inflammation in the gingival soft tissues overlying the bone. In the case of gingivitis, the bone is not affected and therefore is diagnosed clinically, not radiographically. Gingivitis may then progress to periodontitis where a pocket forms that allows for bacteria to move further into the tissues and release toxins that can damage the tissues including bone, or they may cause a local host inflammatory reaction that in turn may damage tissues as well. Periodontitis is classified as either chronic (localized or generalized), aggressive (localized or generalized), a manifestation of systemic disease, necrotizing, or as abscesses of the periodontium and combined periodontic-endodontic lesions. Both extrinsic and intrinsic factors such as complex relationships between microorganisms in dental biofilm (plaque) and the immuno-inflammatory response of the host, the

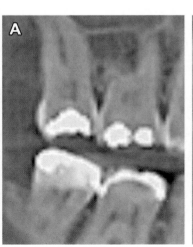

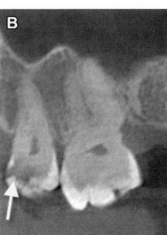

Fig. 4. CBCT cropped images demonstrate the limitations of caries diagnosis using this modality. (*A*) A low-resolution CBCT image with metallic restorations does not allow for diagnosis of caries due to artifact and lower-quality image. (*B*) A higher-resolution CBCT image with no metal artifact shows large caries at the arrow. Diagnosis of larger caries is possible on CBCT with higher-quality images with less artifact.

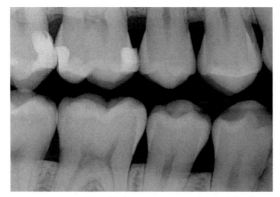

Fig. 5. Bitewing radiograph shows the normal level of the periodontal bone, not more than 2 mm from the CEJ.

influence of genetic factors, environmental and/or acquired conditions, such as smoking and other systemic diseases contribute to the disease process.[11,12] There are at least 16 diseases that may manifest periodontitis.[13]

Radiographic Findings

Radiographically, normal crestal bone levels are seen within 1 to 2 mm of the cemento-enamel junction (CEJ) of the teeth (**Fig. 5**). The shape of the crest may vary from rounded to flat. The radiographic signs of periodontitis include generalized shape change at the crest, crestal bone loss (horizontal and/or vertical), widening of the periodontal ligament (PDL) space, and bone loss in the furcation space. Contributing factors to periodontal disease may be identified radiographically as well, such as presence of calculus, overhanging restorations, tooth impactions, and dental crowding. These may cause retention of plaque, which creates a situation whereby gingivitis may occur and may progress to periodontitis. Several different modalities may be used to identify periodontal disease. Panoramic imaging may be useful as an overall screening tool to evaluate the general bone levels with respect to the dentition but will not provide detail of the dental alveolar relationship (**Fig. 6**). Periapical and bitewing

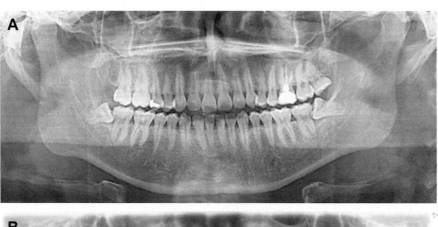

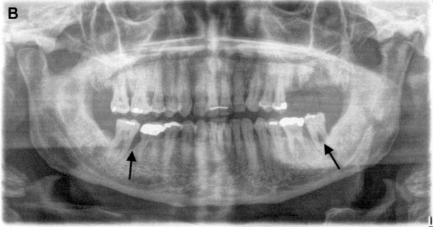

Fig. 6. Panoramic images demonstrate the periodontal bone levels in (*A*) normal and (*B*) a patient with generalized periodontal disease with furcation involvement (bone loss) in the molars (*arrows*).

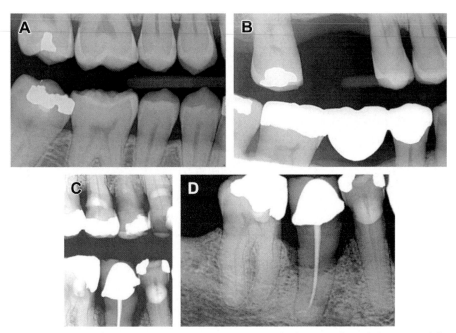

Fig. 7. Images show the use of bitewing and periapical radiographs for periodontal diagnosis: (A) a horizontal bitewing demonstrating normal crestal bone, (B) a horizontal bitewing demonstrates periodontal disease, (C) a vertical bitewing can be used if the bone loss is extensive and cannot be included in the horizontal bitewing field of view, and (D) a periapical radiograph can be used to evaluate moderate to severe lesions that cannot be completely evaluated on vertical bitewings.

radiographs have been considered to play an important role for periodontal diagnosis and treatment planning[14] (Fig. 7). Bitewing radiographs are the standard dental images used for evaluating the crestal bone between the teeth due to the geometry of image acquisition being parallel to the occlusal plane. This allows for an accurate view of the relationship of the tooth structures to the bone. Bone loss in the root furcation area is one example of that relationship. Periapical images help identify any disruption or widening of the PDL space surrounding the tooth (Fig. 8). Three-dimensional imaging such as CBCT at higher resolution may provide both bone levels and assessment of the PDL space; however, lower-resolution scans may not be useful for evaluation of the PDL spaces (Fig. 9). CBCT imaging provides accurate analysis of furcation involvement,[15,16] morphology of vertical bone defects, and root morphology, which are important in treatment planning and tooth prognosis.

Treatment

Periodontitis is a complex disease process and treatment is dependent on the severity, location, and the prognosis of the teeth within the periodontium. Maintenance of healthy periodontal tissues may involve a variety of treatments, including

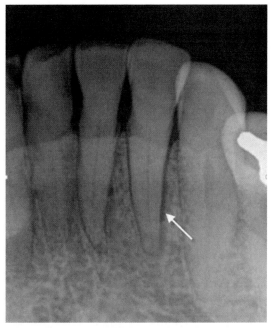

Fig. 8. Periapical radiograph of the anterior mandibular teeth shows widening of the lateral PDL space (arrow). This appearance can be seen in cases of orthodontic movement, periodontal bone loss with mobility of teeth, and malignancy growing within the PDL.

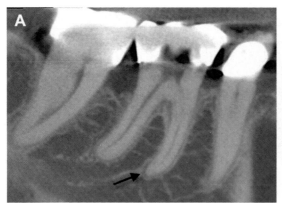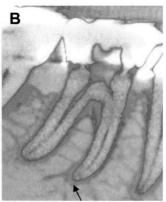

Fig. 9. High-resolution small field-of-view CBCT (*A*) sagittal cross section shows a widened periapical PDL space (*arrow*), suggestive of early periapical inflammation, and (*B*) inversion and colorization of the image in software helps in the visualization of the apical PDL widening (*arrow*).

deep cleaning known as scaling and root planing, localized or systemic antibiotic therapy, and surgical procedures, such as gingival and bone grafting.

PULPAL AND PERIAPICAL DISEASE
Definition

Pulpal and periapical diseases are multiple entities that are a sequela of pulp death. Apical periodontitis (periapical rarefying osteitis) is an inflammatory condition of the apical peri-radicular tissues that is caused by microbial infestation of the tooth's root canal system. An apical granuloma or cyst is the result of chronic apical periodontitis.[17] A granuloma is considered a collection of granulomatous tissue with a well-developed fibrous capsule that is attached to the root surface. An apical or radicular cyst is a true epithelial-lined cyst resulting from chronic apical periodontitis. Condensing osteitis, also known as periapical sclerosing osteitis, represents an increase in lamellar bone in response to low-grade persistent infection.[18]

Etiology

Dental caries is the most common cause of pulpal inflammation. Invasion of microorganisms into the pulp system causes necrosis of the pulpal tissues, which seep into the periapical tissues through the apical foramen, or through the lateral dentinal canals into the lateral periradicular tissues. In the early stages of the disease process, diagnosis is based on clinical signs and symptoms. Chronic apical periodontitis then may lead to formation of a granuloma or cyst. Differentiation between the 2 is most accurate via histologic examination[19];

however, radiographically it may be very difficult to differentiate the 2 entities.

Radiographic Findings

The earliest radiographic changes occur when bacterial colonization of the internal root canal system occurs leading to the breakdown of the tissues surrounding the apex of the root. The widening of the apical periodontal ligament (PDL) space on a periapical radiograph marks the initial radiographic changes of the periapical inflammation.[16] As the disease progresses, disruption of the lamina dura occurs, leading to a periapical radiolucency, which can be appreciated on an intraoral radiograph and may be referred to as rarefying osteitis (**Fig. 10**). Chronic apical periodontitis will result in formation of an apical granuloma/

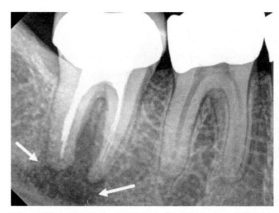

Fig. 10. Periapical radiograph of a mandibular molar shows apical rarefying osteitis/apical periodontitis on a previously endodontically treated tooth (*arrows*).

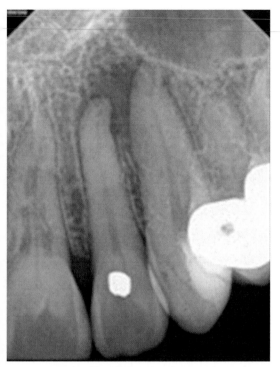

Fig. 11. Periapical radiograph of a maxillary lateral incisor shows periapical osteitis suggestive of an apical cyst or granuloma.

cyst that presents as a well-defined radiolucency at the apex of the tooth (**Fig. 11**). There may or may not be a corticated outline. In some cases, root resorption may occur from long-standing inflammatory pathology. Expansion of the lesion is common but the epicenter remains at the tooth apex. In some cases as a result of chronic inflammation, the adjacent bone may respond by forming sclerotic bone that can be seen as condensing osteitis (**Fig. 12**). Initial radiographic evaluation for periapical disease is best achieved with plain-film dental techniques, such as panoramic or periapical images. Two-dimensional imaging, however, does have its limitations with respect to detection of periapical lesions. Studies have shown[20] that the cortical bone must be eroded to detect the lesion on periapical radiographs. CBCT has proven to be very useful in detecting periapical changes, and recently has been cited to be more accurate at detecting apical lesions than periapical radiographs[21] (**Fig. 13**). However, the convenience of intraoral dental images and lower radiation still make them the initial choice for diagnosis. In cases with clinical signs and no radiographic correlation on 2-dimensional images, CBCT is the next choice for further evaluation. CBCT also may aid in evaluating the epicenter and extension of lesion in bone, canal, and root morphology; root resorptions; and tooth fractures. MR imaging is not indicated in diagnosis of pulpal and periapical disease.

Treatment

The treatment of apical periodontitis is conventionally by root canal therapy. Complete removal of the pulpal tissue within the pulp chamber and root canal system is performed, the chambers are decontaminated and filled with gutta percha. In the case in which the tooth is not restorable, extraction may be indicated.

PERICORONITIS
Definition

Inflammation occurring around the crown of a partially erupted tooth is known as pericoronitis. It most commonly presents in partially erupted mandibular third molars.

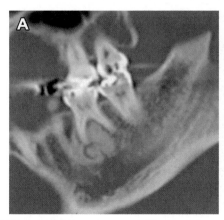
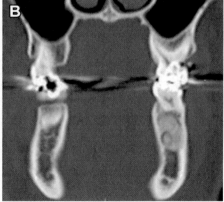

Fig. 12. CBCT sagittal (A) and coronal (B) views show periapical condensing (sclerosing) osteitis related to the mandibular left fist molar.

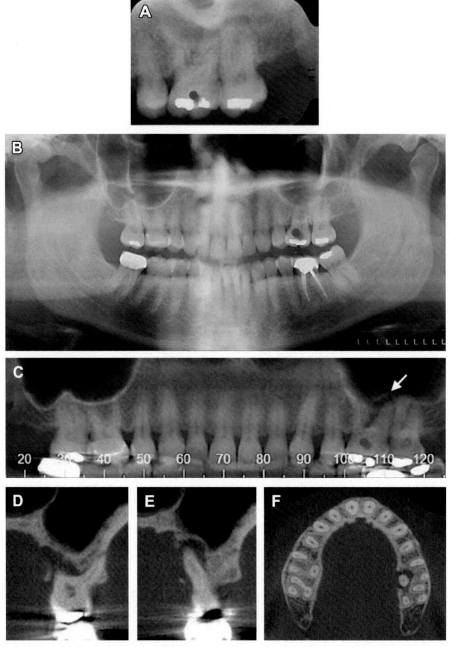

Fig. 13. A series of plain-film imaging and CBCT reformats shows the efficacy of these images for evaluation of the same periapical lesion. (*A*) Periapical radiograph shows the tooth in question marked with a red dot, no visible pathology noted. (*B*) Panoramic radiograph of the same patient, no significant pathology seen associated with the tooth. (*C*) CBCT panoramic reconstruction shows a small opaque line in the sinus (*arrow*), suggestive of elevated periosteum. (*D–F*) Cross-sectional and axial reformats show clearly an apical cyst associated with the palatal root that was not seen on the 2-dimensional imaging.

Etiology

Trapping of food particles in the gingival tissue overlying the partially erupted tooth creates a source of inflammation. This inflammation can then spread into the surrounding bone.

Radiographic Findings

Radiographically the area may include no bony change, loss of trabeculation, localized rarefaction with or without sclerosis, or even osteomyelitis.[22] Commonly, the lesion will present as a small rarefaction with thick sclerotic borders at the distal aspect of the crown of an impacted molar (**Fig. 14**). If there is dilation of the distal aspect of the third-molar follicle due to infection, this is called the "paradental cyst of the third molar." Imaging of pericoronitis may vary from a simple intraoral radiograph of the tooth to more advanced imaging to evaluate the spread of infection. The standard dental imaging, such as periapical or panoramic radiographs, may be used to identify the origin of the infection. A CBCT will show the lesion in 3 dimensions, which helps to evaluate the faciolingual characteristics, including the integrity of the cortices and the relationship of the lesion to surrounding structures, such as the inferior-alveolar canal in the mandible or the sinus in the maxilla. More advanced imaging, such as CT with contrast or MR imaging is useful to evaluate the spread of the infection into potential surrounding spaces.

Treatment

Extraction of the impacted tooth is indicated in the case of pericoronitis. Antibiotic therapy is often used in conjunction with surgery.

OSTEOMYELITIS
Definition

The inflammation of bone and bone marrow is known as osteomyelitis. The process can occur in any bone including the maxillofacial complex, but is more common in the mandible than the maxilla.

Etiology

The origin of the infection may be within the bone or adjacent soft tissues.[2] Osteomyelitis is often classified by its duration; acute versus chronic.[23] Osteomyelitis usually starts as an acute infection and may develop into a chronic condition. Osteomyelitis of the jaws is most often caused by a bacterial focus that can originate from odontogenic infection, periodontal disease, extraction sites, foreign bodies, or fracture sites. As the pyogenic organisms enter the bone marrow, an inflammatory response is generated and the endosteal surface of the cortical bone is resorbed, which can further progress to loss of cortical bone. Osteomyelitis is often described as a continuum. The acute phase is caused by spread of infection into the bone marrow. Clinically the patient typically will exhibit symptoms such as pain, swelling, fever, and lymphadenopathy. Purulent drainage may or may not be present.

Radiographic Findings

Radiographically at its earliest stages there may be minimal changes seen in the bone. An ill-defined area of decreased density may be appreciated on 2-dimensional intraoral images. If the process progresses to the periosteum, the disruption of the membrane can cause new bone to be laid down, known as a "periosteal reaction" or "periosteal new bone formation" (**Fig. 15**). This radiographic finding is characteristic of osteomyelitis but might not always be present. The most pathognomonic feature of osteomyelitis radiographically is the presence of

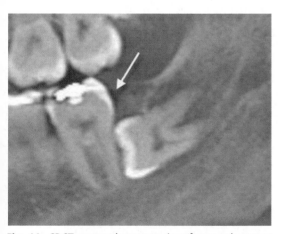

Fig. 14. CBCT cropped panoramic reformat shows an impacted third molar with a clinical presentation of pericoronitis. Bone rarefaction is noted superior to the crown of the impacted tooth (*white arrow*), suggestive of inflammation.

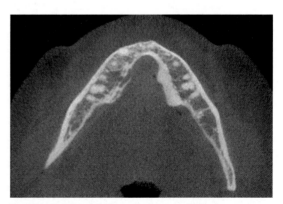

Fig. 15. CBCT axial view of the mandible shows osteomyelitis affecting the right mandibular torus (compare the rarefied appearance to the normal cortical bone of the left torus). This dense bone is more susceptible to developing osteomyelitis due to its decreased vascularity.

bony sequestra. These are small segments of bone that have become isolated due to necrosis of the surrounding bone.[23] In the later stages of acute osteomyelitis, sclerosis at the periphery may be detected as well as small sequestra within the region (**Fig. 16**). Chronic osteomyelitis may present radiographically different from acute osteomyelitis. Cortical erosion, mixed osteopenia with sclerosis, and periosteal reaction are among the late radiographic findings, along with possible soft tissue swelling.[23,24]

Although initial examination may occur with 2-dimensional dental images, CBCT and multi-detector CT (MDCT) are more appropriate for an accurate diagnosis and evaluation of the bone. CBCT can define the bone pattern and extent of the affected area. MDCT images provide the fine bone detail and can identify the source of infection and sequestra. MR imaging is useful and allows for early detection of osteomyelitis and can assess the extent of the disease. The early findings for acute osteomyelitis

are usually low signal intensity on T1-weighted images and a high signal on T2-weighted and STIR sequences.[2] For chronic osteomyelitis, there will be low signal with both T1-weighted and T2-weighted images. A sequestrum will have a low signal intensity with T1-weighted or STIR sequences, whereas the surrounding tissue will have a high signal with T2-weighted or STIR sequences. Nuclear medicine images can also diagnose early osteomyelitis and can detect active disease.[22] Three-phase bone scintigraphy with 99mTc-labeled methyl diphosphonate is mainly used to detect osteomyelitis. FDG-PET has proven to be useful in diagnosing chronic osteomyelitis.[2,23] **Table 1** shows a summary of the different modalities and their findings with respect to osteomyelitis.

Treatment

The treatment of osteomyelitis is often with long-term systemic antibiotic therapy, which may occur

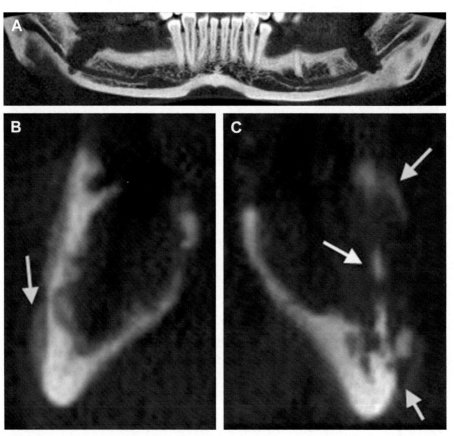

Fig. 16. CBCT (*A*) panoramic reformat of a patient with bilateral osteomyelitis of the posterior mandible shows nonhealed third-molar extraction sockets. (*B*) Coronal cross section of the right posterior mandible shows periosteal new bone formation (*yellow arrow*). (*C*) Coronal cross section of the left posterior mandible shows periosteal new bone formation (*yellow arrows*) and bone sequestration (*white arrow*).

Table 1	
Radiographic findings of osteomyelitis	
Imaging Modality	**Main Findings**
Conventional radiograph	Acute: Ill-defined areas of osteopenia Chronic: Periosteal reaction (onion-skin), mixed density areas changing to more sclerotic over time, sequestrum
MDCT	Chronic: Periosteal reaction, mixed density areas, cortical erosion, sequestrum, blurred fat planes, soft tissue gas, sinus tracts
MR imaging	Acute: T1W, low signal intensity; STIR or T2W, high signal intensity; with gadolinium: enhanced area of granulation tissue around sequestrum Chronic: T1W and T2W and STIR, low signal intensity
Bone scan	Focal areas of hyperperfusion, hyperemia, and bone uptake

Abbreviations: MDCT, multidetector computed tomography; STIR, short-T inversion recovery; T1W, T1-weighted; T2W, T2-weighted.

in conjunction with hyperbaric oxygen treatment. Surgery is often indicated, particularly in the chronic osteomyelitis cases.

SPACE INFECTIONS
Definition

The spread of odontogenic infection into the neighboring spaces surrounding the maxillofacial complex is known as a space infection. These infections are of great concern due to the proximity to areas that can create life-threatening complications. The potential spaces formed by fascial planes give a pathway to areas such as the oropharynx and hypopharynx, orbits, and cavernous sinus among others.

Etiology

Odontogenic infection leads to the spread of the infection into the surrounding spaces. This may

originate from a tooth in either the maxilla or mandible. Space infections caused by dental infection in the mandibular molars tends to start in the submandibular space due to the position of the mandibular molar apices inferior to the mylohyoid muscle. Space infections caused by dental infections in the mandibular premolars or anterior teeth tend to start in the sublingual space, as these apices are located superior to the mylohyoid muscle. Bacterial spread from the odontogenic source travels through the spaces formed by the facial planes. Although modern antibiotic therapy has reduced the occurrence of these "space infections" the morbidity and mortality remain.[25] Complications, such as respiratory obstruction, may occur due to swelling in the floor of the mouth; that is, Ludwig angina, trismus, edema, and abscess formation. In addition, abscess formation in or around the parapharyngeal tonsils, retropharynx, or epiglottis may also cause airway obstruction. Another complication of odontogenic infection is an orbital abscess. This is most commonly seen in maxillary odontogenic infections, particularly those that involve the maxillary sinus. The danger of these infections is the potential retrograde spread into the brain causing cavernous sinus thrombosis, meningitis, cerebritis, brain abscess, or even death.

Radiographic Findings

Initial imaging with plain-film dental images, such as periapical radiographs or panoramic imaging, may help in identifying the odontogenic source of infection. These findings have been discussed in previous sections. CBCT may aid in identifying the source and potential effect on the airway, such as asymmetry, but is not appropriate for soft tissue imaging. **Fig. 17** shows a case of pericoronitis that spread into the parapharyngeal space and created an airway asymmetry detected on CBCT. Comprehensive imaging of odontogenic space infections is achieved by conventional CT with soft tissue windows or possibly MR imaging to thoroughly evaluate the soft tissues involved. Contrast-enhanced CT can indicate the location and the relation of the infections to neurovascular structures (**Fig. 18**). Abscesses appear low in density with an enhanced rim.

Treatment

Space infections can pose life-threatening situations if not addressed immediately. Establishing an airway or preventing its closure is of utmost

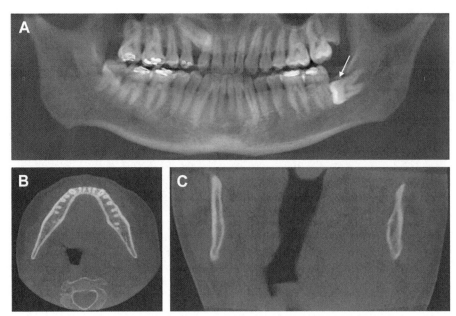

Fig. 17. CBCT (*A*) panoramic reformat of a patient with a clinical presentation of pericoronitis on the mandibular left third molar (*arrow*). (*B*) On the axial view, a soft tissue asymmetry in the shape of the oropharyngeal airway due to the submandibular space and parapharyngeal space infection caused by the inflammation is noted. (*C*) Coronal view further demonstrates the airway lumen asymmetry. (*Courtesy of* Dr Christopher Daniels, Santa Rosa, CA.)

importance. Removal of the source of infection by surgical means and antibiotic therapy is indicated.

SUMMARY

Odontogenic infection can appear in patterns ranging from dental caries to severe space infections. Dental imaging encompasses a wide variety of imaging modalities to aid in diagnosis and determination of the origin of infection. **Table 2** shows a summary of the imaging studies used for the different types of infection. Early diagnosis is the key to preventing serious complications of dental infection.

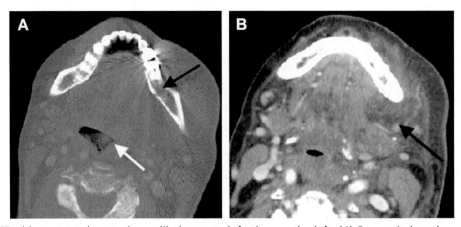

Fig. 18. CT with contrast shows submandibular space infection on the left. (*A*) Bone window shows the area where the infected tooth in the mandible was extracted (*black arrow*) and the deviation of the airway (*white arrow*). (*B*) Soft tissue window depicts the low attenuation in the submandibular space representing the fluid collection. Stranding of the fat in the fat planes and in the subcutaneous layer is a typical radiographic appearance. (*Courtesy of* Dr Andrew Cheung, Oak Ridge, TN.)

Table 2
Indications for imaging studies

Indication	Primary	Alternatives/Additional Info
Caries	Conventional radiographs	CBCT more accurate in detecting the extent
Periodontal disease	Conventional radiographs	CBCT provides more accurate analysis of root furcation areas, vertical bone defects, and root morphology
Pulpal and periapical disease	Conventional radiographs	CBCT can detect small periapical changes, root resorptions, and fractures
Pericoronitis	Conventional radiographs	CBCT provides 3D visualization and able to detect integrity of cortices
Osteomyelitis	MDCT/MR imaging/nuclear bone scan	MR imaging and bone scans allow for early detection
Space infections	MDCT/MR imaging	Contrast-enhanced CT can locate the lesions and their relationship with neurovascular structures

Abbreviations: CBCT, cone-beam computed tomography; CT, computed tomography; MDCT, multidetector computed tomography; 3D, 3-dimensional.

REFERENCES

1. White SC, Pharoah MJ. Oral radiology principles and interpretation. 7th edition. St Louis (MO): Elsevier Mosby; 2014. p. 314–32.
2. Hegde AN, Mohan S, Pandya A, et al. Imaging in infections of the head and neck. Neuroimaging Clin N Am 2012;22(4):727–54.
3. Gonzalez-Beicos A, Nunez D. Imaging of acute head and neck infections. Radiol Clin North Am 2012;50(1):73–83.
4. Hayeri MR, Ziai P, Shehata ML, et al. Mimics: from cellulitis to necrotizing fasciitis. Radiographics 2016;36:1888–910.
5. Dental caries (tooth decay) in adults (age 20 to 64) NIDCR, DATA & statistics. Available at: https://www.nidcr.nih.gov/DataStatistics/FindDataByTopic/DentalCaries/DentalCariesAdults20to64.htm. Accessed May 1, 2017.
6. Featherstone JD, Doméjean S. Minimal intervention dentistry: part 1. From 'compulsive' restorative dentistry to rational therapeutic strategies. Br Dent J 2012;213:441–5.
7. Wenzel A. Radiographic display of carious lesions and cavitation in approximal surfaces: advantages and drawbacks of conventional and advanced modalities. Acta Odontol Scand 2014;72(4):251–64.
8. Park YS, Ahn JS, Kwon HB, et al. Current status of dental caries diagnosis using cone beam computed tomography. Imaging Sci Dent 2011;41(2):43–51.
9. Featherstone JDB. Remineralization, the natural caries repair process—the need for new approaches. Adv Dent Res 2009;21:4–7.
10. Ari G, Cherukuri S, Namasivayam A. Epigenetics and periodontitis: a contemporary review. J Clin Diagn Res 2016;10(11):ZE07–9.
11. Lindroth AM, Parl YJ. Epigenetic biomarkers: a step forward for understanding periodontitis. J Periodontal Implant Sci 2013;43:111–20.
12. Kornman KS. Mapping the pathogenesis of periodontitis: a new look. J Periodontol 2008;79(Suppl 8):1560S–8S.
13. Armitage GC. Periodontal diagnoses and classification of periodontal diseases. Periodontology 2000 2004;34:9–21.
14. Corbet EF, Ho DK, Lai SM. Radiographs in periodontal disease diagnosis and management. Aust Dent J 2009;54(Suppl 1):S27–43.
15. Qiao J, Wang S, Duan J, et al. The accuracy of cone-beam computed tomography in assessing maxillary molar furcation involvement. J Clin Periodontol 2014;41:269–74.
16. Walter C, Kaner D, Berndt DC, et al. Three-dimensional imaging as a pre-operative tool in decision making for furcation surgery. J Clin Periodontol 2009;36:250–7.
17. Zero DT, Zandona AF, Vail MM, et al. Dental caries and pulpal disease. Dent Clin North Am 2011;55(1):29–46.
18. Marimen D, Green TL, Walton RE, et al. Histologic examination of condensing osteitis. J Endod 1992;18(4):196.

19. Rosenberg PA, Frisbie J, Lee J, et al. Evaluation of pathologists (histopathology) and radiologists (cone beam computed tomography) differentiating radicular cysts from granulomas. J Endod 2010; 36(3):423–8.

20. Bender IB. Factors influencing the radiographic appearance of bony lesions. J Endod 1982;8: 161–70.

21. Weissman J, Johnson JD, Anderson M, et al. Association between the presence of apical periodontitis and clinical symptoms in endodontic patients using cone-beam computed tomography and periapical radiographs. J Endod 2015;41(3): 1824–9.

22. Ohshima A, Ariji Y, Goto M, et al. Anatomical considerations for the spread of odontogenic infection originating from the pericoronitis of impacted mandibular third molar: computed tomographic analyses. Oral Surg Oral Med Oral Pathol Oral Radiol Endod 2004;98(5):589–97.

23. Lee YJ, Sadigh S, Mankad K, et al. The imaging of osteomyelitis. Quantitative Imaging Med Surg 2016;6(2):184–98.

24. Calhoun JH, Manring MM, Shirtliff M. Osteomyelitis of the long bones. Semin Plast Surg 2009;23(2):59–72.

25. Bali RK, Sharma P, Gaba S, et al. A review of complications of odontogenic infections. Natl J Maxillofac Surg 2015;6(2):136–43.

Imaging of Benign Odontogenic Lesions

William C. Scarfe, BDS, FRACDS, MS, Shiva Toghyani, DDS, MS*, Bruno Azevedo, DDS, MS

KEYWORDS

- Benign odontogenic cysts • Benign odontogenic tumors • Panoramic radiography • Cone beam CT
- Multidetector CT • MR imaging

KEY POINTS

- Odontogenic cysts and tumors of the jaws originate from remnants of the tooth-forming organ within the alveolus of the maxilla and mandible.
- Odontogenic cysts arise from the epithelium whereas tumors can arise from odontogenic epithelium, ectomesenchyme, or a combination of these tissues.
- Image interpretation requires a description of radiographic presentation according to location in relation to the dentition, radiologic pattern, and identification of disease-specific imaging features.
- Dental panoramic or maxillofacial cone beam CT provides sufficient imaging for most benign odontogenic lesions. Multidetector CT, with or without contrast, and MR imaging is only indicated if there is suspicion of extraosseous soft tissue extension or malignancy.
- A radiologic differential diagnosis is developed based on an understanding of the relative incidence, demographic presentation, and specific imaging features of benign odontogenic lesions.

INTRODUCTION

Most lesions within the jaws are inflammatory in origin, related to the ultimate sequelae of pulpal necrosis of the tooth (see Shaza Mardini and Anita Gohel's article, "Imaging of Odontogenic Infections," in this issue). Other benign lesions may arise from the remnants of the histologic embryonic structures associated with odontogenesis within the tooth-bearing areas of the jaws (dental alveolus). These structures include (1) ectodermal or epithelial cells, giving rise to ameloblasts forming the peripheral components of the crown, and (2) ectomesenchymal cells, giving rise to the odontoblasts, producing dentine and cementum, and the dental papilla, giving rise to the tooth-supporting apparatus (periodontium). Two types of benign entities can arise from these tissues: odontogenic cysts (of either developmental or inflammatory origin) and odontogenic tumors.[1]

Odontogenic cysts are epithelial lined cavities whose lumen can consist of air, fluid, or semifluid material. Cysts are derived from odontogenic epithelium or entrapped remnants within the bone or peripheral gingival tissue. The pathologic classification of odontogenic cysts is based on the origin of the epithelial lining.[1,2] Odontogenic tumors may also be ectodermal in origin or, in addition, may arise from mesenchymal (dental papilla or dental sac) tissue or simultaneously from both tissues. Some odontogenic tumors produce dental calcifications and, therefore, present as mixed high/low-attenuation entities.[3]

ORAL AND MAXILLOFACIAL IMAGING OF BENIGN LESIONS

Although CT and MR imaging are common in medical practices and hospitals, in-office cone beam CT (CBCT) units offer fast volumetric

Radiology and Imaging Sciences, Department of Surgical & Hospital Dentistry, University of Louisville, 501 South Preston Street, Louisville, KY 40202, USA
* Corresponding author.
E-mail address: s0togh01@louisville.edu

Radiol Clin N Am 56 (2018) 45–62
http://dx.doi.org/10.1016/j.rcl.2017.08.004

radiologic.theclinics.com

acquisition with a smaller office footprint, reduced per-scan cost, higher resolution, and significant dose savings compared with multidetector CT (MDCT). Another advantage is that the viewing software provides dental image formatting capabilities with particular application to the visualization of benign odontogenic lesions.[4] MDCT units also have dental software modules (eg, DentaScan [GE Healthcare, Chicago, Illinois]); however, these are usually purchased at additional cost.[5]

Postprocessing Protocols

All dental software programs allow for the creation of a simulated reformatted dental panoramic image (Fig. 1). Reformatted panoramic and cross-sectional images allow visualization of pathology in relation to the teeth and important anatomic structures, such as the inferior alveolar canal (IAC), also referred to as the mandibular canal,

and the maxillary sinuses. The position of the IAC can be traced through the mandible on the panoramic and transaxial views using software (see **Figs. 1D and E**). This feature is valuable when the IAC is obscured or displaced by pathology.[4,6]

IMAGING FEATURES OF ODONTOGENIC CYSTS AND BENIGN TUMORS OF THE JAWS

An important feature differentiating odontogenic from nonodontogenic entities is their location within the jaws. Odontogenic lesions of the jaw bones arise from the remnants of odontogenic apparatus and, therefore, are associated with the teeth or have an epicenter within the dental alveolus and, in the mandible, are usually superior to the IAC. Lesions location can be described according to position relative to the tooth and include periapical, pericoronal (for unerupted teeth), and inter-radicular. Nonodontogenic lesions involve

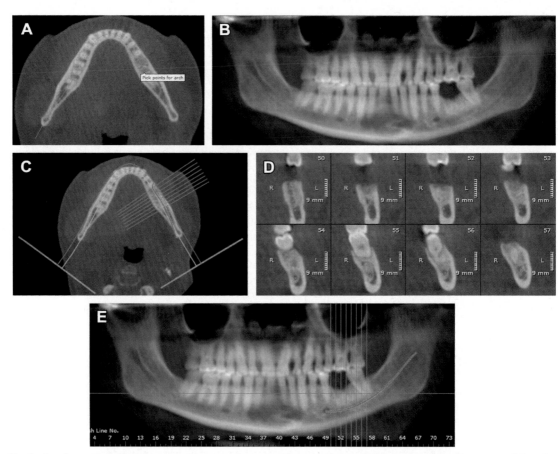

Fig. 1. A reformatted dental panoramic image is created by selecting multiple nodes along the curve of the alveolar process in an axial image (A). The nodes are connected by a curved transaxial plane or spline. Spline thickness may be adjusted from 15 mm to 20 mm to create a ray sum simulated panoramic image (B). Transaxial images are generated perpendicular to the spline (C) producing sequential cross-sectional images (D) related to the panoramic image by a reference numbering system (E). The location of the IAC can be traced on the panoramic and transaxial views using software (D, E).

the alveolus or teeth only after substantial growth. When odontogenic lesions expand, they often displace the IAC in the mandible or, in the maxilla, expand superiorly. Maxillary lesions are usually separated from the floor of the sinus by a cortical boundary unless the lesion becomes secondarily infected or exhibits aggressive features.[5,7]

Benign odontogenic lesions of the jaws usually present a well-defined, sometimes cortical margin. The outline may be (1) circular or oval, particularly with odontogenic cysts due to the hydraulic expansion effect, (2) irregular, especially with large benign odontogenic tumors, or (3) scalloped in between the roots of the teeth. Most odontogenic cysts are hyp attenuating with no internal structure. Long-standing cysts may develop internal dystrophic calcification. Odontogenic tumors are more likely to have a multilocular appearance with internal septa. Odontogenic tumors may produce calcified material, such as enamel, dentin or cementum, which appears as hyperattenuating areas within the lesion. Benign lesions of the jaw are slow-growing and tend to displace adjacent structures, such as IAC, sinus borders, teeth, and boundaries of the bone. Benign entities usually preserve the cortical margins; however, they can perforate the cortices if they reach considerable size.[8–10]

Although location and radiologic pattern may assist to identify odontogenic conditions, intraosseous nonodontogenic lesions may also demonstrate similar benign radiographic features, including well-defined borders, the presence of cortication, and the ability to expand the cortices and displace adjacent anatomic structures.[2,11]

THE RADIOLOGIC DIAGNOSIS OF ODONTOGENIC CYSTS AND TUMORS

Three approaches exist to developing a radiologic differential diagnosis. The pathologic or surgical sieve uses a list (often memorized using a pneumonic) to organize types of processes and develop a taxonomy of possible diagnosis.[12] Histologic typing relies on listing possible entities according to the tissue from which they originate. Both approaches rely on an extensive knowledge base and do little to assist the practicing radiologist rule out entities or include possibilities, particularly when details regarding patient presentation are often missing from the referral prescription. Oral and maxillofacial (OMF) radiologists, who comprise a subspecialty of dentistry, often use a radiographic pattern approach. This scheme relies on describing the primary imaging characteristics of the lesion and then categorizing the appearance into a group with the same features. Once

categorized, secondary and tertiary imaging characteristics, together with clinical presentation and demographics, are used to develop a list of 3 or 4 possible conditions – a working or differential diagnosis. For surgeons, an impression stating "imaging findings consistent with odontogenic cyst or tumor" is insufficient. Although a dentigerous cyst (DC) (odontogenic cyst) and an odontogenic keratocyst (OKC) may both appear as hypoattenuating pericoronal, unilocular, well-defined entities, their management varies greatly. The DC is enucleated whereas the OKC either marsupialized, if large or removed with wide margins because of its high recurrence rate. The presence of secondary radiographic features, such as satellite cyst extensions in the lesion periphery, can explain the more likely occurrence of the OKC.[10]

The differential diagnosis of odontogenic cysts and tumors is based on radiographic pattern recognition according to degree of attenuation, location in relation to the tooth or within bone, shape, and an understanding of the similarities of presentation of nonodontogenic cysts and tumors. The following provides a review of odontogenic cysts and tumors found in the jaws categorized by radiographic presentation. **Table 1** provides a brief list of nonodontogenic conditions with similar radiographic appearance.[8]

Low-Attenuating Lesions

Periapical (around the tooth apices)
The most common radiographic pathologies involving the apex of the teeth are inflammatory and referred to collectively as apical periodontitis or periapical rarefying osteitis. Although radiologically similar, they are histologically different (see Shaza Mardini and Anita Gohel's article, "Imaging of Odontogenic Infections," in this issue for more information).

Radicular cyst The radicular cyst (RC), also known as periapical cyst, is the most common cyst found in the jaws. Usually located at the apex of the root of a tooth, the RC initially presents as a loss of a defined sclerotic margin of the socket of the tooth (lamina dura). Most RCs are less than 10 mm in diameter; however, some become very large. Apical lesions greater than 20 mm in diameter are most often RCs.[13] RCs are unilocular (round to ovoid) well-defined lesions, often with a cortical outline unless secondarily infected. Intraoral periapical radiography is adequate in diagnosing RCs. CBCT imaging may be considered for large lesions requiring surgical removal and involving adjacent structures, such as the IAC or the maxillary sinus (**Fig. 2**). As incidental findings on MR imaging, they are typically homogenously isointense

Table 1
Radiographic patterns of odontogenic and nonodontogenic conditions of the jaws

Attenuation	Location	Border	Odontogenic	Nonodontogenic
Low	Periapical	Unilocular	RC, chronic apical periodontitis, periapical scar, incomplete root formation	POD, leukemia, metastasis
	Pericoronal	Unilocular Multilocular	DC, OKC, AMB, AF OKC, AMB	MNTI
	Inter-radicular	Unilocular Multilocular	LPC, BBC, AMB Botryoid odontogenic cyst, OM, OKC	CGCG, SBC
	Intraosseous	Unilocular	Residual cyst	Submandibular salivary gland defect (Stafne), nasopalatine duct cyst, nasolabial cyst, SBC, MM, EG
		Multilocular	OM, GOC	ABC, hemangioma, cherubism, central mucoepidermoid carcinoma
High	Periapical		Odontoma, hypercementosis, CB	Idiopathic osteosclerosis, condensing osteitis, POD/FOD, enostosis, exostosis, osteoid osteoma, OF
	Pericoronal		Odontoma	
	Inter-radicular		Remaining tooth root	
Mixed	Periapical			POD/FOD, OF
	Pericoronal		AOT, CCOT, CEOT, AFO	
	Intraosseous			OF

Abbreviations: ABC, aneurysmal bone cyst; BBC, buccal bifurcation cyst; EG, eosinophilic granuloma; MM, multiple myeloma; MNTI, melanotic neuroectodermal tumor of infancy; SBC, simple bone cyst.

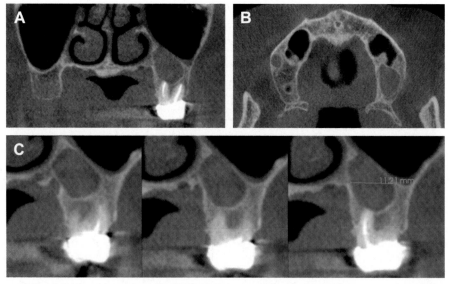

Fig. 2. Coronal (*A*), axial (*B*), and cross-sectional (*C*) CBCT images of a 50-year-old woman referred for implant site assessment show an RC associated with the apex of the palatal root of a previously root canal filled left maxillary second molar. Note the elevation and mild interruption of the floor of the maxillary sinus.

to the surrounding tissue on T1-weighted and homogenously hyperintense on T2-weighted sequences.[11] RCs may displace or resorb the roots of adjacent teeth or displace the inferior border of, or invaginate into, the sinus. Treatment includes extraction or endodontic therapy for the involved tooth. Healing after endodontic therapy may lead to complete or partial resolution of the radiographic appearance. Large RCs that have invaded the maxillary sinus may partially heal by peripheral sclerosis (collapsed or involuting RC) and mimic ossifying fibroma (OF).[11,14]

Periapical scar The success of endodontic (root canal) treatment of an abscess, granuloma, or cyst can be defined according to the stage of healing as healed (clinical and radiographically normal), healing (normal clinical presentation with a relative reduction in attenuation), and active/diseased. Radiographically healing or healed endodontic teeth may present with a residual, albeit smaller, apical hypoattenuation indicative of fibrous connective tissue rather than normal bone, referred to as an apical scar. Occasionally the apical third of a root of a tooth together with an associated intra-alveolar pathology may be surgically removed (apicoectomy) for persistent apical lesions and may exhibit the same low-density area at the apex indicating incomplete healing.

Incompletely formed root apex Permanent tooth formation (range, 3 months to 10 years), root completion (range, 9 years to 25 years), and eruption (range, 6 years to 30 years) occur sequentially for each of the 32 teeth in the dentition. During this time, the tooth follicle undergoing development may resemble a unilocular lesion or periapical area of low attenuation (**Fig. 3**). A small periapical low-density area seen in association with an incompletely formed, blunderbuss-shaped tooth apex is most likely the dental papilla and not periapical pathology.

Odontogenic or nonodontogenic lesions occurring periapically Benign or malignant odontogenic or nonodontogenic pathology may superimpose over or involve the roots of teeth. A positive response to clinical intraoral testing of the associated teeth involving the application of electrical and thermal stimuli (called pulp vitality testing) is suggestive of lesion of nonpulpal inflammatory in origin (see **Table 1**).

Diagnostic pearls
- Periapical hypoattenuating well-defined unilocular entities with nonvital or endodontically treated teeth greater than 20 mm in diameter are most likely RCs.
- RCs may displace teeth and can result in apical root resorption.
- Initially periapical osseous dysplasia (POD) may mimic the radiographic appearance of a small RC, particularly in the anterior and posterior mandible. Positive pulp vitality testing distinguishes POD from the RC. For more information about POD, see Mansur Ahmad and Laurence Gaalaas's article, "Fibro-Osseous and Other Lesions of Bone in the Jaws," in this issue.

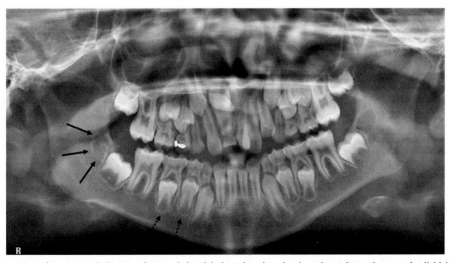

Fig. 3. Conventional panoramic image shows right third molar developing dental tooth crypt (*solid black arrows*) and periapical apexogenesis as solitary, unilocular, and periapical hypoattenuating entities. These conditions are also present on the left (unmarked). Dotted arrows demonstrate developing roots with open apices.

- Irregular asymmetric widening of the peri-odontal ligament (PDL) space along the surface of the root of a tooth may be a sign of localized periodontal disease or malignancy (eg, osteogenic sarcoma). A detailed medical history and possibly a biopsy should be considered.

Pericoronal (around the tooth crown)

Dentigerous cyst DCs are the second most commonly occurring hypoattenuating cyst, after the RC. They present as well-defined unilocular corticated entities developing around the crown of an unerupted tooth (pericoronal). They attach at or near the cementoenamel junction (CEJ) and are also called follicular cysts. They tend to remain unilocular even when large, unlike odontogenic tumors. The most common teeth affected are, in order, the mandibular third molars, maxillary third molars, and maxillary canines. An asymmetric pericoronal space larger than 3 mm is suspicious of cystic degeneration and a biopsy should be considered.[15] DC may result in substantial displacement of the involved tooth and root resorption of adjacent teeth. The DC presents in 1 of 3 radiographic pericoronal patterns: (1) classic, symmetric enveloping of the crown of the unerupted tooth; (2) lateral, arising from the side of a crown, and; (3) circumferential, extension of the lesion below the CEJ (**Fig. 4**). Possible sequelae include secondary infection and conversion of the cystic lining to OKC or a benign odontogenic tumor (unicystic ameloblastoma [AMB]) and, rarely, malignant neoplasm squamous cell carcinoma or mucoepidermoid carcinoma. DCs are often associated with odontomas. On MR imaging, DCs are typically homogenous isointense on T1-weighted and homogenous or heterogeneous hyperintense on T2-weighted MR sequences and may demonstrate rim enhancement on a postgadolinium sequence. The typical treatment is enucleation with extraction of the involved tooth. Recurrence is rare.[11,15]

Odontogenic Keratocyst This lesion was called keratocystic odontogenic tumor (KOT) for a brief time and then was renamed OKC. It arises from the dental lamina and contain keratinized epithelium. It presents as a well-defined corticated entity, most commonly found in the mandibular body or ramus. OKCs may arise pericoronally or within the alveolus (**Fig. 5**). They can displace or resorb teeth and displace the mandibular canal. They usually cause minimal expansion and tend to spread within the intramedullary space "growing in the length of the bone." Unlike the DC, OKC does not expand the bone symmetrically. The lesion often presents with peripheral soft tissue intramedullary extensions, known as daughter cysts that, together with the surgical friability of the lesion, may contribute to a high recurrence. Unlike DCs, they may erode the cortical plate. OKCs are unilocular in nearly half cases and may exhibit sclerotic scalloped borders or present as multilocularity with small (soap-bubble) or larger (honeycomb) loculations. Septae are often thin and curved.

Because OKCs may contain keratin material, on MR imaging OKC appear as heterogeneous hypointense to mildly hyperintense on T1-weighted images. They appear heterogeneous or homogeneous hyperintense on T2. Rim enhancement happens due to focal inflammatory ulceration of the cyst lining. Management includes resection with a large margin, curettage, or marsupialization to reduce the size before removal for larger cysts. Periodic radiographic monitoring annually for the first 5 years is mandatory and periodically every 2 years to 3 years thereafter due to their high rate of recurrence (see **Fig. 5**B) and rapid growth. Multiple OKCs can be associated with basal cell nevus (BCN) syndrome (**Fig. 6**).

Ameloblastoma AMB is a benign, locally aggressive odontogenic tumor, arising from the enamel-forming cells of the odontogenic epithelium. It is the second most common odontogenic tumor, after odontoma. AMB presents as a painless, slow-growing expansion (**Fig. 7**). AMB may arise de novo within the alveolus or pericoronally. AMB may present as unilocular (unicystic) or multilocular lesion. If unilocular, AMB may have faint, disordered septae, often radiating from a common center. Multilocular lesions may appear with either a soap-bubble or occasionally honeycomb pattern. Initial lesions and unicystic variants are usually unilocular and may be radiographically indistinguishable from other solitary unilocular radiolucencies, such as DC and OKC. Internal scalloping and knife-edge resorption of the roots of adjacent erupted teeth are common, as is displacement of unerupted teeth. Larger lesions produce orofacial expansion (unlike DC, which predominantly expands the buccal cortex, and OKC, which has less concentric expansion), isolated cortical perforation or erosion, and displacement and erosion of the lower border of the mandible. The IAC can be, in decreasing frequency, displaced, eroded, or absent. Contrast-enhanced MDCT shows irregular peripheral enhancement, septae, and solid and cystic mural nodule components within the lesion, reflecting the pathologic characteristics of the lesion. On MR imaging, AMB shows internal similar

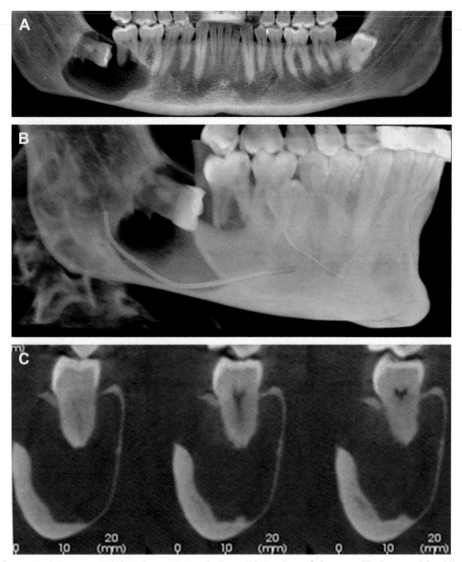

Fig. 4. Reformatted panoramic (*A*), volumetric rendering with tracing of the mandibular canal (*red line*) (*B*) and 1-mm thick/1-mm interval contiguous cross-sectional images (*C*) of a 36-year-old man show a DC surrounding the crown of impacted right third molar, causing mesial displacement of the roots of second molar and resorption of the apices of the first and second molars. The lesion extends beyond the CEJ of the involved tooth due to the significant enlargement.

T1-weighted (low to intermediate signal) and T2-weighted (intermediate to high intensity) signals but on contrast-enhanced T1-weighted images, solid components show hyperintense signal. They exhibit low to intermediate signal intensity on TI-weighted and high signal intensity on T2-weighted images. The recurrence rate is moderately high (up to 15%), especially with multicystic variants. Treatment method depends on radiographic presentation (unicystic vs multilocular), size, anatomic location, histologic variant, and adjacent anatomic involvement; however,

most require resection with wide margins (>1 cm) with or without reconstruction.

The unicystic AMB is a specific variant of AMB that typically occurs in a younger age group and appears as a pericoronal lesion, similar to DC. It may arise from the epithelial lining of an existing cyst or de novo. Most are unilocular and may show scalloping margins if larger. Compared with AMB, they are locally less aggressive and demonstrate less recurrence. Enhancement of mural nodules in T1-weighted images with contrast assists to confirm the diagnosis of this lesion.[2,11]

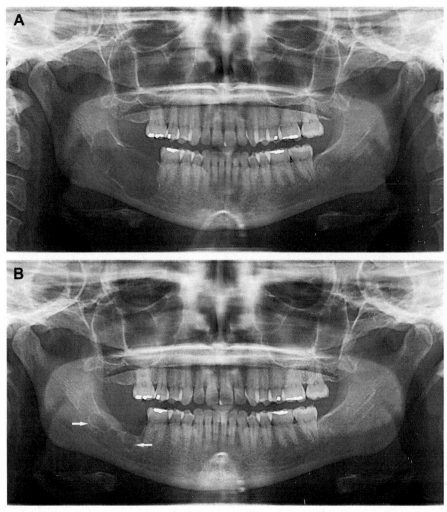

Fig. 5. Presurgical (*A*) and follow-up (*B*) conventional panoramic image of a patient with OKC showing a well-defined low-density lesion with scalloped borders in the right posterior mandible. White arrows show the recurrence of the same lesion 2 years later.

Ameloblastic fibroma The ameloblastic fibroma (AF) is a rare mixed epithelial and ectomesenchymal benign odontogenic tumor arising in childhood or adolescence. This tumor appears as a well-defined corticated low-attenuating lesion without calcification most commonly in the posterior mandible with or without pericoronal involvement (**Fig. 8**). If tooth density structures are seen within the lesion stroma, the lesion can be called ameloblastic fibro-odontoma (AFO). The lesion usually presents as an expansile multilocularity but may be unilocular. Malignant transformation occurs in up to 10% of cases, in particular those younger than 22 years of age. Treatment is enucleation, curettage, excision, or resection, depending on the size of the tumor. A general rule of thumb for diagnosing these lesions is that if it looks like an AMB and occurs in a child, then consider AF.

Diagnostic pearls
- Widening of the pericoronal space greater than 3 mm should increase the degree of suspicion of odontogenic pathology; radiographic follow-up is recommended.
- The DC is the most likely radiologic differential for a lesion with a pericoronal epicenter, lateral, or circumferential unilocular low-attenuating lesion.
- A key differential diagnosis feature for DC is the maintenance of the attachment of the lesion at the CEJ of the involved tooth.
- Differential diagnosis of a pericoronal unilocular lesion must also include OKC and odontogenic tumors (AMB and AF in the younger age group).
- OKCs may look similar to AMB but tend to grow intramedullary within the bone with less expansion.

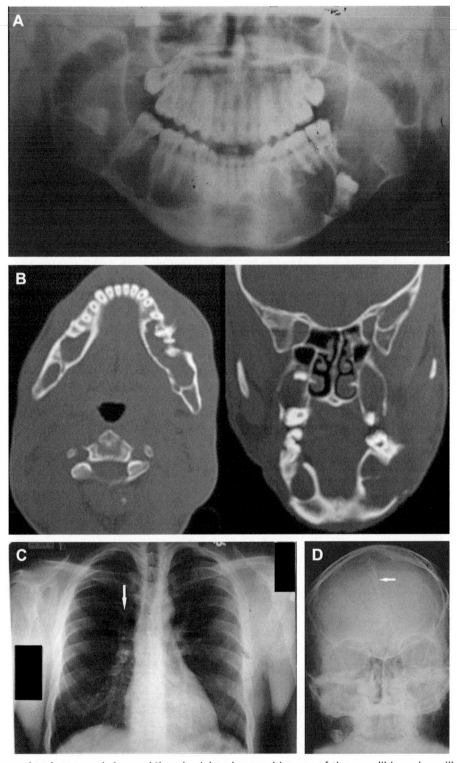

Fig. 6. Conventional panoramic image (*A*) and axial and coronal images of the mandible and maxilla (*B*) show multiple pericoronal multilocular hypoattenuating lesions suggestive of BCN syndrome. BCN is an autosomal dominant disorder with variable expressivity, associated with multiple OKCs, multiple basal cell nevi skeletal abnormalities, and increased incidence of certain neoplasm. Chest radiograph on this patient shows bifid ribs (*white arrow*) (*C*) and frontal skull radiograph demonstrates calcification of falx cerebri (*white arrow*) (*D*). (*Courtesy of Dr George Kushner, University of Louisville School of Dentistry, Louisville, Kentucky*).

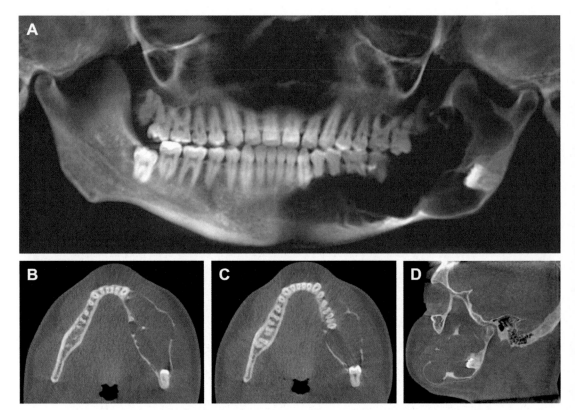

Fig. 7. CBCT reformatted dental panoramic (*A*), axial views of the mandible at the level of midroot (*B, C*), and sagittal view of the left ramus of a 34-year-old patient show a well-defined multilocular expansile lesion with scalloped borders developing pericoronal to the mandibular third molar. Thinning and erosion of the buccal and lingual cortical plates and knife-edge root resorption on the adjacent teeth is visualized. IAC is eroded and is not traceable throughout the lesion. These are radiographic features seen with AMB.

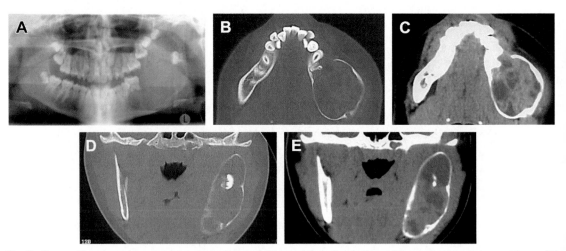

Fig. 8. Conventional panoramic radiography (*A*), axial bone (*B*) and soft tissue (*C*) window, and coronal bone (*D*) and soft tissue (*E*) window multislice CT images of a 14-year-old girl with an asymptomatic large multilocular expansion of the left mandible involving the body, angle, and ramus. Soft tissue images show heterogeneous contents consistent with AF.

- If a pericoronal lesion is multilocular, then DC is ruled out in the radiologic differential diagnosis.
- It is important to describe the mass effect of any pericoronal entity on the IAC to assist in determining the surgical approach.
- For pericoronal multilocular lesions, the presence of a mural nodule on MDCT or CBCT assists in differentiating neoplastic from cystic odontogenic lesions.
- Postoperative yearly clinical and radiographic monitoring of the pericoronal surgical site of all entities except the DC is highly recommended for up to 10 years because of high recurrence rates (up to 25%).
- Periodic CT/CBCT imaging indicating dimensions of the lesion may be requested after marsupialization of OKCs to monitor reduction in size prior to definitive surgery.
- MR or contrast-enhanced MDCT imaging is unnecessary.

Inter-radicular (between the roots of teeth)
Lateral periodontal cyst The lateral periodontal cyst (LPC) is a noninflammatory developmental odontogenic cyst presenting as a well-defined small unilocular low-density lesion in the inter-radicular alveolus associated with the proximal aspects of the roots of teeth. It occurs most commonly in the mandible in the region of the lateral incisor to the second premolar. A multilocular variant is called the botryoid odontogenic cyst. If large, the LPC may displace adjacent teeth. A positive response to pulpal vitality testing of the involved teeth differentiates the LPC from the RC (**Fig. 9**).

Mandibular infected buccal cyst Also known as mandibular infected buccal cyst (MIBC)-molar area, circumferential DC, buccal bifurcation cyst, and juvenile paradental cyst, the MIBC is a rare inflammatory odontogenic cyst presenting as a local swelling on the buccal aspect of the mandibular first or second molars in children. The MIBC may also be associated with pain and local suppuration. The MIBC presents as a well-defined unilocular corticated low-attenuating area and may resorb, displace, or delay the eruption of the involved tooth (**Fig. 10**). Treatment is usually enucleation of the cyst.[9,11]

Odontogenic tumors and cysts Previously described pericoronal odontogenic tumors, such as AMB and OKC, may also arise inter-radicularly.

Nonodontogenic conditions Numerous nonodontogenic cysts as well as osseous and nonosseous tumors may present inter-radicularly with a similar radiographic appearance to the odontogenic conditions previously described (see **Table 1**).

Diagnostic pearls
- Small unilocular inter-radicular lesions are most likely odontogenic cysts (eg, LPC and OKC). Odontogenic tumors (eg, AMB) and nonodontogenic entities (eg, central giant cell granuloma [CGCG] and simple bone cavity [SBC]) should also be considered.
- A clinical and radiographic characteristic feature of MIBC is buccal tilting of the crown of the molar with the roots tipping toward the lingual cortex.
- OKCs with minimal cortical expansion and scalloped borders can mimic SBC; however, OKCs are typically corticated and can displace and resorb teeth.
- Superior inter-radicular extensions of a unilocular scalloped intraosseous lesion are a characteristic radiographic feature of SBC.
- CGCG may cross the mandibular midline.

Intraosseous
Several odontogenic and nonodontogenic (see **Table 1**) cysts and tumor arise from the basal

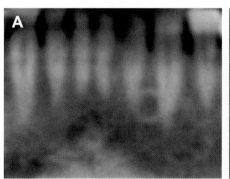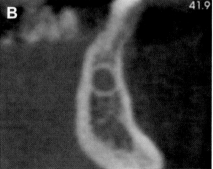

Fig. 9. Reformatted dental panoramic (*A*) and cross-sectional view (*B*) of anterior mandible demonstrate a well-defined corticated low-density inter-radicular lesion consistent with a LPC.

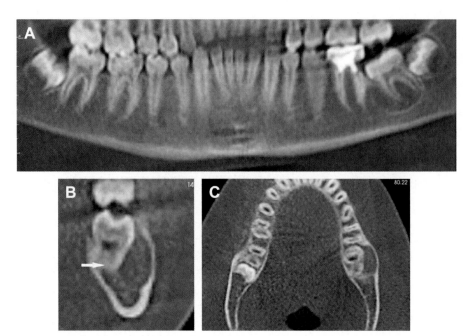

Fig. 10. Reformatted panoramic (*A*), cross-sectional (*B*), and axial view (*C*) show a low-attenuating unilocular lesion adjacent to the buccal aspect of the left mandibular second molar preventing the eruption of this tooth and tipping the tooth roots lingually (*white arrow*) (*B*), consistent with MIBC.

bone of the jaws and many secondarily involve the alveolus and associated dentition.

Ameloblastoma/odontogenic   Keratocyst AMB and OKC may present as solitary, intraosseous lesions unrelated to the root or crown of the adjacent dentition. These entities are described previously.

Residual cyst The residual cyst is an RC found in the alveolus in the area of a missing tooth. It typically presents as a round, unilocular, well-defined, corticated hypoattenuating circular lesion (**Fig. 11**).

Odontogenic myxoma The odontogenic myxoma (OM) is a rare benign odontogenic tumor of ecto-mesenchymal origin with a locally aggressive behavior presenting as a slow-growing painless expansion. OMs occur most frequently in the posterior mandible and occasionally in the ramus, condyle, maxilla, and zygoma. Radiographically, OM is a multilocular hypoattenuating lesion, with well-developed locules and scalloped borders, which may be well defined or ill defined, corticated or noncorticated (**Fig. 12**). Internally the locules are separated by thin septae, arranged at right angles, known as the tennis-racquet or step-ladder pattern. When present, this is considered a characteristic imaging feature of this entity. Septae may also be coarse and curved. Presence of straight septae at the periphery may mimic

periosteal reaction. OM shows a tendency to scallop between the roots. OM does not metastasize but shows a high recurrence rate.

Glandular odontogenic cyst Also known as sialo-odontogenic cyst and polymorphous odontogenic cyst, glandular odontogenic cysts (GOCs) are rare cysts of odontogenic epithelium with aggressive behavior. These cysts are more common in the anterior mandible and anterior maxilla. They appear as a multilocular low-attenuating lesion with a scalloped corticated margin and can cause expansion and perforation of the cortical margin and displace the involved teeth. Recurrence rate is high.

Diagnostic pearls

- A single unilocular round or ovoid hypoattenuating lesion in an edentulous alveolus (without teeth) is most likely a residual cyst. A clinical history and previous dental radiographs can provide useful information in confirming the radiologic impression.
- A differential pneumonic for multilocular lesions of the jaws is *GAMOT-CC* (CGCG, AMB, OM, OKC, traumatic bone cavity, cherubism, and central hemangioma).
- Multilocular jaw entities may demonstrate specific internal septal patterns: OM, tennis-racquet, or step-ladder pattern; CGCG, straight septae at right angles to the periphery

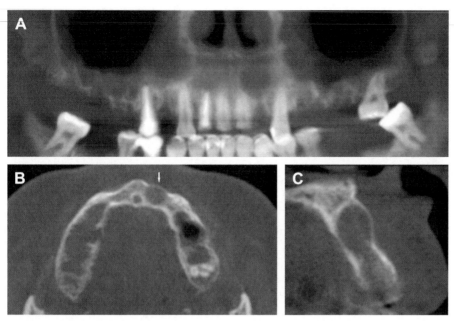

Fig. 11. Reformatted panoramic (*A*), axial (*B*), and cross-sectional (*C*) CBCT images show a round well-defined low-density lesion in the area of missing left lateral incisor, consistent with a residual cyst. Note the tooth socket on (*C*), which was the cause of the lesion prior to extraction.

of the lesion; central hemangioma, thin, and radiating septae like the spokes of a wheel).

- A high index of suspicion should be attributable to certain hypoattenuating jaw entities in children: cherubism, localized Langerhans cell histiocytosis, and central hemangioma
- The shape and location of lesions are highly suggestive of specific nonodontogenic entities: the submandibular salivary gland defect

is a unilocular cortical deficiency superimposed over or below the IAC in the mandibular body; the nasopalatine duct cyst is a unilocular or heart-shaped low-density lesion located in the midline of the maxilla, often between the roots of the central incisors.

- The following conditions are associated with the presence of multiple, often bilateral, hypoattenuating lesions: florid osseous dysplasia

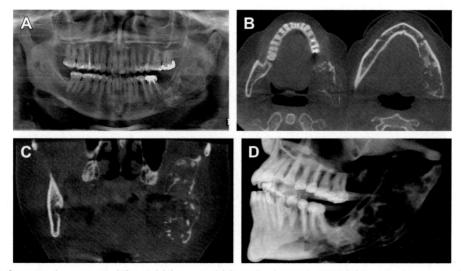

Fig. 12. Reformatted panoramic (*A*), axial (*B*), coronal (*C*), and volumetric CBCT (*D*) images show a poorly-defined multilocular soap-bubble low-density lesion of the left mandibular body and ramus consistent with an OM. Note: sunburst periodontal reaction is an unusual appearance in the OM (*B*).

(FOD), cheubism, multiple myeloma, and BCN syndrome

High-Attenuating Lesions

Periapical

Although a majority of periapical high-attenuating lesions conditions are odontogenic, some nonodontogenic conditions may present with a similar appearance associated with the roots of the teeth (see **Table 1**).

Condensing osteitis Condensing osteitis (also known as periapical sclerosing osteitis) is a term used to describe the appearance of a peripheral hyperattenuating ill-defined intramedullary sclerotic zone associated with concomitant low-attenuating apical epicenter of a nonvital tooth (**Fig. 13**). Most often the PDL space of the involved tooth is widened, and periapical lamina dura is eroded, suggesting chronic apical periodontitis. Condensing osteitis is common, suggests chronic pulpitis of the involved tooth, and necessitates clinical investigation of the pulpal vitality status. Management may involve periodic intraoral radiographic monitoring or, if symptomatic, extraction or endodontic therapy of the involved tooth/teeth.

Odontoma Odontomas are the most common benign odontogenic neoplasm of the jaws with both epithelium and ectomesenchymal origin with mature dental tooth structure formation (enamel, dentin, cementum, and pulp). They present as an asymptomatic well-defined expansive mass, limited to the alveolus, often associated with the failure of eruption of a permanent tooth. Most occur in the second decade and involve unerupted teeth and are discovered incidentally on dental images. Radiographically odontomas present in 1 of 2 hyperattenuating patterns: (1) complex odontoma—a single unorganized amorphous mineralized mass, tending to be round or ovoid with a round or smooth margin having density greater than bone (**Fig. 14**), or (2) compound

odontoma—as multiple small tooth-like structures as a bag of teeth (**Fig. 15**). Both patterns demonstrate a well-defined hypoattenuating periphery that may cause equal buccal and lingual expansion of the cortical plates, displacement or involvement of the IAC, and unerupted tooth displacement. They may occur anywhere in the jaws with compound odontomas more frequently in the anterior maxilla and complex odontomas more frequently in the posterior mandible. Both subtypes may develop pericoronal to an impacted tooth. Uneven dilatation of a pericoronal low-density capsule may represent secondary infection or cystic degeneration to a DC.[1]

Hypercementosis The roots of teeth may develop excessive non-neoplastic proliferation of cementum, usually associated with hyperfunction. Radiographically this appears as either irregular or globular hyperattenuating deposits on the roots of 1 or more teeth with no root resorption. The teeth remain separated from the alveolar bone by a normal PDL space.

Cementoblastoma Cementoblastoma (CB) is a rare ectomesenchymal neoplasm, specifically of cementum, the material covering the root surface of teeth. CB typically presents as an incidental asymptomatic solitary radiographic finding in patients less than 25 years of age, most commonly male, and affecting the mandibular first molar. The associated tooth is usually vital. Radiographically the lesion presents as a large circular sunburst hyperattenuating mass resorbing with the apex of a tooth root. The lesion is surrounded by a low-intensity rim (**Fig. 16**).

Diagnostic pearls
- The location and imaging presentation of numerous nonodontogenic entities adjacent to the periapical region is pathognomonic, such as mandibular tori, torus palatinus, buccal exostoses, idiopathic osteosclerosis,

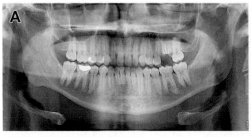
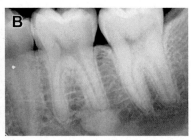

Fig. 13. Conventional panoramic (*A*) and intraoral periapical image (*B*) show an asymptomatic focal hyperattenuating mass with no peripheral hypoattenuating rim adjacent to the distal root of the left mandibular first molar consistent with either idiopathic osteosclerosis or condensing osteitis (pulp related). Pulp vitality testing is recommended to distinguish between the 2 entities.

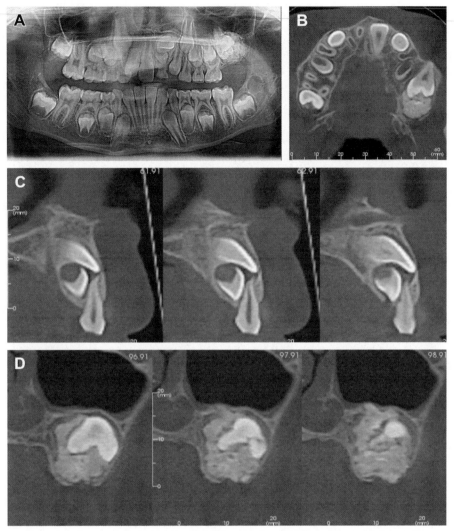

Fig. 14. Cropped conventional panoramic (*A*), axial (*B*), anterior maxillary (*C*), and left maxillary posterior (*D*) cross-sectional images of an 8-year-old girl with a failure of eruption of anterior maxillary tooth show the presence of a complex odontoma associated with the crown of the left unerupted first molar, and a developing supernumerary tooth preventing the eruption of the maxillary left central incisor tooth.

and osseous dysplasia. These entities should be ruled out and differentiated from the odontogenic lesions discussed previously.

Pericoronal

Odontoma Odontomas are often associated with the pericoronal follicle of unerupted and impacted teeth. Odontomas are often associated with the pericoronal follicle of unerupted and impacted teeth. Both compound and complex odontomas may appear as a pericoronal high-attenuating lesion. Compound odontomas occur more frequently in the anterior maxilla, mostly associated with an impacted maxillary canine.

Intra-radicular

Tooth roots The retained roots of an extracted permanent tooth or a retained root of a resorbed primary tooth may appear as a high-attenuating entity in between the roots of teeth.

Mixed High/Low Attenuating

Periapical

Other than complex odontomas, no odontogenic conditions appear as periapical mixed attenuating lesions. The intermediate stage of all fibro-osseous dysplastic lesions (eg, POD, FOD, and OF) may appear radiographically as an apically associated mixed-density lesion and these are reviewed in Mansur Ahmad and Laurence

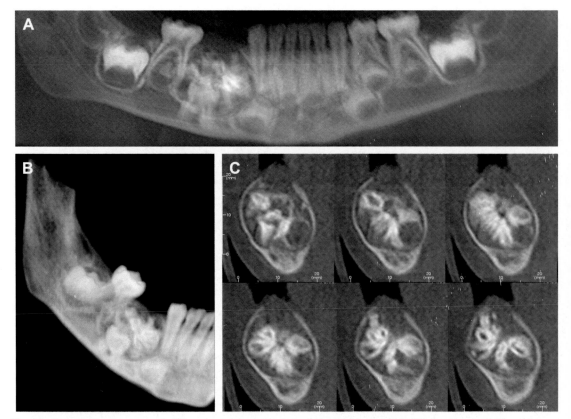

Fig. 15. Reformatted panoramic (A), volumetric rendering of the right mandible (B), and cross-sectional images (C) of a 5-year-old boy with failure of eruption of the permanent right mandibular premolar tooth show the presence of a compound odontoma preventing the eruption of the tooth in that region.

Gaalaas's article, "Fibro-Osseous and Other Lesions of Bone in the Jaws," in this issue.

Pericoronal

All mixed high-attenuating and low-attenuating pericoronal conditions are odontogenic in origin but rare. They include calcifying epithelial odontogenic tumor (CEOT), adenomatoid odontogenic tumor (AOT), AFO, and calcifying cystic odontogenic tumor (CCOT).

Diagnostic pearls

- The lumenal pattern of calcifications in pericoronal mixed attenuating lesions can assist in radiologic differential diagnosis; CEOT and CCOT tend to cluster around the crown of the impacted tooth; the AOT may demonstrate central hyperattenuating homogeneity and a peripheral low-attenuating rim.
- The radiologic differential diagnosis of pericoronal mixed attenuating lesions in the child and adolescent should include odontoma, AOT, CEOT, CCOT, and AFO.

Intraosseous

All entities described under the previously (ie, AOT, CEOT, CCOT and AFO) may present as solitary intraosseous lesions. The mature stage of development of all fibro-osseous dysplastic lesions (eg, POD, FOD, and OF) may appear radiographically as a solitary, intraosseous hyperattenuating lesion. The OF, in particular, is one of the most common nonodontogenic neoplasms to arise in the alveolar bone, generally centered within the non–tooth-bearing areas of the alveolus. These lesions are expansile even when small. These lesions may appear either cystic or largely sclerotic depending on the degree of internal calcification.

WHAT TO INCLUDE IN THE RADIOLOGIC REPORT

With the widespread availability of CBCT in dentistry, it is likely that medical radiologists will be increasingly called on to interpret volumetric datasets taken on patients for the assessment of hitherto dental conditions. It is also common for medical radiologists to confront these lesions as

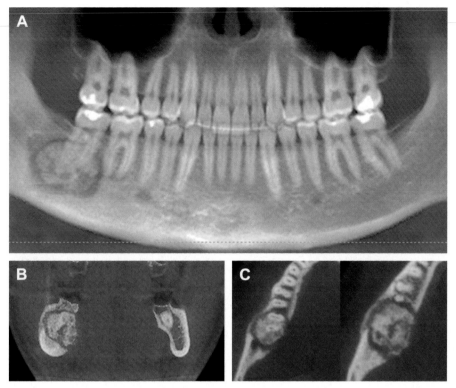

Fig. 16. Cropped reformatted panoramic (*A*), coronal (*B*), and axial (*C*) CBCT images show a well-defined, mixed-attenuation lesion with a hypoattenuating rim, attached to the apices of second right mandibular molar consistent with a CB. (*Courtesy of* Dr Douglas Wallace, Fairfield, Ohio).

an incidental finding on MDCT. To assist referring clinicians in the management of patients with jaw pathology, the essential elements of a radiologic report should include

1 Description of the location, tooth association, shape, periphery, internal aspect of the lesion, and effects on surrounding structures. These are the key diagnostic clues that define aggressive or nonaggressive behavior and assist in developing an accurate treatment plan or surgical approach. Proximity or involvement of the adjacent teeth may influence decisions on removal or retention. In addition, a description of the relationship of the lesion to the maxillary sinus or IAC is critical in determining surgical approach and reducing morbidity.
2 A radiologic differential diagnosis. Specific disease entities should be listed in order of probability. Many jaw entities are commonly detected on dental panoramic or intraoral radiographic images are more familiar to OMF radiologists. In these cases, consulting an OMF radiologist may help hone interpretive skills. A list of board-certified OMF radiologists can be found at https://www.aaomr.org/find-an-omr2#/.

3 Recommendation on whether further imaging (eg, MDCT with contrast or MR imaging or even higher resolution intraoral radiography) should be considered (suggestion), recommended (desirable), or advisable (obligatory).

SUMMARY

Knowledge of the imaging characteristics of common odontogenic pathologies in the jaws is crucial for providing an accurate differential diagnosis. The emerging availability of in-office CBCT, especially for surgeons, allows for comprehensive volumetric assessment of the jaws. This article offers a systematic approach for assessment of the odontogenic cysts and tumors based on the appearance and location of these lesions. Nonodontogenic conditions, which may resemble the odontogenic lesions in the same region, should also be considered in the differential diagnosis.

REFERENCES

1. Bilodeau EA, Collins BM. Odontogenic cysts and neoplasms. Surg Pathol Clin 2017;10(1):177–222.
2. Robinson RA. Diagnosing the most common odontogenic cystic and osseous lesions of the jaws for the

practicing pathologist. Mod Pathol 2017;30(s1): S96–103.

3. Sekerci AE, Nazlim S, Etoz M, et al. Odontogenic tumors: a collaborative study of 218 cases diagnosed over 12 years and comprehensive review of the literature. Med Oral Patol Oral Cir Bucal 2015;20(1): e34–44.

4. Liao R, Sun M, Gu Y, et al. Clinical application of cone beam CT in the treatment of jaw bone cyst. Hua Xi Kou Qiang Yi Xue Za Zhi 2012;30(3):262–6.

5. Koenig LJ. Imaging of the jaws. Semin Ultrasound CT MR 2015;36(5):407–14.

6. Haas LF, Dutra K, Porporatti AL, et al. Anatomical variations of mandibular canal detected by panoramic radiography and CT: a systematic review and meta-analysis. Dentomaxillofac Radiol 2016; 45(2):20150310.

7. Mosier KM. Lesions of the jaw. Semin Ultrasound CT MR 2015;36(5):444–50.

8. Harmon M, Arrigan M, Toner M, et al. A radiological approach to benign and malignant lesions of the mandible. Clin Radiol 2015;70(4):335–50.

9. Meyer KA, Bancroft LW, Dietrich TJ, et al. Imaging characteristics of benign, malignant, and infectious jaw lesions: a pictorial review. AJR Am J Roentgenol 2011;197(3):W412–21.

10. Avril L, Lombardi T, Ailianou A, et al. Radiolucent lesions of the mandible: a pattern-based approach to diagnosis. Insights Imaging 2014;5(1):85–101.

11. Bharatha A, Pharoah MJ, Lee L, et al. Pictorial essay: cysts and cyst-like lesions of the jaws. Can Assoc Radiol J 2010;61(3):133–43.

12. Kramer IR, Pindborg JJ, Shear M. The WHO histological typing of odontogenic tumours. A commentary on the second edition. Cancer 1992;70(12): 2988–94.

13. Zain RB, Roswati N, Ismail K. Radiographic evaluation of lesion sizes of histologically diagnosed periapical cysts and granulomas. Ann Dent 1989; 48(2):3–5, 46.

14. Johnson NR, Gannon OM, Savage NW, et al. Frequency of odontogenic cysts and tumors: a systematic review. J Investig Clin Dent 2014;5(1):9–14.

15. Costa FW, Viana TS, Cavalcante GM, et al. A clinicoradiographic and pathological study of pericoronal follicles associated to mandibular third molars. J Craniofac Surg 2014;25(3):e283–7.

Malignant Lesions in the Dentomaxillofacial Complex

Susan M. White, DDS

KEYWORDS

• CBCT imaging • Dental imaging • Mandible • Maxilla • Paranasal sinuses • Malignancy

KEY POINTS

• Malignancies in the maxillofacial complex may mimic the symptomatology of benign dental disease, sinusitis, and temporomandibular joint disorders.
• Plain film radiography, cone beam CT, or sinus CT imaging may be the initial imaging study conducted of undiagnosed maxillofacial malignancies.
• The dentition, periodontium, and alveolar ridge are common sites of infection and postsurgical changes that should be distinguished in their clinical context from malignant changes.

INTRODUCTION

The contents of this text emphasize the effect of malignant changes on hard tissue structures of the maxillofacial complex, including the periodontium, maxilla, mandible, and sinuses. Malignant pathologies are characterized according to the manner of osseous involvement: (1) primary malignancies arising within the maxilla or mandible, (2) local osseous invasion of adjacent epithelial or soft tissue tumors, (3) malignancies spread to the maxillofacial complex via the hematopoietic or lymphatic system, and (4) metastases from distant primary tumors. The malignancies affecting the maxillofacial structures represent a broad spectrum of disease, with widely varying management and prognosis. Most malignancies, however, presenting in the head and neck region are squamous cell carcinomas (SCCs) arising within the muscular surfaces of the pharynx, larynx, paranasal sinuses, oral cavity, and nasal cavity. Many benign pathologies may mimic the radiographic features of malignancies, particularly in an area of the body prone to infection and inflammation, such as the oral cavity and paranasal sinuses.

IMAGING PROTOCOLS

The imaging techniques emphasized in this article include conventional radiographs and cone beam CT (CBCT) imaging, commonly used in dentomaxillofacial imaging, and bone-window multidetector CT (MDCT) imaging, standard for sinus evaluation. These techniques allow examination of detailed, initial osseous changes of occult malignancies, including lytic or osteoblastic changes, cortical disruption, or periodontal ligament (PDL) space changes. CBCT imaging allows manipulation of orientation that can more precisely characterize the pattern of bone loss in relationship to the dentition. MDCT imaging may better characterize lesions with soft tissue windowing and contrast enhancement but is limited by the fixed orientation of reconstructed images.

In known malignancies, MDCT and MR imaging allow for evaluation of tumor extension in the soft tissue, lymph node evaluation, and staging of the disease for appropriate treatment planning. MR imaging also allows for an assessment of bone marrow involvement before lytic or sclerotic changes are radiographically apparent.

Disclosure: The author has nothing to disclose.
Private Practice, 8 Brenda Lane, Merrimack, NH 03054, USA
E-mail address: susanwhite@ucla.edu

Radiol Clin N Am 56 (2018) 63–76
http://dx.doi.org/10.1016/j.rcl.2017.08.005
0033-8389/18/© 2017 Elsevier Inc. All rights reserved.

Fluorodeoxyglucose (^{18}FDG) PET/CT imaging may be used in cases of suspected disseminated disease (not limited to the head and neck region), including multiple myeloma (MM), metastatic disease, and extranodal lymphoma.

NORMAL ANATOMY

The normal anatomic features of the dental and maxillofacial structures are outlined in Mohammed Abbas Husain's article, "Dental Anatomy and Nomenclature for the Radiologist"; and Mitra Sadrameli and Mel Mupparapu's article, "Oral and Maxillofacial Anatomy," in this issue. A review of dental anatomy is provided in Mohammed Abbas Husain's article, "Dental Anatomy and Nomenclature for the Radiologist," in this issue, whereas overall maxillofacial anatomy is outlined in Mitra Sadrameli and Mel Mupparapu's article, "Oral and Maxillofacial Anatomy," in this issue.

COMMON CLINICAL AND RADIOGRAPHIC FEATURES OF MALIGNANCIES ON DENTAL AND OSSEOUS STRUCTURES
Clinical Changes

Clinical signs and symptomatology may be entirely absent or may present as a clinically identifiable mass or lump, ulceration, oral cavity leukoplakia/erythroplakia, nasal congestion or airway obstruction, epistaxis, anosmia, paresthesia/anesthesia/dysesthesia (especially a numb chin), dental/temporomandibular joint [TMJ]/sinus pain, or, in advanced high-grade malignancies, hemorrhage, rapid onset of tooth mobility, fever, malaise, and weight loss.

Radiographic Changes

A majority of malignancies involving bone in the maxillofacial region present as an ill-defined lytic change radiographically, whereas a minority demonstrate an osteoblastic component with or without periosteal reaction. The maxillofacial region is a unique anatomic area of the body that often demonstrates inflammatory and postsurgical changes. Bone loss around teeth has many causes other than malignancy, including periapical granulomas or cysts, root fractures, furcational bone loss, and vertical alveolar defects (**Fig. 1**). The irregular PDL space widening of malignancies is ragged, often not centered on the apex and not associated with obvious dental pathology. Malignant periosteal bone is characteristically aggressive (**Fig. 2**). A summary of radiographic changes suspicious for malignancies is included in **Box 1**.

REVIEW OF DIAGNOSTIC CRITERIA

The diagnostic criteria that suggest a malignancy in the maxillofacial complex are outlined in previous section and in **Box 1**. Lesions detected in the maxillofacial complex suspicious for malignancy on plain film or CBCT imaging usually require fine-needle aspiration, biopsy, and/or advanced imaging for better characterization to establish a diagnosis.

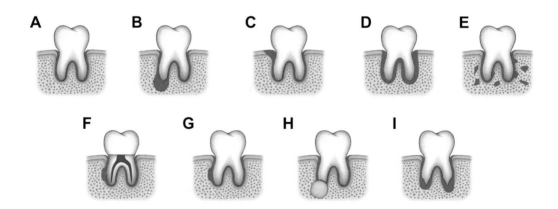

Fig. 1. The images show the different tooth-related changes seen with malignancy on dental imaging. (*A*) Normal PDL space. (*B*) Periapical pathology (granuloma or cyst) centered at a root apex. (*C*) Periodontal bone loss, originating from the alveolar crest, forming a vertical defect. (*D*) Generalized PDL space widening (occlusal trauma or scleroderma). (*E*) Irregular PDL space widening and ragged, lytic changes in trabecular bone. (*F*) Midroot PDL space widening in endodontically treated tooth with a post, suggestive of a root fracture. (*G*) Midroot PDL space widening in vital tooth with no inflammatory etiology, suspicious for malignancy. (*H*) Sharp root resorption, associated with benign, space-occupying lesions. (*I*) Spiking resorption of roots associated with aggressive or malignant lesions.

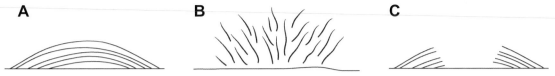

Fig. 2. The following graphics demonstrate the appearance of periosteal reaction associated with malignancies in the jaws. (*A*) Lamellar or onion skin periosteal reaction, is more indicative of a low-grade, chronic irritation. (*B*) A spiculated or sunray periosteal reaction is consistent with an aggressive benign or malignant lesion. (*C*) Codman triangle refers to lack of bone formation in the central portion of lamellar periosteal reaction, consistent with an aggressive lesion.

PRIMARY OSSEOUS MALIGNANCIES
Osteosarcoma (Osteogenic Sarcoma)

Epidemiology
Osteosarcoma is the second most common primary malignancy found in bone, after plasma cell tumors, accounting for approximately 30% of skeletal lesions.[1] Osteosarcoma usually presents at the metaphyseal regions of long bones, in skeletally immature pediatric and adolescent patients. Gnathic osteosarcoma represents 4% to 8% of cases, peaking in the third to fourth decades.[2] Osteosarcomas in the maxillofacial complex show a predilection for men and affect the mandible slightly more than the maxilla. Mandibular lesions often involve the alveolar ridge and posterior mandibular body, whereas maxillary lesions are noted in the alveolar ridge, sinus floor, and palate. Secondary osteosarcoma is a separate entity, usually presenting in older adults, and associated with an underlying condition, such as Paget disease, fibrous dysplasia, radiation or bone infarcts.

Prognosis
Survival rates for primary osteosarcomas, arising de novo, have improved over the past several decades,[3] but the prognosis for osteosarcomas secondary to Paget disease remains poor.[4] The prognosis for postirradiation osteogenic sarcomas is similar to that for de novo tumors.[5] Gnathic osteosarcomas have a better prognosis than those in the appendicular skeleton and typically do not metastasize to regional lymph nodes or distant sites.[2] Instead, local recurrence (maxilla > mandible) is the primary cause of mortality. Survival rates improve from 12% to 20% to 60% to 70% when treatment protocol includes both surgical resection and a chemotherapy regimen.[2]

Clinical presentation
Osteosarcomas usually present with pain and may include other nonspecific complaints of jaw swelling, loosening of teeth, paresthesia, mucosal erythema, or ulceration.

Radiographic appearance
Radiographically, the initial signs of osteosarcoma may be subtle. Early diagnosis of gnathic lesions is usually made by detection of irregular, asymmetric PDL space changes in a young patient (**Fig. 3**).

Advanced osteosarcomas may demonstrate both osteoblastic and osteolytic components. Osteosarcomas typically develop within the intramedullary bone, with eventual expansion, cortical disruption, periosteal bone formation, and a soft tissue mass (**Fig. 4**). The margins are typically ill defined. The osteoid matrix within medullary bone often includes granular or sclerotic bone. Periosteal bone reaction usually forms perpendicular to the underlying cortex, in a haphazard fashion with sunray spicules. Rare subtypes include juxtacortical osteomas (eg, parosteal or

---

Box 1
Malignant features on conventional and CT imaging in the maxillofacial region

- Irregular widening of the PDL space
- Spiking resorption of roots
- Irregular destruction of the lamina dura
- Extensive bone destruction around teeth without tooth displacement
- Delayed healing of extraction sockets
- Ill-defined, permeative periphery
- Destruction of cortical borders
- Loss of mandibular canal cortication
- Multifocal, ragged radiolucent foci or rarefaction in trabecular bone
- Osteoblastic changes with bone destruction
- Sunray or spiculated periosteal reaction
- Codman triangle periosteal reaction
- Widening of neural foramina, particularly the greater/lesser palatine foramina for masses along the CN V2 distribution and the mental and mandibular foramina for masses along the CN V3 distribution.
- Widening of the pterygopalatine fossa

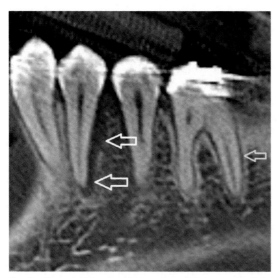

Fig. 3. Chondroblastic osteosarcoma in a young adult. Oblique sagittal CBCT. Asymmetric PDL space widening at the distal surface of #20 (*white arrows*), with no inflammatory etiology. Normal PDL space (*yellow arrow*).

periosteal) that originate within the periosteum and do not invade the underlying medullary bone.[6]

Chondrosarcoma

Epidemiology

Chondrosarcoma is a malignancy of mesenchymal origin, arising within bone, with a wide age distribution, peaking in the fourth to sixth decades. Men and women are affected equally. Although chondrosarcomas comprise approximately one-quarter of malignant skeletal tumors,[7] these lesions only rarely present in the head and neck, comprising only 0.1% of head and neck neoplasms.[8] The base of the skull is most frequently involved. In the dentomaxillofacial complex, the condylar head, coronoid process, and anterior maxilla are most frequently involved.

Prognosis

Chondrosarcomas in the maxillofacial region are often low grade and demonstrate slow, progressive growth.[9] Distant metastasis and lymph node involvement are rare. Higher-grade chondrosarcomas, however, may metastasize and are associated with a poor 10-year survival rate.[7] In the head and neck region, resectability of the tumor is the primary indicator of prognosis.[10]

Clinical presentation

When the TMJ is the site of origin, trismus or joint dysfunction may be present. In a low-grade tumor, a hard joint mass may be appreciated by the patient for multiple years. Intraorally, a painless swelling or mass, without ulceration, may be the presenting sign.[5]

Radiographic appearance

Chondrosarcomas may demonstrate radiologic features similar to osteosarcoma, including a soft tissue mass with internal calcifications, and sometimes sunray spiculated periosteal bone formation. Tumors are usually mixed density. The nature of the periphery demonstrates a wide variability. Low-grade tumors may have well-defined or even corticated margins. Higher-grade lesions have infiltrative, ill-defined borders. Similar to other malignancies in the maxillofacial region, irregular PDL space widening may be appreciated. In the TMJ area, and destruction of the temporal bone may be appreciated.

Malignant Ameloblastoma

Epidemiology

Malignant ameloblastoma (MA) is a rare malignancy of middle-aged adults in the oral and

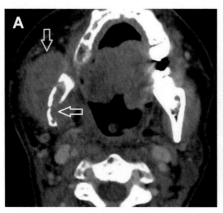
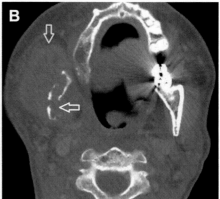

Fig. 4. High-grade osteosarcoma, with soft tissue mass (*yellow arrow*) in right masticator space and lytic changes in ramus (*white arrow*). Axial CECT (*A*) and bone-window MDCT (*B*). (*Courtesy of* Philip Chapman, MD, Birmingham, AL.)

maxillofacial region. This entity is defined in terms of behavior in which there is tumor spread to the lower aerodigestive tract, including the lungs.[11] There is debate as to whether MA constitutes a true malignancy and if the pulmonary lesions arise from inhaled tissue rather than metastasis.

Prognosis
The prognosis has been difficult to assess due to the rarity of this lesion; 10-year survival rates as high as 89% in young adults have been reported.[12]

Clinical presentation
Patients may present with a jaw swelling or with chest pain as the primary symptom.[13]

Radiographic appearance
MA is radiologically and histologically indistinguishable from benign ameloblastoma (described in William C. Scarfe and colleagues', "Imaging of Benign Odontogenic Lesions," in this issue) and should be differentiated from carcinoma ex ameloblastoma, an extremely rare lesion arising from malignant transformation of a preexisting benign ameloblastoma. MA is well corticated with clear margins, whereas carcinoma ex ameloblastoma is expected to demonstrate infiltrative changes.

SECONDARY INVASION FROM SOFT TISSUE MALIGNANCY

Secondary malignant invasion of bone in the dentomaxillofacial complex most often arises from SCC originating in the overlying mucosal epithelium. It is possible, however, for malignancies of many adjacent structures to invade the underlying bone, including minor salivary glands (MSGs), fibroblasts, melanocytes, skeletal or smooth muscle, adipose tissue, vascular endothelium, and neural tissue (**Box 2**). Due to their rarity and similar radiographic features, only a subset of these malignancies is discussed.

Squamous Cell Carcinoma

Epidemiology
SSC accounts for greater than 90% of all head and neck malignancies.[14] The oral cavity, nasopharynx, and oropharynx are more commonly affected than the nasal cavity and paranasal sinuses. SSC in the oral and maxillofacial region is most common in the fifth to seventh decades, with a male predilection. There has been a recent increase, however, in incidence of oropharyngeal SSC among young adults (<30 years) in Western countries.[15]

Prevalence may vary widely between populations, following lifestyle practices.[14] Common risk factors for head and neck SSC include tobacco,

---

> **Box 2**
> **Malignancies of the maxillofacial region that may secondarily invade bone**
>
> - Squamous cell carcinoma (90%)
> - MSGMs
> - Sinonasal undifferentiated carcinoma
> - Small cell carcinoma
> - Malignant melanoma
> - Esthesioneuroblastoma
> - Fibrosarcoma
> - Malignant peripheral nerve sheath tumor
> - Rhabdomyosarcoma
> - Leiomyosarcoma
> - Liposarcoma
> - Angiosarcoma

alcohol, betel quid, human papilloma virus (HPV) infection, and exposure to molten heavy metals and wood dust (particularly for paranasal sinus SSC).[16] HPV DNA has been detected in approximately 50% to 85% of oropharyngeal SSC,[15] often in younger patients.

The most common sites of SSC in the maxillofacial region include the ventral or lateral surfaces of the tongue and the floor of the mouth. SCC involving the mandible often originates from the gingiva or floor of the mouth, whereas those involving the maxilla often originate from the maxillary sinus.[1]

Prognosis
The prognosis of SSC in the maxillofacial region generally remains poor due to advanced staging of the disease at the time of diagnosis. Survivors frequently exhibit considerable morbidity, including disfigurement, distorted speech, difficulty swallowing, loss of taste, and xerostomia.[14]

Clinical presentation
Clinical features of squamous cell carcinoma in the oral cavity include a soft tissue mass, erythroplakia developing into leukoplakia, rolled or indurated borders, ulceration, pain, foul smell, trismus, loosening of teeth, and hemorrhage. SSC originating in the attached gingiva may be confused with soft tissue changes in advanced periodontal disease. SSC originating within the maxillary sinuses may mimic sinusitis and present with pain, nasal congestion, or anosmia. Patients with advanced disease may complain of epitasis or paresthesia.

Imaging recommendations
Early invasion of the alveolar ridge may best be appreciated in high spatial resolution periapical

radiographs or CBCT imaging. Advanced lesions are evaluated with both (1) CBCT or bone-window MDCT to assess the involvement of bone and (2) MR imaging, contrast-enhanced CT (CECT), and/or PET imaging to assess the extent of the heterogeneously enhancing soft tissue mass and lymph node involvement.

Radiographic appearances

Initial presentation may be a breach in cortication of the alveolar crest, border of the maxillary sinus, mandibular body, or ramus (**Fig. 5**). Areas of cortical destruction may develop multiple lytic lesions within the underlying medullary cavity that may coalesce to form a larger, saucer-shaped lesion over time. The adjacent dentition may demonstrate irregular PDL space widening or appear to float in the surrounding soft tissue. Extensive, permeative bone destruction may lead to a pathologic fracture or obliteration of the mandible with a large, poorly marginated soft tissue mass (**Fig. 6**).

Minor Salivary Gland Malignancies

Epidemiology

MSGs are located in the submucosa of the hard and soft palate, buccal, labial, and lingual mucosa, the floor of the mouth, and the mucoperiosteal lining of the paranasal sinuses as well as the tonsils, larynx, and trachea. MSG neoplasms often present in the third to seventh decades of life, with a slight female or no gender predilection. Approximately half of MSG tumors arise on the hard palate, whereas a quarter present on the mucosal

surface of the lips, 10% to 15% in the buccal mucosa, and the remaining in other mucosal surfaces of the paranasal sinuses or upper aerodigestive tract.[17] MSG malignancies (MSGMs) comprise approximately half of MSG tumors.[18] Most benign neoplasms of MSGs are pleomorphic adenomas, whereas the most common malignancies are mucoepidermoid carcinomas and adenoid cystic carcinomas.

Prognosis

MSGMs are a heterogeneous group of malignancies with varying prognosis. Adenoid cystic carcinomas have a particular tendency for vascular spread and perineural invasion via the greater palatine foramen and carry a poorer prognosis.[19] Tumors in the sinonasal region tend to be more advanced when discovered and also carry a poorer prognosis than MSGMs originating in the hard palate.[20] Long-term follow-up of adenoid cystic carcinoma is recommended, given a tendency for late recurrence.

Clinical presentation

MSGMs originating within the oral cavity are more likely to be detected early due to direct visualization. These entities typical presentation is a hard, slowly growing lump, usually at the hard palate, buccal mucosa, or lip, with or without pain. Perineural involvement of the trigeminal nerve (cranial nerve [CN] V) may result in sensory deficits. In the hypopharynx or larynx, a growing tumor may result in airway obstruction, hoarseness, or dysphagia. In the paranasal sinuses or nasal cavities, however, MSGMs may remain undetected for an extended period of time. The presenting symptoms of nasal obstruction, drainage, and/or sinus pain mimic sinusitis. Therefore, the initial detection of sinonasal MSGMs may be due to malignant radiologic features noted on a sinus CT scan.

Imaging recommendations

In known MSGMs, MR imaging is recommended to determine the full extent of soft tissue infiltration and perineural tumor spread. Depending on their histologic grade, MSGMs may demonstrate smooth or ill-defined margins on MR imaging. T1 imaging with contrast and fat-suppression is optimal for assessment of CN V2 involvement.[19]

Radiographic appearance

Radiologically, an MSGM presents as a soft tissue mass, with a round or lobulated contours, in the oral cavity, nasal cavity, paranasal sinuses, or pharyngeal airway. Malignancy is suspected if destruction or erosion of the adjacent hard palate, alveolar ridge, or sinus borders is appreciated (**Fig. 7**). In addition, asymmetric widening or

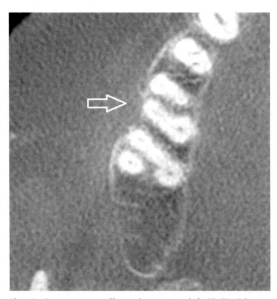

Fig. 5. Squamous cell carcinoma, axial CBCT. Disruption of alveolar cortex buccal to #2 and #3 (*arrow*).

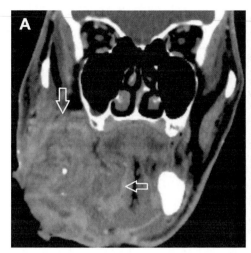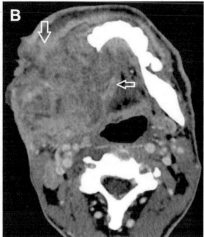

Fig. 6. Squamous cell carcinoma. Complete destruction of right mandible with heterogeneously enhancing soft tissue mass (*arrows*). (*A*) Coronal CECT; (*B*) Axial CECT. (*Courtesy of* Philip Chapman, MD, Birmingham, AL.)

osseous destruction of the greater palatine foramen, the pterygopalatine fossa, and/or the inferior orbital fissure are consistent with perineural tumor spread (see **Fig. 7**B).

Rhabdomyosarcoma

Epidemiology

Rhabdomyosarcomas are a rare malignancy of skeletal muscle but warrant special mention because they are the most common soft tissue sarcoma and most common sinonasal tumor in the pediatric population and young adults.[21] In children, head and neck rhabdomyosarcoma commonly involve the orbit.[22] In young adults, the head and neck region accounts for approximately one-quarter of sites, with approximately half in the paranasal sinuses and the remainder in the nasal cavity or infratemporal fossa.[23]

Prognosis

The prognosis of head and neck rhabdomyosarcoma depends on age of the patient, location and size of the tumor, and histologic subtype.[24,25] Risk factors for a poorer prognosis include adult patient (>20 years), alveolar subtype, sinonasal location, large tumors (>5 cm), and positive surgical margins.[24] Disseminated disease with distant metastasis at the time of diagnosis is common (60%) in adult rhabdomyosarcoma.[24] In contrast, orbital cases of rhabdomyosarcoma in the pediatric population have a 10-year survival rate of 77%.[25]

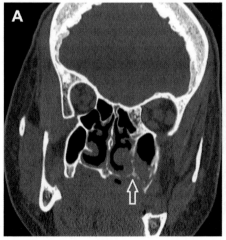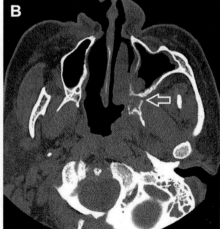

Fig. 7. Basal cell adenocarcinoma with perineural tumor spread. (*A*) Coronal MDCT. Soft tissue mass in left maxillary sinus with osseous destruction of sinus and hard palate (*arrow*). (*B*) Axial MDCT. Lytic changes in left pterygopalatine fossa (*arrow*). (*Courtesy of* Philip Chapman, MD, Birmingham, AL.)

Clinical presentation

Pediatric cases often present with proptosis, limited eye movement, and/or vision loss.[24] When rhabdomyosarcoma presents in the nasal cavities or paranasal sinuses, however, presenting symptoms may mimic sinusitis or dental disease, resulting in a delayed diagnosis.

Imaging recommendations

CT and MR imaging is similar to other malignancies and allows for mapping locoregional extension but does not often aid in diagnosis.[26] Full-body PET/CT imaging is often performed in adult patients due to the high rate of distant metastasis.[24]

Radiographic appearance

In the dentomaxillofacial region, radiographic features are nonspecific and include disruption of the sinus floor or alveolar ridge cortication, irregular PDL space widening, and multiple lytic foci within the trabecular bone (**Fig. 8**).

HEMATOPOIETIC AND LYMPHOID MALIGNANCIES
Multiple Myeloma

Epidemiology

MM is a monoclonal malignant proliferation of plasma cells and is the most common primary bone malignancy in adults.[27–29] Middle-aged to elderly adults are typically affected, ranging from the fifth to ninth decades, with a male predilection. The etiology is unknown. Lesions may be (1) a single, solitary lytic lesion, (2) multifocal disseminated disease involving more than one bone, or (3) extramedullary solitary lesions within the soft tissues. Solitary lesions are known as plasmacytomas and eventually transition to the disseminated form (approximately 70% within 20 months).[27]

Overall, approximately 80% to 85% of patients with medullary plasmacytomas progress to MM.[28] Skull lesions are present in approximately half of cases, whereas the mandible is involved in 15% to 20% of cases.[30] Within the mandible, the angle, ramus, and posterior mandibular alveolar ridge are favored.[1]

Prognosis

Until recently, the prognosis of MM patients remained poor. In the early 2000s, most institutions reported a 5-year survival rate of 25%.[5] Due to improvements in the chemotherapy regimen, recent 5-year survival rates have improved: 66% in patients less than 50 years, 52% in patients 50 years to 69 years, and 31% in patients greater than 70 years.[31]

Clinical presentation

Patients with MM often present with bone pain, fatigue, weight loss, and/or fever. Anemia or hypercalcemia may be detected in the disseminated form of disease but not solitary plasmacytomas.[28] In approximately half of patients, Bence Jones protein is detected in the urine. When lesions present in the dentomaxillofacial region, the patient is often asymptomatic but may complain of dental or TMJ pain, swelling, paresthesia.[29]

Imaging recommendations

MM lesions are best appreciated on CBCT and bone-window MDCT imaging. When a single plasmacytoma is suspected, full-body [18]FDG PET/CT may be conducted to rule out other sites of involvement and disseminated disease.[27]

Radiographic appearance

The disseminated form of disease demonstrates multiple, small, ragged or ovoid, noncorticated punched-out lesions, often in the calvarium, that

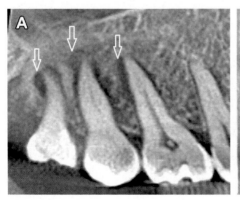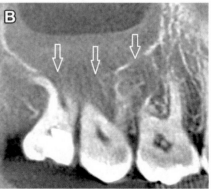

Fig. 8. Rhabdomyosarcoma, undiagnosed recurrence in adult man with dental pain in right maxillary arch. Oblique sagittal CBCT views. (*A*) Irregular PDL space widening (*arrows*). (*B*) Interruption of sinus floor (*arrows*) with soft tissue thickening.

are pathognomonic for MM. They arise within the medullary bone and may grow in size to scallop the endosteal surface of cortical bone or disrupt it (Fig. 9).[16] If MM presents as a rarefaction at the apices of teeth, it may mimic periapical disease. The 2 may be distinguished, however, because MM usually presents with multiple other lesions within the jaw not localized to an apex. A solitary plasmacytoma in the mandible forms a larger, radiolucent lesion with thinning, mild expansion, and eventually disruption of the cortical plates. Within the mandible, it may be undiagnosed at the time of imaging and mistaken for metastatic disease (Fig. 10).

Non-Hodgkin Lymphoma

Epidemiology

Non-Hodgkin lymphoma (NHL) is the second most common neoplasm of the head and neck region, aside from SCCs.[32] The age distribution is broad, peaking in the sixth decade, with a slight male predilection. NHL represents a broad spectrum of malignancies involving the lymphoreticular system. Head and neck NHL is subdivided into nodal and extranodal sites.[19] Approximately 20% of NHLs in the head and neck area include masses outside of lymph nodes, with the incidence increasing in recent years.[16,33] Common extranodal sites in the maxillofacial region include Waldeyer ring, the paranasal sinuses, the nasal cavity, the hard palate, and the posterior mandible, although any site may be affected.

Prognosis

Prognosis for NHL patients is widely variable and depends on age of the patient, the number of extranodal sites, and the stage of the disease.

An age of greater than 60 years, greater than 1 extranodal site, and stage III/IV disease are all indicative of poor prognosis.[19]

Clinical presentation

A patient with head and neck NHL may present with a known neck mass or lymphadenopathy. Some classes of NHL present with fever, night sweats, or weight loss. Low-grade indolent lymphomas, including mucosa-associated lymphoid tissue lymphomas may be initially present asymptomatically. Nodal NHL is characterized by multiple, enlarged, non-necrotic nodes which may be palpable. Extranodal NHL often presents as a large, enhancing tonsillar mass or as an infiltrative mass anywhere throughout the maxillofacial region, imitating several other malignancies.

Imaging recommendations

After diagnosis, the imaging protocol of known head and neck NHL may include [18]FDG PET/CT to determine the full extent of extranodal involvement. This has proved more sensitive than CECT imaging.[33]

Radiographic appearance

Radiographically, the early osseous changes of NHL within bone are lytic and ill defined. The overall morphology of the bone is typically preserved, although the cortex often demonstrates multiple lytic foci (Fig. 11). The affected trabecular bone demonstrates generalized, irregular rarefaction. Within the alveolar ridge, lymphomas are known to invade and irregularly widen the PDL space.[16] Generally, no periosteal reaction is appreciated. An adjacent soft tissue mass may be appreciated within the maxillary sinuses or oral cavity.

METASTASES
Epidemiology

Aside from direct locoregional spread of SSC, metastatic lesions to the jaws are the next most common malignancy that may involve the osseous tissues of the dentomaxillofacial complex.[11] The mandible is 5 times more likely to present with a metastatic lesion than the maxilla. The primary tumor is typically a carcinoma, spreading via a hematogenous route, most commonly from the breast, kidney, lung, prostate, thyroid, or colon. When a metastatic lesion is detected in the mandible, the primary site is most often unknown.[11]

Prognosis

The detection of metastases in the bones of the maxillofacial complex represents stage IV disease

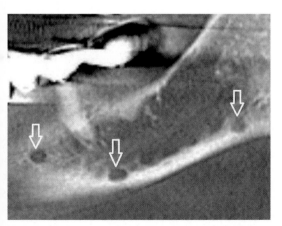

Fig. 9. MM, undiagnosed and asymptomatic. Oblique sagittal CBCT view. Multiple punched out lesions with endosteal scalloping (arrows). (Courtesy of Mohammed Abbas Husain, DDS, Los Angeles, CA.)

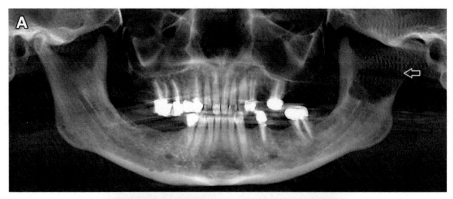

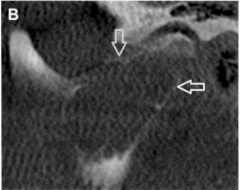

Fig. 10. Plasmacytoma, undiagnosed with left TMJ pain. (A) Panoramic reconstruction from CBCT scan. Large lytic lesion at left ramus/TMJ (arrow). (B) Axially corrected sagittal oblique CBCT view. Thinning, expansion and cortical destruction of condylar neck, posterior border of ramus (white arrow), and sigmoid notch (yellow arrow).

and usually indicates poor prognosis. An esti-mated two-thirds of patients with metastases to the jaws succumb to their disease in less than 1 year.[11]

Clinical Presentation

Malignant disease of unknown primaries may be detected due to a patient complaint of a nonheal-ing extraction socket; unusual and rapid loosening

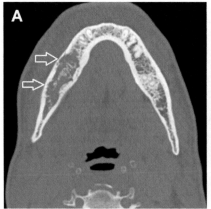

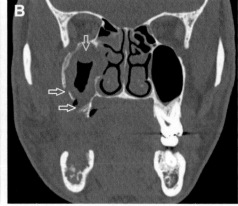

Fig. 11. T-cell lymphoma. (A) Axial bone-window MDCT. Permeative, lytic changes in right mandible (arrows). (B) Coronal bone-window MDCT. Cortical disruption of maxillary sinus (white arrows) and associated soft tissue thickening (yellow arrow), with signs of superimposed inflammatory change. (Courtesy of Philip Chapman, MD, Birmingham, AL.)

of teeth; or dental, sinus, or TMJ pain. Other cases may be noted only as incidental, asymptomatic findings on a radiograph.

Imaging Recommendations

When a metastatic lesion is suspected, a bone scan or PET/CT scan is recommended to assess the degree of dissemination and, if necessary, locate the primary.

Radiographic Appearance

Radiographically, metastatic lesions to the bone are nonspecific and may demonstrate osteolytic or osteoblastic features. Osteolytic metastases may vary from a single, poorly defined radiolucent lesion to a generalized, permeative, moth-eaten change within the bone (**Fig. 12**). Some primaries, in particular prostate or breast, yield mixed-density metastases with an osteoblastic component. This osteoblastic component may feature sunray spiculated periosteal reaction, and irregular, sclerotic changes in the medullary bone (**Fig. 13**).

DIFFERENTIAL DIAGNOSIS
Periapical and Periodontal Disease

As discussed previously, bone loss and PDL space widening around the dentition is a common phenomenon (see **Fig. 1**; **Fig. 14**).

Patterns of bone loss of PDL space widening consistent with periapical or radicular disease include

1. Bone loss centered at the apex, where the contents of a necrotic pulp come in contact with the trabecular bone

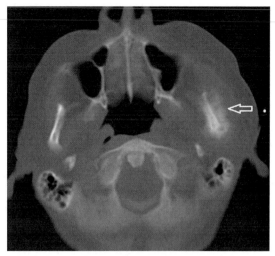

Fig. 13. Metastatic breast cancer. Axial bone-window MDCT view. Osteoblastic changes and spiculated, sun-ray periosteal reaction at the left ramus (*arrow*).

2. PDL space widening at the termination of a post in an endodontically treated tooth
3. Evidence of sclerotic reaction in the surrounding alveolar bone, particularly in larger or chronic lesions

Patterns of bone loss consistent with periodontal disease include

1. Extension apically from the alveolar crest, where a vertical defect is broadest

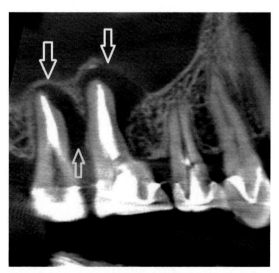

Fig. 14. Malignancy differential diagnosis: persistent periapical disease. Oblique Sagittal CBCT view. Apical rarefaction with sclerotic border (*white arrows*). Endoperio defect extending to alveolar crest (*yellow arrow*).

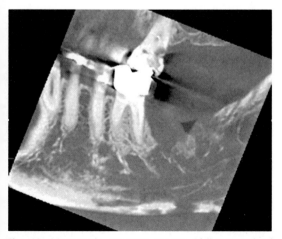

Fig. 12. Metastatic prostate cancer. Oblique sagittal CBCT view. Infiltrative, lytic changes in the trabecular and cortical bone of the left posterior mandible.

2. Bone loss centered at the furcational areas of posterior teeth, continuous with the oral cavity
3. Bone loss explained by a precipitating phenomenon (eg, overhanging restoration)

Periapical and Florid Osseous Dysplasia

Periapical osseous dysplasia is a non-neoplastic fibro-osseous condition, in which normal bone is replaced by fibrous tissue, then amorphous bone. In early stages, the lesions are entirely radiolucent and present at the apex or apical third of teeth (**Fig. 15**). The teeth may be vital, raising suspicion of pathology other than periapical disease. Periapical osseous dysplasia lesions frequently affect vital teeth in the anterior mandible in middle-aged African or Asian women.

Florid osseous dysplasia may simulate a low-grade osteosarcoma in the mixed-density stage, because amorphous bone develops within radiolucent lesions (**Fig. 16**). Secondary infection is a known complication of florid osseous dysplasia, obscuring the clearly demarcated periphery, further complicating the diagnosis.

Secondary Infection of Benign Cyst or Tumor

Secondary infection of a benign odontogenic cyst or tumor in the jaws may feature cortical disruption and irregular, ill-defined lytic changes (**Fig. 17**). These secondarily infected space-occupying lesions may be confused with malignancies. The probability of superimposed inflammatory changes far outweighs malignancy in the jaws.

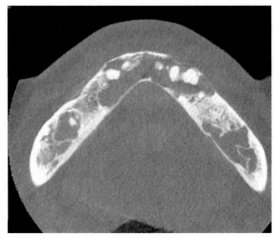

Fig. 16. Malignancy differential diagnosis: florid osseous dysplasia. Axial CBCT view. Multiple, large lytic foci with amorphous radiopacities in the mandible, with sclerotic cortication.

Calcium Pyrophosphate Dihydrate Deposition Disease of the Temporomandibular Joint

Calcium pyrophosphate dihydrate deposition disease is an arthropathy in which calcium pyrophosphate dihydrate crystals are deposited in the joint space. The calcifications within the joint space are often fine, granular, and evenly distributed. Advanced cases of this condition may mimic chondrosarcoma of the TMJ when destruction of the temporal bone and condylar head are appreciated (**Fig. 18**).

Osteoradionecrosis

Osteoradionecrosis (ORN) is a complication of radiation therapy, when the mandible is positioned in

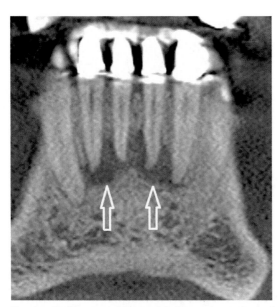

Fig. 15. Malignancy differential diagnosis: periapical osseous dysplasia. Coronal CBCT view. Noncorticated apical rarefaction in vital teeth (*arrows*).

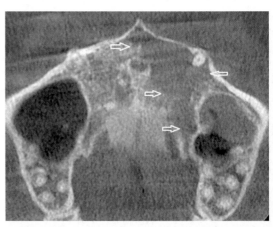

Fig. 17. Malignancy differential diagnosis: secondarily infected odontogenic keratocyst. Axial CBCT view. Ill-defined, lytic changes in left anterior maxilla, extending posteriorly to the hard palate (*arrows*).

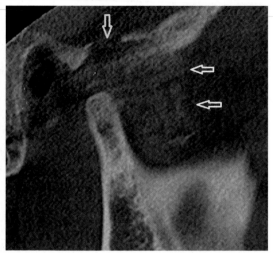

Fig. 18. Malignancy differential diagnosis: CPPD. Sagittal CBCT view. Delicate, granular mass surrounding the right TMJ (*white arrows*). Destruction of temporal bone (*yellow arrow*).

the field of the beam, usually exposed to doses exceeding 60 Gy. Radiographically, ORN closely resembles the irregular, multifocal lytic changes of many malignancies in the dentomaxillofacial region (**Fig. 19**). Isolated segments of cortical bone may be sequestered. In advanced cases, pathologic fracture may be present. Distinguishing ORN from a recurrence of osteolytic malignancies in the oral cavity may not be possible radiographically. A history of radiation therapy and clinical evidence of exposed, necrotic bone are necessary for diagnosis.

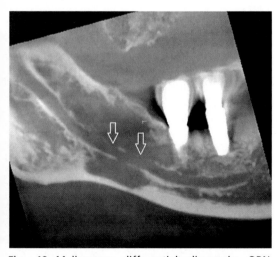

Fig. 19. Malignancy differential diagnosis: ORN. Sagittal CBCT view. Lytic trabecular and cortical changes in the posterior right mandible, with focal disruption of the IA canal (*arrows*). (*Courtesy of* Sotirios Tetradis, DDS, Los Angeles, CA.)

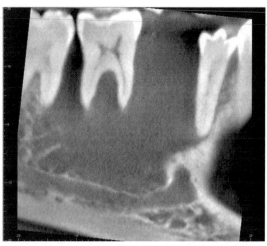

Fig. 20. Malignancy differential diagnosis: giant cell granuloma. Sagittal CBCT view. Permeative, lytic changes in right posterior mandible, with destruction of alveolar crest and floating dentition. (*Courtesy of* Sanjay Mallya, DDS, Los Angeles, CA.)

Central Giant Cell Granuloma

Central giant cell granulomas are benign, reactive lesions, usually involving the mandible with variable radiographic presentation. Slow-growing lesions may be multilocular, with clear, sclerotic margins. Aggressive central giant cell granulomalesions may demonstrate little internal structure, erode cortices, and mimic malignancies (**Fig. 20**).

SUMMARY

Malignancies affecting the osseous structures of the dentomaxillofacial region are a heterogeneous group of lesions that may be subdivided into (1) primary osseous malignancies, (2) secondary invasion of bone from locoregional spread, (3) hematopoietic and lymphatic malignancies, and (4) metastatic disease. Many of these malignancies may simulate the clinical presentation of dental, sinus, or TMJ diseases. Initial observation of malignant osteolytic or osteoblastic changes to the hard tissues of the dentomaxillofacial complex may aid in the early detection of occult malignancies.

REFERENCES

1. Weber A, Bui C, Kaneda T. Malignant tumors of the mandible and maxilla. Neuroimaging Clin N Am 2003;13(3):509–24.
2. George A, Mani V. Gnathic osteosarcoma: review of literature and report of two cases in maxilla. J Oral Maxillofac Pathol 2011;15(2):138–43.

3. Gill J, Ahluwalia M, Geller D, et al. New targets and approaches in osteosarcoma. Pharmacol Ther 2013; 137(1):89–99.

4. Ruggieri P, Calabro T, Montalti M, et al. The role of surgery and adjuvants to survival in Pagetic osteosarcoma. Clin Orthop Relat Res 2010;468(11): 2962–8.

5. Neville B, Damm D, Allen C, et al. Bone Pathology. In: Neville B, Damm D, Allen C, et al, editors. Oral & maxillofacial pathology. 3rd edition. St Louis (MO): Elsevier; 2009. p. 660–4.

6. Sawair FA, Cheng J, Hao N, et al. Periosteal osteosarcoma of the jaw bones: a clinicopathological review. Oral Med Pathol 2007;12(1):3–10.

7. Giuffrida A, Burgueno J, Koniaris L, et al. Chondrosarcoma in the United States (1973 to 2003): an analysis of 2890 cases from the SEER database. J Bone Joint Surg Am 2009;91(5):1063–72.

8. Koch B, Karnell L, Hoffman H, et al. National cancer database report on chondrosarcoma of the head and neck. Head Neck 2000;22:408–25.

9. Larheim TA, Westesson P-L, editors. Maxillofacial imaging. Berlin: Springer; 2006.

10. Lee SY, Lim YC, Song MH, et al. Chondrosarcoma of the head and neck. Yonsei Med J 2005;46(2):228–32.

11. Sciubba JJ, Eversole LR, Slootweg PJ. Odontogenic / amelobastic carcinomas. In: Barnes L, Eveson JW, Reichart P, et al, editors. World Heath Organization Classification of Tumors. Pathology and Genetics of Head and Neck Tumours. Lyon: IARC Press; 2005. p. 287–9.

12. Rizzitelli A, Smoll N, Chae M, et al. Incidence and overall survival of malignant ameloblastoma. PLoS One 2015;10(2):e0117789.

13. Bi R, Shen L, Zhu X, et al. Malignant Amelobastoma (metastatic ameloblastoma) in the Lung: 3 cases of misdiagnosis as primary lung tumor with a unique growth pattern. Diagn Pathol 2015;10:123.

14. Rekha R, Reddy MVV, Reddy PP. Epidemiological studies of head and neck cancer in South Indian Population. Res Cancer Tumor 2013;2(2):38–44.

15. Attner P, Du J, Nasman A, et al. The role of human papilloma virus in the increased incidence of base of tongue cancer. Int J Cancer 2010;126(12):2879–84.

16. White S, Pharoah M. Malignant diseases. In: White S, Pharoah M, editors. Oral radiology: principles & interpretation. 7th edition. St Louis (MO): Elsevier; 2014. p. 427–51.

17. Yih W, Kratochvil F, Stewart J. Intraoral minor salivary gland neoplasms: review of 213 cases. J Oral Maxillofac Surg 2005;63(6):805–10.

18. Vaidya A, Pantvaidya G, Metgudmath R, et al. Minor salivary gland tumors of the oral cavity: a case series with review of the literature. J Cancer Res Ther 2012;8(Suppl 1):S111–5.

19. Koenig L, editor. Diagnostic imaging: oral & maxillofacial. Salt Lake City (UT): Lippincott Williams & Wilkins; 2011.

20. Strick MJ, Kelly C, Soames JV, et al. Malignant tumours of the minor salivary glands–a 20 year review. Br J Plast Surg 2004;57(7):624–31.

21. Kumar V, Abbas AK, Fausto N, et al, editors. Robbins basic pathology. 8th edition. Philadelphia: Elsevier; 2007.

22. Ahmed A, Tsokos M. Sinonasal rhabdomyosarcoma in children and young adults. Int J Surg Pathol 2007; 15:160–5.

23. Lee J, Lee M, Lee B, et al. Rhabdomyosarcoma of the head and neck in adults: MR and CT findings. AJNR Am J Neuroradiol 1996;17:1923–8.

24. Erkul E, Pinar D, Yilmaz I, et al. Rare adult sinonasal embryonal rhabdomyosarcoma with optic involvement. Otolaryngology 2012;2(3):3–5.

25. Torres-Peña JL, Castrillo AIR, Mencía-Gutiérrez E, et al. Nasal cavity or alveolar paranasal sinus rhabdomyosarcoma with orbital extension in adults: 2 cases. Plast Reconstr Surg Glob Open 2015;3(6): 1–3.

26. El Sanharawi A, Coulibaly B, Bessede JP, et al. Paranasal sinus rhabdomyosarcoma: a rare tumor of poor prognosis. Eur Ann Otorhinolaryngol Head Neck Dis 2013;130(1):26–9.

27. An SY, An CH, Choi KS, et al. Multiple myeloma presenting as plasmacytoma of the jaws showing prominent bone formation during chemotherapy. Dentomaxillofac Radiol 2013;42(4):20110143.

28. Kamal M, Kaur P, Gupta R, et al. Mandibular plasmacytoma of jaw - A case report. J Clin Diagn Res 2014;8(8):20–1.

29. Baad R, Kapse S, Rathod N, et al. Solitary plasmacytoma of the mandible: a rare entity. J Int Oral Health 2013;5(3):97–101.

30. Witt C, Borges A, Klein K, et al. Radiographic manifestations of multiple myeloma in the mandible: a retrospectic study of 77 patients. J Oral Maxillofac Surg 1997;55(5):450–3.

31. Pulte D, Redaniel M, Brenner H, et al. Recent improvement in survival of patients with multiple myeloma: variation by ethnicity. Leuk Lymphoma 2014;55(5):1083–9.

32. Harnsberger H, Bragg D, Osborn A, et al. Non-Hodgkin's lymphoma of the head & neck: CT evaluation of nodal and extranodal sites. AJR Am J Roentgenol 1987;149(4):785–91.

33. Paes F, Kalkanis D, Sideras P, et al. FDG PET/CT of extranodal involvement in Non-Hodgkin lymphoma and Hodgkin disease. Radiographics 2010;30: 269–91.

Imaging of Radiation- and Medication-Related Osteonecrosis

 CrossMark

Sanjay M. Mallya, BDS, MDS, PhD*, Sotirios Tetradis, DDS, PhD

KEYWORDS

- Osteoradionecrosis • Medication-related osteonecrosis • Osteonecrosis • Radiation therapy
- Antiresorptive medication

KEY POINTS

- Osteonecrosis of the jaws is a consequence of prior radiation therapy or certain antiresorptive medications.
- The diagnosis of osteonecrosis is made clinically, based on the presence of devitalized exposed bone.
- Radiologic imaging, often with CT, is essential in identifying risk modulators, defining disease extent, and the assessing impact of the disease on adjacent structures to guide management.
- Imaging appearances of osteoradionecrosis and medication-related osteonecrosis encompass a broad spectrum, ranging from lytic to mixed to sclerotic osseous changes.

INTRODUCTION

Bone is a specialized connective tissue that provides structural support and a microenvironment that facilitates several physiologic functions, including production of red and white blood cells, and calcium homeostasis. The cellular elements of bone include osteoblasts (bone forming), osteoclasts (bone resorbing), and osteocytes. The dynamic nature of bone is manifested in its constant structural adaptation to mechanical forces, local disease, and systemic hormonal influence. Continual turnover of bone is a net result of a regulated balance between osteoblastic and osteoclastic activity. External insults, such as therapeutic ionizing radiation, and pharmacologic interventions, such as antiresorptive agents, often disrupt this balance. In the jaws, such altered bone homeostasis is further complicated by the oral cavity environment and the presence of

teeth—the inflammatory diseases of teeth (dental caries, periodontal disease), and traumatic disruptions of the oral mucosa serve as portals of infection and subsequent bone inflammation, increasing the risk for pathologic consequences of osteoradionecrosis (ORN) or medication-related osteonecrosis (MRON). Both of these conditions have debilitating effects on the integrity of the jaw bone with structural and functional consequences that significantly impair the quality of life.

The term osteonecrosis broadly refers to devitalization of bone and consequent lytic changes. At some sites, such as the femoral head, osteonecrosis is often a consequence of altered vascular supply leading to avascular (aseptic) necrosis. Although altered perfusion may partly contribute to their pathogeneses, it is important to recognize that ORN and MRON are considered discrete entities that differ from such areas of avascular necrosis. Moreover, despite the

Disclosure: Dr S. Tetradis has served as a consultant from Amgen. This work was supported by grant support from the NIH/NIDCRDE019465 (ST).
Section of Oral and Maxillofacial Radiology, School of Dentistry, University of California Los Angeles, 10833 Le Conte Avenue, Los Angeles, CA 90095-1668, USA
* Corresponding author.
E-mail address: smallya@ucla.edu

Radiol Clin N Am 56 (2018) 77–89
http://dx.doi.org/10.1016/j.rcl.2017.08.006

similarities in their therapy-related causation, ORN and MRON are separate entities, characterized by distinctive but frequently overlapping clinical and radiographic manifestations, and are managed by different therapeutic approaches.

OSTEORADIONECROSIS
Definition

ORN is a late complication of radiation therapy and occurs when an area of irradiated bone becomes devitalized. ORN is defined as an area of exposed irradiated bone tissue that fails to heal over a period of 3 months, without residual or recurrent tumor; and when other causes of osteonecrosis have been excluded.[1] There is now increasing recognition that such necrotic changes could occur in the bone even before mucosal breakdown is clinically evident, emphasizing the importance of imaging in the diagnostic workup of this condition.

Pathogenesis, Epidemiology, and Risk Factors

The pathogenesis of ORN is not understood completely. Initial theories proposed that mucosal trauma allowed for bacterial entry and subsequent osteomyelitis.[2] There is now evidence that microbes are contaminants, and do not have a causal role in ORN.[1] A widely accepted model is that radiation-induced microvascular changes create a state of hypoxia, hypovascularity, and hypocellularity, thereby disturbing normal bone homeostasis, and leading to a chronic, nonhealing wound.[1] Recent data emphasize the potential role of radiation-induced fibrosis to ORN development—where radiation-induced cell damage triggers a cascade of chronic inflammation and deregulated fibroblastic activity around the blood vessel walls, exacerbating a chronic fibrotic response in both the bone and the overlying mucosa.[3]

ORN can develop anytime after radiation therapy, and typically manifests 6 to 12 months after radiation treatment. However, the time to onset is variable, ranging from months to years. The incidence of ORN with current therapeutic delivery systems is approximately 5% to 7%, and is similar with conventional radiotherapy, intensity-modulated radiation therapy, and brachytherapy.[4] ORN occurs more frequent in the mandible than the maxilla, and is thought to reflect the relatively lower vascularity in the mandible. Furthermore, the mandible is more often in the path of radiation delivery. Although rare, maxillary osteonecrosis may develop, and most often occurs secondary to irradiation for nasopharyngeal cancer.

ORN risk is modulated by several factors (**Box 1**). An important primary determinant is the total radiation dose—ORN is unlikely to occur

Box 1
Factors that increase osteoradionecrosis risk

- Total radiation dose, greater than 60 Gy
- Proximity of neoplasm to bone
- Larger size of the therapeutic field
- Concomitant chemotherapy
- Poor oral hygiene
- Smoking
- Alcohol abuse
- Dental extractions and other surgical manipulations of the irradiated area
- Trauma from dentures and dental appliances

when the delivered radiation dose is less than 60 Gy, and is rare when the dose is less than 50 Gy. At doses above 66 Gy, ORN risk is increased 11-fold. Besides dose, ORN risk is modulated by other aspects of the radiation delivery protocol, including field size, concomitant chemotherapy, and proximity of the neoplastic lesion to bone. Notably, contemporary approaches to deliver radiation, such as intensity-modulated radiation therapy, offer the advantage of limiting "hot-spots" of high radiation dose deposition in the jaw. Other crucial modifiers of ORN modifier of ORN risk are the presence of carious teeth or periodontal disease, or trauma from dental extractions, and from ill-fitting dentures.

Clinical Manifestations and Disease Staging

ORN manifests as exposed bone in an area of prior therapeutic irradiation that fails to heal over a period of 3 months, without residual or recurrent tumor; and when other causes of osteonecrosis have been excluded. The presenting symptoms are nonspecific and vary from pain, often neuropathic in nature, paresthesia along the course of the inferior alveolar nerve, trismus, bad breath, and formation of fistulas, often with purulent discharge. Notably, ORN-related symptoms can develop even several years after radiation treatment. ORN is often precipitated by an injury, for example, tooth extraction, or by infection from caries or periodontal disease, emphasizing the importance of evaluating these changes in the diagnostic workup of ORN.

Small areas of clinically evident bone exposure may be asymptomatic and remain stable for months, and can be adequately managed by conservative approaches. Often, the region of bone exposure progresses, and is complicated by repeated episodes of superimposed bacterial infection and osteomyelitis. The tissue destruction may result in skin fistulas, and may be severe enough to cause facial disfigurement.

Current staging or scoring systems are based on response to hyperbaric oxygen therapy, the extent of the osseous necrotic changes, and clinical and radiologic parameters.[1,5–9] In the absence of a universally accepted staging system, the system proposed by Store and Boysen[9] is a convenient and effective tool for the diagnostic radiologist to communicate disease status to the referring provider (**Box 2**).

Diagnostic Imaging Objectives and Protocols

The diagnosis of ORN is established based on a positive history of irradiation and exclusion of other causes of necrotic bone exposure. Often, the diagnosis of ORN can be made based on history and clinical findings. ORN management seeks to remove the necrotic tissue, and allow for physiologic repair.

The goals of imaging the patient with suspected or established ORN are listed in **Box 3**. Specifically, imaging seeks to identify potential precipitating causes of ORN, such as dental or periodontal disease. Furthermore, imaging aims to evaluate the extent of ORN, and its impact on the integrity of the bone and vital anatomic boundaries.

Considering that the diagnostic assessments are almost all related to hard tissue alterations, conventional radiography and CT are the preferred imaging modalities. Typically, the initial radiographic examinations include conventional dental

---

Box 2
Store and Boysen's classification of osteoradionecrosis

Stage	Criteria
0	Mucosal defects only
I	Radiologic evidence of necrotic bone with intact mucosa
II	Positive radiographic findings with denuded bone intraorally
III	Clinically exposed radionecrotic bone, verified by imaging, skin fistulas, and infection

From Store G, Boysen M. Mandibular osteoradionecrosis: clinical behaviour and diagnostic aspects. Clin Otolaryngol Allied Sci 2000;25(5):378; with permission.

Box 3
Objectives of imaging for suspected or established osteoradionecrosis

- Evaluate teeth and periodontal structures for potential sources of inflammation.
- Detect radiographic bone lysis before clinical bone exposure.
- Detect presence and define extent of lytic bone changes.
- Detect cortical destruction in the jaw.
- Detect periosteal bone formation.
- Evaluate mandibular bone integrity and assess the risk for pathologic fracture.
- Evaluate the integrity of the mandibular canal.
- Evaluate the integrity of the nasal cavity and maxillary sinus.
- Rule out the presence of recurrent malignancy.

---

and panoramic radiographs to provide detailed evaluation of the teeth, periodontal ligament, and surrounding alveolar bone. If clinical bone exposure is detected, or when lytic changes are detected on conventional imaging, multiplanar imaging is indicated to better assess the severity of bone loss and its impact on the adjacent structures, and is accomplished by either cone-beam CT (CBCT) or multidetector CT (MDCT) imaging.

Depending on the extent of the bone changes, limited to medium field of view CBCT is usually adequate. Given the marked variation of the jaw bone trabecular density and architecture, the clinically unaffected contralateral side must be included in the examination for comparison. When assessment of the adjacent soft tissue is indicated, MDCT imaging should be selected. The imaged MDCT volume must encompass the maxillofacial region, starting at the frontal sinuses and extending through the mandible, with axial reconstructions parallel to the dental occlusal plane, using both soft tissue and bone algorithms. Reformations in the coronal and sagittal planes are useful to better depict the effects on the mandibular canal and sinus borders.

Radiographic Appearances of Osteoradionecrosis

Patients with prior irradiation of the head and neck are typically monitored periodically for ORN development. Often, the presenting symptoms may be nonspecific in nature, with no clinically evident bone exposure, and in these cases imaging is an important component to detect early, and frequently, preclinical ORN. When bone exposure is evident, and the clinical presentation is consistent with ORN, imaging is warranted to assess the extent of the disease and its impact on the surrounding vital structures, and on the integrity of the jaw.

Typically, the first line of diagnostic imaging of the patient with suspect ORN is accomplished with dental periapical and panoramic radiography. These techniques are readily available, relatively inexpensive and convenient, and deliver a minimal radiation dose to the patient.[10] Initial changes of ORN are manifested as subtle areas of altered trabecular architecture and rarefaction. Given that dental infection is often a precipitating factor in ORN development, the teeth should be examined closely for signs of caries, and periodontal and periapical inflammations (**Fig. 1**A). Notably,

widening of the periodontal ligament space along the mandibular tooth roots is a common finding in the irradiated mandible,[11] and in the absence of adjacent bone destruction, it requires no management. As the disease progresses, frank lytic bone destruction becomes radiographically evident, and produces a patchy radiolucent appearance with radiodense islands of necrotic bone, or sequestrum, contrasted against the radiolucent lytic changes (see **Fig. 1**B). The extent of bone destruction may be severe enough to compromise the integrity of the mandible and lead to a pathologic fracture. It is important to recognize that the radiographic manifestation of ORN is not specific, and must be differentiated from other causes of bone necrosis, osteomyelitis, and recurrent malignancy.

Although panoramic radiography is appropriate as the initial radiographic evaluation of the ORN

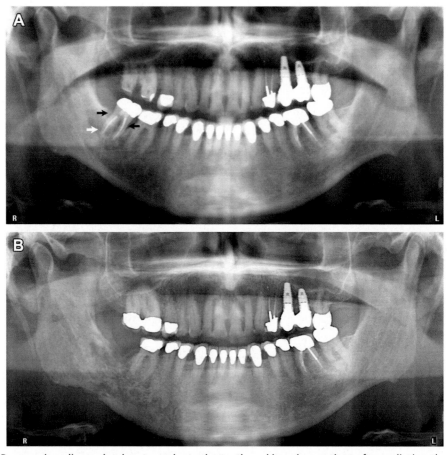

Fig. 1. (*A*) Panoramic radiograph taken to evaluate the teeth and jaws in a patient after radiation therapy shows presence of periodontal bone loss around the mandibular second molar (*black arrows*). A periapical radiolucency is present at the distal root of the tooth (*white arrowhead*), suggestive of local microbial infection and inflammation, and potentially early osteoradionecrosis. (*B*) Panoramic radiograph of same patient taken 2 years later shows extensive patchy and irregular lytic changes in the right posterior mandible extending to partly destroy the cortical borders of the mandibular canal, and the inferior mandibular cortex.

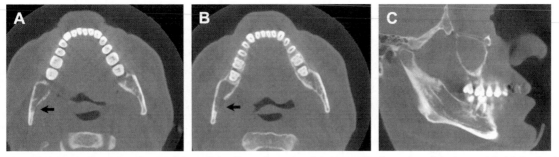

Fig. 2. (*A, B*) Axial sections show erosion of the lingual cortex of the mandibular ramus (*black arrows*). (*C*) Sagittal section shows lytic lesions in the mandibular body with loss of mandibular canal cortication.

patient, it is limited by its 2-dimensional nature, and often underestimates the extent of the osseous changes, relative to CT.[12] Thus, when the clinical suspicion is high, and panoramic radiography is inconclusive, CT is the imaging modality of choice. Indeed, CT imaging better depicts cortical destruction, central necrosis, and sequestration and, in general, provides a better assessment of the extent and impact of the bony changes (**Figs. 2–4**).[12] Both CBCT and MDCT are adequate to provide information on osseous changes. CBCT, especially when performed with

limited field of view protocols, provides high-resolution imaging of the teeth and periodontal structures, and is more sensitive than conventional 2-dimensional imaging for detection of dental disease.[13] However, the contrast resolution of CBCT is inadequate to provide detailed assessment of soft tissue changes. Certain clinical situations dictate the need for soft tissue imaging, including superimposed osteomyelitis and cellulitis, or a soft tissue mass that may represent recurrent malignancy. In such scenarios, contrast-enhanced MDCT imaging should be the modality of choice.

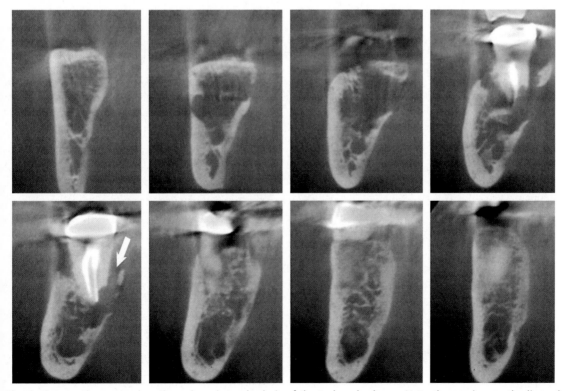

Fig. 3. Consecutive coronal sections show irregular lysis of the trabecular bone. Note the erosion on the lingual cortex. A troughlike defect is noted along the root surface and with partial sequestration of bone of the lingual plate (*arrow*).

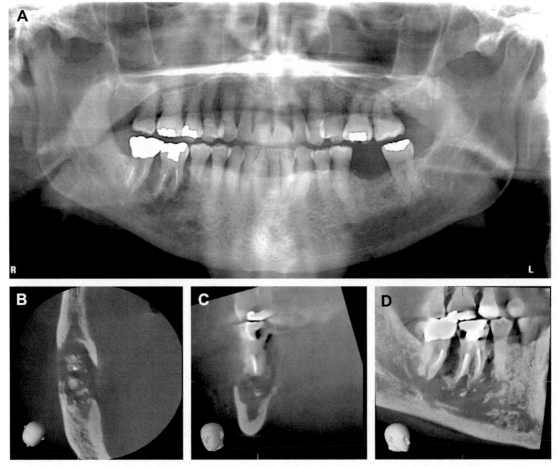

Fig. 4. (*A*) Panoramic radiograph of a patient with clinically evident bone exposure in the mandibular right molar region shows irregular lysis around the mandibular first molar. (*B, C*) Axial and coronal sections show extensive cortical erosion on the buccal and lingual plates, with small bony sequestrae. (*D*) Sagittal section shows extent of the lesion inferiorly to the mandibular cortex and ablation of the mandibular canal cortex.

MR imaging can depict early ORN-induced changes in the bone marrow, before its clinical manifestation. This entity is detected as a reduced intensity of the bone marrow signal on T1-weighted MR imaging, and as an increase in bone marrow signal intensity, on T2-weighted images.[14,15] MR imaging also depicts cortical erosions and changes in the adjacent soft-tissues.[14,15] However, because most of the diagnostic objectives are met with CBCT or MDCT imaging, application of MR imaging to the routine ORN diagnostic workup has been limited.

MEDICATION-RELATED OSTEONECROSIS OF THE JAWS
Definition

Medication-related osteonecrosis of the jaws (MRONJ) is osteonecrosis that develops in association with antiresorptive or antiangiogenic therapy.[16] Antiresorptive therapies are used to manage skeletal-related events associated with bone metastases (such as from the breast, prostate, and lung cancers), and the lytic lesions of multiple myeloma. In addition, antiresorptive agents are used to decrease fracture risk in patients with osteoporosis or to manage other bone diseases, such as Paget's disease and fibrous dysplasia of McCune-Albright syndrome. As with ORN, these necrotic lesions typically manifest as areas of nonhealing, exposed bone. To clarify its difference from other causes of exposed bone, the American Academy of Oral and Maxillofacial Surgery has developed specific diagnostic criteria, as detailed in **Box 4**.[16]

Pathogenesis, Epidemiology, and Risk Factors

The most recognized risk factor for MRONJ development is prior antiresorptive therapy, either with bisphosphonates or the RANK-ligand inhibitor, denosumab. Other antiangiogenic drugs have been implicated, but MRONJ results less frequently with them. The risk of developing MRONJ is primarily dependent on the indication for its use. In cancer patients, treatment with the bisphosphonate, zolendronate, or with the RANK-ligand inhibitor denosumab increases the risk of MRONJ by 50- to 100-fold, relative to cancer patients treated with placebo. Contemporary estimates for MRONJ development after zolendronate therapy range from 0.7% to 6.7%.[16] Likewise, the risk with denosumab therapy ranges from 0.7% to 1.9%.[16] In contrast with cancer patients, the risk for developing MRONJ among patients with osteoporosis after either denosumab or zolendronate therapy is considerably lower, and ranges from 0.001% to 0.010%.[17] This reflects an MRONJ risk that is more than 100 times lower than that in cancer patients, and emphasizes that MRONJ development correlates with the total antiresorptive dose.

The pathophysiology of MRONJ remains to be fully elucidated. Its association with antiresorptive medications suggests a central role of osteoclastic inhibition that leads to an imbalance in bone turnover. An altered immune response, inhibition of angiogenesis, increased risk for infection, and direct toxicity of antiresorptive medications on soft and hard tissues of the oral cavity have also been proposed to underlie disease pathogenesis. Like ORN, local inflammation and surgical trauma are thought to precipitate the development of MRONJ.[16,17]

Clinical Manifestations and Disease Staging

To facilitate disease stratification, the American Academy of Oral and Maxillofacial Surgery has defined criteria for staging of preclinical and clinical MRONJ. This staging system (**Table 1**) is also used to direct appropriate medical, conservative, and radical surgical intervention, and thus provides the radiologist with a clinically relevant tool to communicate disease severity and complications to the referring clinician.

Table 1
Staging of medication-related osteonecrosis of the jaws

Stage	Exposed or Necrotic Bone	History and Clinical Findings
At risk	No clinical evidence	
Stage 0	No clinical evidence	Nonspecific clinical and radiographic findings
Stage 1	Exposed and necrotic bone, or fistulae that probes to bone	Asymptomatic with no evidence of infection
Stage 2	Exposed and necrotic bone, or fistulae that probes to bone	Associated with infection, Pain and erythema in the region of the exposed bone with or without purulent drainage
Stage 3	Exposed and necrotic bone, or fistulae that probes to bone	Pain, infection, and ≥1 of the following: • Exposed, necrotic bone extending beyond the region of alveolar bone resulting in pathologic fracture • Extraoral fistula, oroantral or oronasal communication • Lytic changes that extend to the inferior border of the mandible or sinus floor

Adapted from Ruggiero SL, Dodson TB, Fantasia J, et al. American Association of Oral and Maxillofacial Surgeons position paper on medication-related osteonecrosis of the jaw–2014 update. J Oral Maxillofac Surg 2014;72(10):1938–56.

Diagnostic Objectives of Imaging

The diagnosis of MRONJ is essentially based on historical and clinical data. Imaging is an important component of the overall workup to monitor and manage patients at risk for MRONJ, or with established MRONJ. Specifically, imaging seeks to identify precipitating factors such as dental or periodontal disease. Furthermore, imaging aims to evaluate the extent of MRONJ to facilitate its staging and subsequent management.

As with ORN, most the diagnostic tasks evaluate hard tissue alterations, and conventional radiography and CT are adequate in most patients with suspect or established MRONJ. Initial radiographic examinations include conventional dental and panoramic radiographs that serve to detect dental disease and screen at-risk patients. CBCT and MDCT protocols are identical to those as described for ORN.

Imaging of the Patients at Risk, or with Suspect or Established Medication-Related Osteonecrosis of the Jaws

Patients being managed for osteoporosis with antiresorptive therapy are at a much lower risk for MRONJ development.[17] When asymptomatic, they do not require any imaging beyond that directed to evaluating dental and periodontal disease. Such imaging is often accomplished at the dentists' offices with conventional intraoral and panoramic imaging.

High-dose antiresorptive treatment, used to manage skeletal metastases, carries a much higher risk for MRONJ development. Patients on these treatment regimens benefit from regular dental examinations, including clinical evaluation, intraoral and panoramic radiographs as appropriate, and limited to medium field of view CBCT imaging that encompasses the entire jaw being imaged for comparison purposes, and is often useful in identifying potential dental disease, that increase the risk for MRONJ (Fig. 5). Imaging of these asymptomatic patients provides a baseline to monitor future subtle changes that may permit early detection of necrotic bone changes. When clinical changes suggest establishment of MRONJ (stages 1–3), imaging is indicated to assess the extent of the changes, and the potential for complications such as pathologic fracture or disruption of the nasal cavity and maxillary sinus (Fig. 6). Although MR imaging has the potential to contribute to early preclinical detection of disease, its use for the care of the MRONJ patient is limited.

Spectrum of Radiologic Appearances of Medication-related Osteonecrosis of the Jaws

Initial panoramic and intraoral radiographs are essential to provide an overall assessment of the dental arches. Frank necrotic changes may be visualized, although their extent is likely less than the true lesion (see Fig. 6). As described, panoramic radiography is limited by its 2-dimensional nature, and may underestimate the presence or

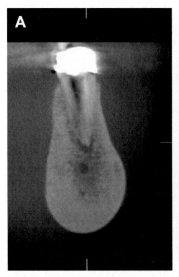
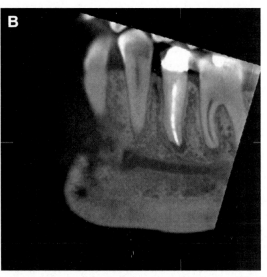

Fig. 5. (A, B) Coronal and sagittal cone-beam computed tomography sections through the mandibular premolar show intense sclerosis that alters the trabecular pattern of the mandibular body, and widening of the apical periodontal ligament, indicating potential residual odontogenic inflammation.

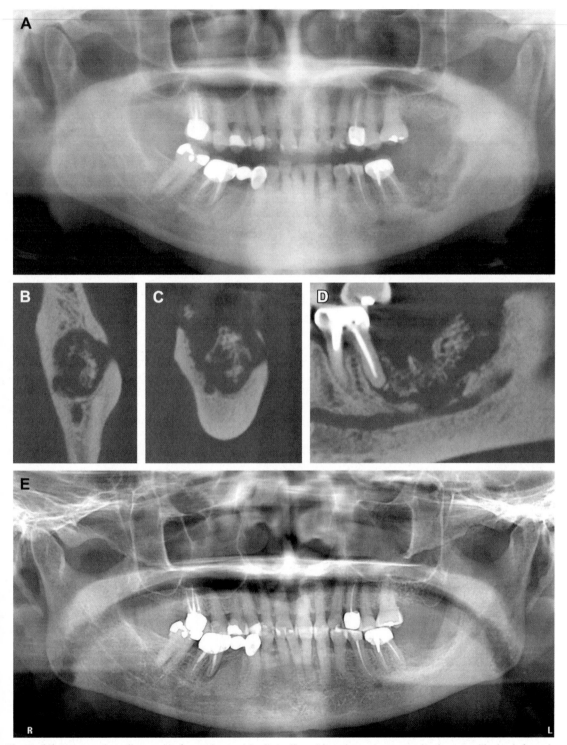

Fig. 6. (*A*) Panoramic radiograph of a patient with clinically evident bone exposure in the mandibular left molar region shows irregular bone destruction that extends into the ascending ramus, and inferiorly to the mandibular canal. (*B–D*) Axial, coronal, and sagittal sections demonstrate marked cortical erosion on the buccal and lingual plates, with multiple small bony sequestrate, and loss of the cortication of the mandibular canal. Note the extent of the lesion inferiorly to the mandibular cortex and ablation of the mandibular canal cortex. (*E*) Panoramic radiograph taken 2 years after conservative management shows osseous healing at the previously necrotic site in the left mandibular molar and retromolar region.

extent of necrosis. Ambiguous results on this imaging should trigger more advanced imaging, with CT, either CBCT or MDCT. However, in certain clinical situations the radiologist should anticipate the need for soft tissue imaging, in which case contrast-enhanced MDCT imaging or MR imaging is the imaging modality of choice.

Radiographic changes include lytic and sclerotic changes. Lytic changes are apparent as initially as areas of altered trabecular architecture and density that progress to frank, patchy radiolucent bone destruction with cortical erosion and marked bone destruction. The lytic changes may extend to disrupt anatomic boundaries of the maxillary sinus and nasal cavity, neurovascular canals, and the cortical boundaries of the mandible with consequent pathologic fracture. Nonhealing extraction sockets or surgical defects should be identified. Of note, lytic and sclerotic changes are often seen even in the absence of frank bone exposure, emphasizing the need to consider the clinical and radiographic data for appropriate staging of the disease. Notably, recognition of stage 0 MRONJ is particularly important—50% of patients with stage 0 disease progress to more advanced MRONJ disease.[18,19]

Sclerotic changes in MRONJ manifest as localized to widespread diffuse osteosclerosis. These changes may be marked and involve the entire height of the mandibular body (**Fig. 7**). Often, the sclerotic changes are accompanied by periosteal bone formation, and this can be exuberant and cause anatomic expansion of the mandible (**Fig. 8**). As the necrotic changes progress and coalesce, they isolate islands of necrotic bone sequestra.

Although the radiographic appearance of ORN and MRONJ can overlap, in general the prominent osteoclastic activation and attenuation of osteoblastic function during ORN result in a rarefying appearance with loss of cortical outlines and trabecular density. In contrast, osteoclastic inhibition in MRONJ produces an overall increased trabecular and cortical density with frequent pronounced periosteal bone formation.

Lytic lesions of MRONJ must be differentiated from recurrent malignancy, or metastatic lesions in the jaw. Both MRONJ and malignancy have similar destructive appearances, often with periosteal bone formation. The periosteal new bone formation in MRONJ is regular, typically paralleling the existing cortex. In contrast, periosteal bone formation in metastatic malignancies is more often disorganized, with radiating spicules of new bone that are perpendicular to the existing cortex. Given that a large subset of patients with MRONJ are managed for metastatic bone disease, this distinction is particularly important (**Fig. 9**). Finally, these patients may receive periodic PET with fludeoxyglucose F 18/CT examinations (**Fig. 10**) and interval analyses on the bony changes may provide important information of the nature of the MRONJ lesion.

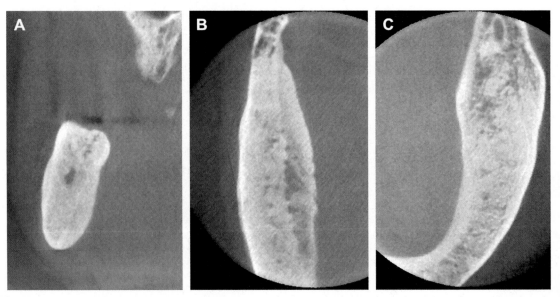

Fig. 7. (*A–C*) Cone-beam computed tomography sections demonstrate marked alteration of normal trabecular pattern with intense sclerosis and effacement of the trabecular pattern.

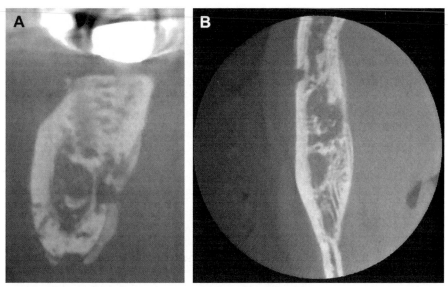

Fig. 8. (A, B) Cone-beam computed tomography sections demonstrate patchy bony destruction, cortical erosion, and periosteal bone formation. Note the layers of periosteal bone that are parallel to the cortical plate.

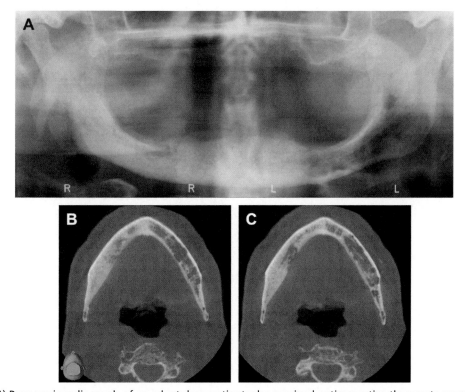

Fig. 9. (A) Panoramic radiograph of an edentulous patient who received antiresorptive therapy to manage bone lesions of multiple myeloma shows intense sclerosis that extends through the right mandibular body. Patchy lytic lesions with endosteal cortical erosion are present in the left mandibular body, and likely represent bony lesions of multiple myeloma. (B, C) Axial cone-beam computed tomography sections demonstrate the extent of the sclerotic changes that characterize antiresorptive therapy, and the lytic changes of multiple myeloma.

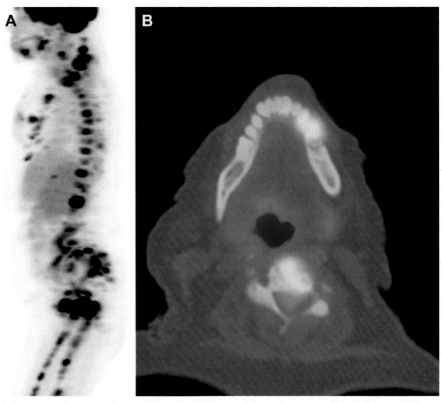

Fig. 10. (A) Full body PET with fludeoxyglucose F 18 imaging to evaluate a patient with multiple metastases to the bone and pleura shows 2 areas of increased uptake in the jaws. (B) Axial fused PET-computed tomography image shows the area of increased uptake in the mandibular body. Note also the increased uptake in the cervical vertebra.

SUMMARY

ORN and MRONJ are 2 distinct entities with different etiologies. Although they share some radiographic features, understanding their pathogenesis and their radiographic subtleties as well as obtaining a good patient history should facilitate diagnosis and differentiation from other similar appearing entities, such as osteomyelitis.

REFERENCES

1. Marx RE. Osteoradionecrosis: a new concept of its pathophysiology. J Oral Maxillofac Surg 1983; 41(5):283–8.
2. Meyer I. Infectious diseases of the jaws. J Oral Surg 1970;28(1):17–26.
3. Delanian S, Lefaix JL. The radiation-induced fibroatrophic process: therapeutic perspective via the antioxidant pathway. Radiother Oncol 2004;73(2):119–31.
4. Peterson DE, Doerr W, Hovan A, et al. Osteoradionecrosis in cancer patients: the evidence base for treatment-dependent frequency, current management strategies, and future studies. Support Care Cancer 2010;18(8):1089–98.
5. Glanzmann C, Gratz KW. Radionecrosis of the mandibula: a retrospective analysis of the incidence and risk factors. Radiother Oncol 1995;36(2):94–100.
6. Epstein JB, Wong FL, Stevenson-Moore P. Osteoradionecrosis: clinical experience and a proposal for classification. J Oral Maxillofac Surg 1987;45(2): 104–10.
7. Notani K, Yamazaki Y, Kitada H, et al. Management of mandibular osteoradionecrosis corresponding to the severity of osteoradionecrosis and the method of radiotherapy. Head Neck 2003;25(3):181–6.
8. Schwartz HC, Kagan AR. Osteoradionecrosis of the mandible: scientific basis for clinical staging. Am J Clin Oncol 2002;25(2):168–71.
9. Store G, Boysen M. Mandibular osteoradionecrosis: clinical behaviour and diagnostic aspects. Clin Otolaryngol Allied Sci 2000;25(5):378–84.
10. White SC, Mallya SM. Update on the biological effects of ionizing radiation, relative dose factors and radiation hygiene. Aust Dent J 2012;57(Suppl 1):2–8.
11. Chan KC, Perschbacher SE, Lam EW, et al. Mandibular changes on panoramic imaging after head and neck radiotherapy. Oral Surg Oral Med Oral Pathol Oral Radiol 2016;121(6):666–72.

12. Store G, Larheim TA. Mandibular osteoradionecrosis: a comparison of computed tomography with panoramic radiography. Dentomaxillofac Radiol 1999;28(5):295–300.

13. Fayad MI, Nair M, Levin MD, et al. AAE and AAOMR joint position statement: use of cone beam computed tomography in endodontics 2015 update. Oral Surg Oral Med Oral Pathol Oral Radiol 2015; 120(4):508–12.

14. Chong J, Hinckley LK, Ginsberg LE. Masticator space abnormalities associated with mandibular osteoradionecrosis: MR and CT findings in five patients. AJNR Am J Neuroradiol 2000;21(1): 175–8.

15. Hermans R. Imaging of mandibular osteoradionecrosis. Neuroimaging Clin N Am 2003;13(3): 597–604.

16. Ruggiero SL, Dodson TB, Fantasia J, et al. American Association of Oral and Maxillofacial Surgeons position paper on medication-related osteonecrosis of the jaw–2014 update. J Oral Maxillofac Surg 2014; 72(10):1938–56.

17. Khan AA, Morrison A, Hanley DA, et al. Diagnosis and management of osteonecrosis of the jaw: a systematic review and international consensus. J Bone Miner Res 2015;30(1):3–23.

18. Bedogni A, Fusco V, Agrillo A, et al. Learning from experience. Proposal of a refined definition and staging system for bisphosphonate-related osteonecrosis of the jaw (BRONJ). Oral Dis 2012;18(6):621–3.

19. O'Ryan FS, Khoury S, Liao W, et al. Intravenous bisphosphonate-related osteonecrosis of the jaw: bone scintigraphy as an early indicator. J Oral Maxillofac Surg 2009;67(7):1363–72.

Fibro-Osseous and Other Lesions of Bone in the Jaws

Mansur Ahmad, BDS, PhD*, Laurence Gaalaas, DDS, MS

KEYWORDS

- Fibro-osseous lesions • Periapical osseous dysplasia • Cherubism • Paget disease
- Central giant cell granuloma • Fibrous dysplasia

KEY POINTS

- Fibro-osseous lesions in the jaws are a group of similar-appearing conditions. Some of these conditions are quite common in the jaws; others are rare.
- Fibro-osseous lesion pathophysiology varies widely from simple dysplasia to reactive lesions to formal neoplasms. Management of these conditions can range from monitoring to jaw resection.
- The histopathologic features of fibro-osseous lesions can be similar. Therefore, imaging findings are crucial to arrive at a definitive diagnosis.
- Clinical information, for example, age, gender, and race of the patient, are important factors that help in arriving at a diagnosis of similar-appearing fibro-osseous lesions.

INTRODUCTION

Fibro-osseous lesions and other lesions of the bone in the jaws are a group of similar-appearing conditions[1,2] that can be confusing to the radiologist whose primary focus is pathology other than in the jaws. Some conditions are quite common; others are rare. Furthermore, lesion pathophysiology varies widely from simple dysplasia to reactive lesions to formal neoplasms. This mix of etiology dictates that management can range from monitoring with the contraindication of biopsy to cosmetic surgical revision to systemic management with medications to exploratory surgical "diagnosis" to full resection. Like imaging findings, the histopathologic appearance of these altered tissues is in many cases similar appearing as well[3] and, accordingly, imaging findings are heavily relied on to make a definitive diagnosis. As oral and maxillofacial radiologists, our experience focusing on pathology of the jaws and face have taught us to recognize the key imaging findings and patient demographics linked to these conditions. It is our goal to articulate these features in a manner that will not only help any radiologist or clinician arrive at the correct radiographic diagnosis, but recognize when the radiographic diagnosis may fully dictate the definitive diagnosis and, ultimately, direct the patient toward correct management, be it aggressive surgery or simple monitoring.

FIBRO-OSSEOUS LESIONS
Periapical Osseous Dysplasia

As the name indicates, periapical osseous dysplasia (POD) is typically found in the periapical regions of the jaws, most commonly in the mandibular arch. In previous literature, this condition has been named as periapical cemental dysplasia, periapical cementoosseous dysplasia, periapical cementoma, or periapical fibrous dysplasia. Currently, the preference is to use the

Disclosure Statement: The authors have nothing to disclose.
Department of Diagnostic and Biological Sciences, University of Minnesota School of Dentistry, Minneapolis, MN 55455, USA
* Corresponding author.
E-mail address: ahmad005@umn.edu

Radiol Clin N Am 56 (2018) 91–104
http://dx.doi.org/10.1016/j.rcl.2017.08.007

radiologic.theclinics.com

term POD, because there is no conclusive evidence of the presence of cementum-like tissues in the dysplasia.[4] This condition has histologic features of abnormal and disorganized production of bone. Typically, the histologic features are composed of cellular mesenchymal tissues and collagen fibers in a bed of woven bone, laminar bone and cementum-like entities.[5] The ratio of these components varies as the lesion matures through the 3 radiographic stages: (1) completely radiolucent stage, (2) mixed radiolucent and radiopaque stage, and (3) densely radiopaque stage with a thinned radiolucent rim.[6]

Patient demographics

POD has classic demographic representation.[7,8] A typical patient with POD is a middle-aged black woman. Typical age is around 40 years. Females are about 9 times more likely to have POD compared with males. Blacks are about 3 times more likely than whites are. The occurrence of this condition is rare in patients under the age of 20 years. Usually, there are no signs or symptoms associated with the teeth. The condition is frequently identified on radiographs acquired for other clinical reasons.

Imaging features

Classical radiographic features of the early stage of this condition is a low-density area around the apices of mandibular anterior teeth, very similar in appearance to a routine periapical cyst or granuloma associated with an infected tooth (**Fig. 1**). Usually, the teeth are noncarious, without any restorations, and without any endodontic (root canal) treatment. A dental clinical examination could often reveal the pulp tissues of the involved teeth to be vital, without evidence of infection or necrosis. Despite the clinical tests revealing the tooth as being vital, such a tooth may be erroneously treated endodontically, and therefore may contain evidence of endodontic fillings.[9] The border of the lesion is often well-defined, and can have uneven corticated margins. The surrounding bone may display increased trabecular density. At an early stage, the lesion is usually oval or circular. As the condition enlarges, the shape often becomes irregular, but mostly remains limited to the region of the root apices. The internal content of the lesion changes as the condition progresses. At the early stage, the lesion is uniformly radiolucent, mimicking an inflammatory lesion of pulpal origin. In the second stage, mostly homogeneous radiopacity with irregular margins is seen around the core of this lesion. At the late or mature stage, the lesion is almost completely radiopaque, with homogeneous density, and often has an undulating irregularly thin or sometimes vague radiolucent band, surrounded by an outer corticated margin. The adjacent teeth are not displaced. The roots of the adjacent teeth are often not resorbed. Larger lesions may on occasion cause thinning and expansion of the cortical plates, mostly in the buccal orientation.

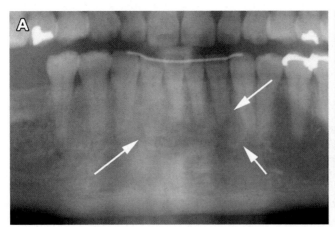 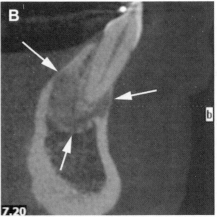

Fig. 1. (A) Cropped panoramic radiograph of a 40-year-old African American female patient shows mixed density lesions (*arrows*) in the periapical region of the anterior mandibular teeth consistent with periapical osseous dysplasia, stage III. The lesions are difficult to visualize because of superimposition of the blurred spine image over the anterior jaws. (B) Sagittal cone-beam computed tomography sections of the mandibular anterior region demonstrate mixed density lesions (*arrows*) with preservation of peripheral lucent rims of variable thickness and definition. Portions of the buccal and lingual cortical plates are thinned. A secondarily infected lesion may demonstrate increased width and definition of the peripheral lucent band, but not to the extent of secondary idiopathic or simple bone cavity formation. In this case, cross-sectional imaging greatly aids visualization of the lesions and subsequent diagnosis.

There are several variations of POD. The lesions limited to a few teeth are termed focal POD. Widespread involvement of the jaws, occupying 3 or 4 jaw quadrants, is termed florid osseous dysplasia[10,11] (**Fig. 2**). When the lesion is limited to only 1 jaw, the mandible is more likely to be involved than the maxilla. Large florid lesions can displace the mandibular alveolar canal or floor of the maxillary sinus. In the late stages of some lesions, idiopathic bone cavities form with florid osseous dysplasia. In such cases, the homogeneous radiopacities are surrounded by wide areas of well-defined radiolucency with noncorticated or thinly corticated borders. Lesions or portions of lesions that become secondarily infected many times demonstrate thickening and increased definition of the outer radiolucent band surrounding the internal calcification that can act as a "nidus" of sequestra.[12,13] In these cases of secondary infection, the thickening of the radiolucent band does not typically reach the extent of the secondary idiopathic bone cavities.

Management
Diagnosis of POD or its variants is achieved by clinical and radiographic findings. Histopathologic examination of POD or its variants is not recommended, primarily owing to concern about reduced vascularity of the altered bone and associated secondary infection from any surgical procedures. Furthermore, histopathologic findings may be equivocal for other fibro-osseous lesions, such as fibrous dysplasia and central ossifying fibroma, leading the clinician to reference imaging findings

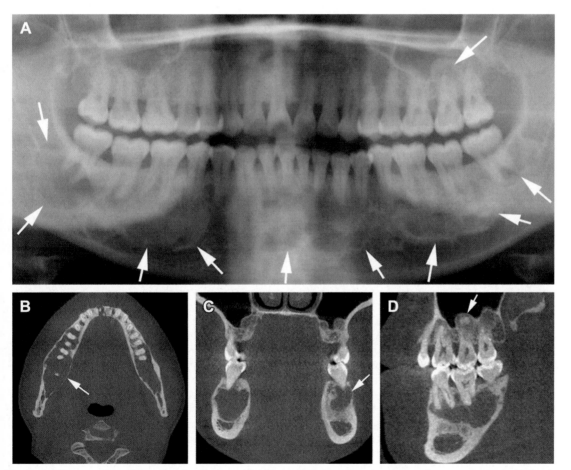

Fig. 2. (*A*) Panoramic radiograph of a 42-year-old African American female patient demonstrates mixed density bony lesions (*arrows*) in the periapical regions of the teeth throughout the mandible and much of the maxilla. The findings are consistent with florid osseous dysplasia, stage III. A larger lucent region in the right posterior mandible indicates secondary idiopathic or simple bone cavity formation. (*B–D*) Axial, coronal, and sagittal cone-beam computed tomography sections of the same patient imaged at a later date revealing extent of florid osseous dysplasia (*arrows*). (*B*) Expansion of the larger lucent areas indicating continued bone cavity formation. Persistent mixed density lesions are visible in the anterior mandible and posterior maxilla periapical regions of teeth.

for definitive diagnosis.[7] POD does not require any treatment, unless the lesions are secondarily infected.[14] The primary complication of POD and its variants is chronic low-grade osteomyelitis when the alveolar bone is exposed owing to biopsy, tooth infection, tooth extraction, or resorption of the alveolar bone owing to pressure from dentures. Ideal management of patients with POD is to maintain excellent oral hygiene to prevent the need for root canal treatment or extraction. Secondary formation of idiopathic bone cavities is typically monitored unless the lesions become very large and create a risk for pathologic bone fracture.

Fibrous Dysplasia

Fibrous dysplasia is a developmental condition with tumorlike behavior, and is often considered a hamartoma. In the bone affected by fibrous dysplasia, the cancellous bone is replaced by a combination of fibrous and abnormal bone. Clinically, fibrous dysplasia may affect only 1 bone (monostotic) or multiple bones (polyostotic).[15]

Patient demographics
A patient affected with polyostotic fibrous dysplasia is usually is child under 10 years age with cutaneous and endocrine disturbances. On completion of skeletal development, the proliferation of fibrous dysplasia becomes slow or static. The proliferation may reinitiate when a patient becomes pregnant or is under hormone therapy, for example, oral contraceptives. The polyostotic form associated with McCune–Albright syndrome is found almost exclusively in females.[16] The monostotic form does not have sexual predilection. Mandibular lesions are mostly monostotic. Maxillary lesions are often polyostotic, involving the adjacent craniofacial bones.

Imaging features
Fibrous dysplasia is most common in the maxilla, and is mostly unilateral.[15] The margin of the lesion is striking: a gradual blending of the lesion to the normal trabecular pattern without signs of cortication. Only in the early stages, there may be a hint of corticated margin.[7,17] Owing to the lack of clear margins, the extent of involvement can be difficult to discern on a radiographic image. The classic radiographic appearance is described as "ground glass," or a grainy appearance of the trabecular bone. In early stages, the lesion is mixed to low density rather than the classical ground glass appearance. Radiographic features have also been described as "orange peel" or "cotton wool" mixed density appearance. Cross-sectional images reveal significant expansion of the cortical outline of the bone (**Fig. 3**). Such expansion is frequently nonconcentric and maintains some normal morphology of the affected bone, unlike the expansion of benign tumors. Adjacent structures, for example, the teeth, sinus floor, orbital floor, or nasal wall are often displaced.[18] Unlike most odontogenic cysts or benign tumors, the mandibular canal may be displaced superiorly.[19] Because this lesion frequently affects younger patients, tooth eruption is commonly impaired. Some radiographic features mimic Paget disease, which is a condition that affects a markedly older population. Fibrous dysplasia has a reputation of appearing especially confusing or even aggressive/malignant on MR images compared with computed tomography or other radiographic findings. On T1-weighted MR imaging, fibrous dysplasia has low to intermediate signals depending on the ratio of fibrous and mineralized contents.[17,20] On T2-weighted images, the fibrous component has bright signal. The signal intensity increases with gadolinium, because the fibrous component is well-vascularized.[20]

Management
The diagnosis of fibrous dysplasia can be attained by clinical and radiographic features. The ground glass appearance and lack of defined margin are often hallmark findings of fibrous dysplasia. Although the appearance may be similar to Paget disease, age of the patient is an exclusion criterion. Histologic findings are similar to Chinese script writing, with a curvilinear trabecular pattern. Histopathologic findings may be equivocal for other fibro-osseous lesions, such as POD and central ossifying fibroma, leading the clinician to reference imaging findings for definitive diagnosis. Small fibrous dysplasia lesions can be surgically resected. Larger lesions, particularly the ones that approach critical structures, may require surgical recontouring to achieve cosmetic benefits. In many patients, the surgery may be postponed until the patient reaches skeletal maturity, and when the growth of fibrous dysplasia ceases. To limit the growth of well-vascularized fibrous dysplasia, radiation therapy has been attempted. However, radiation therapy carries the risk of sarcomatous transformation. Even without radiation therapy, sarcomatous transformations have been detected in a small percentage of patients of craniofacial fibrous dysplasia.[21,22] Especially confusing or aggressive/malignant mixed signal craniofacial bony lesions noted on MR imaging evaluations of patients fitting fibrous dysplasia demographics may be cross-evaluated with computed tomography or other radiographic examinations to confirm the diagnosis.

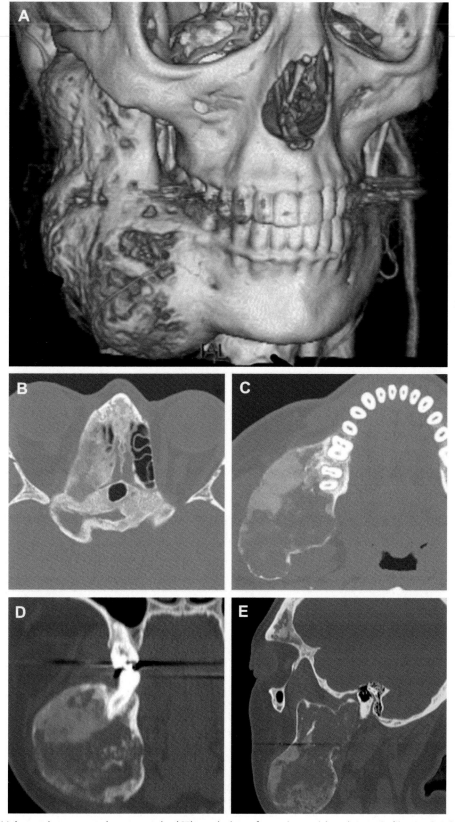

Fig. 3. (*A*) Volumetric computed tomography (CT) rendering of a patient with polyostotic fibrous dysplasia superficially evident in the right mandible. (*B*) Axial CT section demonstrating nonconcentric expansion of the right

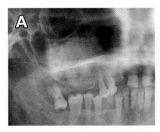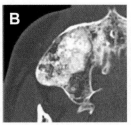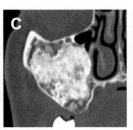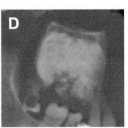

Fig. 4. (*A*) Cropped panoramic radiograph of an ossifying fibroma right maxilla shows mostly concentric expansion and suggestions of a peripheral lucent band surrounding heterogeneous calcification are common to the late stage of the condition. (*B–D*) Axial, coronal, and sagittal cone-beam computed tomography sections showing mostly rounded expansion of the lesion into the right maxillary sinus. A lucent band visible throughout most of the periphery of the lesion surrounding heterogeneous calcification distinguish this neoplasm from a large, collapsing radicular cyst, which would have peripheral thickened calcification and central radiolucency. (*Courtesy of* Phillip Chapman, MD, Birmingham, AL.)

Ossifying Fibroma

Although this lesions has radiographic and histologic features similar to bony dysplasias, this is a true neoplasm of fibro-osseous contents. Unlike a fibrous dysplasia, the margin of the ossifying fibroma is well-defined. Histologically, the tumor contains varying amount of fibrocellular and mineralized tissues. This neoplasm can be classified into 2 broad categories: (1) ossifying fibroma of odontogenic origin (cementoossifying fibroma), and (2) juvenile/aggressive ossifying fibroma, a rare and aggressive tumor.[21]

Patient demographics
Ossifying fibroma affects mostly women in their third and fourth decades of life.[23] The condition primarily seen in patients of Caucasian descent, followed by patients of African descent. The mean age range of juvenile form of ossifying fibroma is 8.5 to 12.0 years, and without any sexual predilection. A variant of the juvenile condition, psammomatoid juvenile ossifying fibroma, is also seen without sexual predilection, but found in an age group of 16 to 33 years.[24]

Imaging features
Ossifying fibromas are often asymptomatic, and discovered on radiographs acquired for other reasons. At the initial stage, the lesion is primarily radiolucent. As the tumor enlarges, the lesion assumes a mixed density appearance. In the late stage, a thin radiolucent soft tissue capsule surrounds the mineralized component.[23] This tumor is exclusive to the jaws, and most commonly found in mandibular posterior region. On the maxillary arch, this may occur in areas anterior to the premolars. Adjacent teeth may show signs of resorption. A few radiographic features help to differentiate this lesion from fibrous dysplasia. Unlike fibrous dysplasia, a thin radiolucent band separates ossifying fibroma from the neighboring bone. The expansion of the cortical plates in ossifying fibroma is mostly concentric, as expected from a benign tumor. Superior displacement of the mandibular canal is not common. In the maxillary arch, the displacement of the maxillary sinus is common, sometimes occupying almost the complete volume of the maxillary sinus (**Fig. 4**). When invading into the maxillary sinus, the ossifying fibroma can appear similar to a large, collapsing radicular cyst associated with a prior infected tooth that has also occupied the sinus. Interestingly, histologic findings can be confused with a collapsing radicular cyst. These lesions have low to high signal intensity on T1-weighted MR imaging.[25] Postgadolinium MR imaging may reveal uniform contrast enhancement for a mixed appearance.[20]

Management
Conservative surgical resection or curettage is the treatment of choice.[26] The presence of a fibrous capsule allows easy removal of the tumor.

portion of the ethmoid bone, sphenoid body, and nasal bones. The right ethmoid air cells have been almost completely remodeled and replaced by grainy-appearing heterogeneous bone. The degree of involvement of the nasal and left portion of the ethmoid bone is not well-appreciated owing to the poorly defined, blending borders of this condition. (*C–E*) Axial, coronal, and sagittal CT sections of the right mandible show expansion that seems to be concentric in the coronal view, but is confirmed otherwise in the axial and sagittal views. Note the variable appearance of the altered trabecular bone from a more uniform radiopaque "ground glass" appearance laterally to a more radiolucent appearance with irregular calcifications medially and superiorly. (*Courtesy of* Phillip Chapman, MD, Birmingham, AL.)

Recurrence of lesions has been reported. Therefore, follow-up imaging is needed to rule out recurrence.[27] Malignant transformation has not been reported. Similar to POD and fibrous dysplasia, histopathologic findings may be equivocal for other fibro-osseous lesions, leading the clinician to reference imaging findings for definitive diagnosis. The characteristic appearance of peripheral calcification (no peripheral lucent rim) at the border of the mixed density, collapsing radicular cyst in the maxillary sinus plus a history of tooth extraction may save a patient unnecessary surgery, despite similar histopathologic findings between these entities.

LESIONS OF BONE
Central Giant Cell Granuloma

Although this lesion appears as a neoplasm, controversy does exist as to whether this is a reactive lesion of unknown stimulus. Therefore, other names, for example, giant cell reparative granuloma or giant cell lesion, have also been used. The feature of "reparative" is not conclusive.

Patient demographics
Central giant cell granuloma (CGCG) is often seen in patients in their first to third decades of life, but has also been seen in patients as old as 80 years of age. This lesion is more common in females. Most of the lesions are seen in mandible, with only about one-third occurring in the maxilla. Typically asymptomatic, the lesion may also be associated with pain or paresthesia. The growth of the lesion is usually slow and without pain. A variant of CGCG grows rapidly, causes pain, and resorbs the roots of the adjacent teeth. These aggressive lesions have a tendency to recur after surgical removal.

Imaging features
Radiographically, CGCG can be a unilocular or multilocular radiolucent defect appearing in the posterior regions of the mandible.[28] In younger patients, the lesion is most frequently in the area anterior to the molars, often crossing the midline of the mandible. In the maxilla, the lesion in younger patient is seen in the anterior area of the jaw. Small lesions are usually unilocular. When the lesion is multilocular, the septa are typically ill-defined and wispy.[4] The margins of the lesion are scalloped, and the wispy septa are almost at right angles to the border (**Fig. 5**). Such orthogonal junction of the septa and the lesion border is a characteristic radiographic finding of CGCG. In larger lesions, irregular expansion of the cortical bone is common and may be massive. These lesions may also cause significant root resorption.[29,30] Displacement of the adjoining teeth is a common radiographic finding. T1-weighted images see CGCG are of homogeneous intermediate signal intensity. Postgadolinium MR imaging can have enhanced contrast intensity.[20]

Management
Surgical resection is usually conservative, with risk of recurrence. Recurrence is usually more common with maxillary lesion.[31] Most of the lesions can be surgically enucleated. Resection of the jaw may be needed. Follow-up imaging is recommended to rule out recurrence. Lesions are occurring after the second decade of life may be related to hyperparathyroidism (brown tumor of hyperparathyroidism). Therefore, older patients should be tested for serum calcium and parathyroid hormone levels.

Aneurysmal Bone Cyst

This expansile osteolytic condition is a reactive lesion of the bone, although it may have radiographic features of an aggressive benign tumor. Histologically, the lesion has poorly calcified woven bone separated by fibrous septa and osteoclast-type giant cells. This vascular-rich lesion is mostly radiolucent.

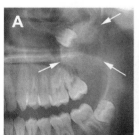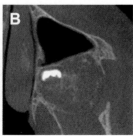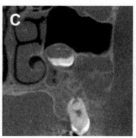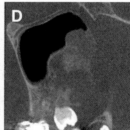

Fig. 5. (A) Cropped panoramic radiograph of a central giant cell granuloma (*arrows*) left posterior maxilla shows that the lesion has displaced the developing third molar tooth superiorly into the maxillary sinus. (*B–D*) Axial, coronal, and sagittal cone-beam computed tomography sections demonstrate irregular expansion into the sinus superiorly and mediolateral irregular expansion of the maxillary alveolus. Note the ill-defined septa that meet the border at right angles. (*Courtesy of* Anita Gohel, BDS, PhD, Columbus, OH.)

Patient demographics

Most patients affected with aneurysmal bone cyst (ABC) are younger than 30 years age, although it may occur at any age.[32] There is no sexual predilection, but females may have slight predominance. The lesion is characterized by rapid buccal growth, with occasional pain and tenderness. The lesion may affect either jaw. The mandible has a higher incidence of ABC, where the lesion has a tendency to be in the posterior segment, including the ramus.[33]

Imaging features

Most ABC lesions are circular and well-defined, consistent with the vascular nature of the lesion. Larger lesions may have evidence of ill-defined wispy septa, similar to the radiographic features of the CGCG (Fig. 6). The orthogonal junction of wispy septa with the cortical bone is also a feature of ABC. Therefore, radiographic features of CGCG and ABC may be identical. On a cross-sectional image, balloonlike expansion of ABC may help in differentiating it from CGCG. Displacement and resorption of teeth are common. Rapid and significant expansion of the bone may also lead to pathologic fracture. T2-weighted MR imaging can be helpful in diagnosis where ABC has a high signal intensity with a fluid level.[20,34]

Management

Because the radiographic features of ABC is identical to CGCG, an aspirational biopsy with hemorrhagic content leads to the diagnosis of ABC.[35] The lesion is usually treated by surgical curettage or enucleation. Extensive surgical resection may also be needed. Recurrence rate is moderate to high after conservative curettage. Owing to the as high as 60% recurrence rate, follow-up imaging is needed.

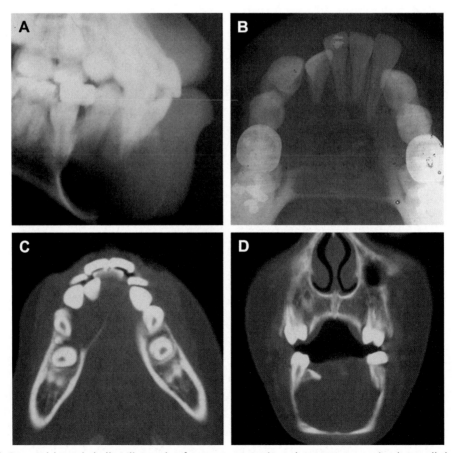

Fig. 6. (A) Cropped lateral skull radiograph of a teen-age patient demonstrates a circular, well-defined, and expansive lesion of the anterior mandible. (B) Mandibular occlusal radiograph shows displacement of the anterior teeth and the presence of faint septa within the lesion. (C) Axial computed tomography (CT) hard tissue section through the mandible shows displacement of the right posterior teeth. (D) Coronal CT soft tissue section through the anterior mandible shows artifact from metallic dental restorative material partially obscures visualization of faint, internal septa. (Courtesy of Brad J. Potter, DDS, MS, Denver, CO.)

Cherubism

Cherubism is a rare, autosomal-dominant developmental condition that causes significant bilateral expansion of the jaws, giving a clinical appearance of round faces of angels or cherubs as portrayed in Renaissance paintings. Most cases are bilateral, often involving both the jaws. Rarely, unilateral lesions have been encountered. Histologically, the lesions of cherubism are identical to giant cell granuloma.

Patient demographics

Cherubism is a disease of childhood that stabilizes or regresses with age. Early lesions have been seen in patients as young as 1 year old. Typically, the diagnosis is made between the ages of 2 and 3 years. A mild form of cherubism may not be detected until the patient reaches the age of 10 to 12 years. The enlargement of the jaws continues until puberty. The radiolucent defects persist into adulthood.[36] The male to female ratio is 2:1.

Imaging features

Radiographic diagnosis of cherubism is rather easy and straightforward. Presence of bilateral, well-defined, multilocular radiolucent defects rules out any other odontogenic cyst or benign tumors. The lesions frequently resemble CGCGs. Most frequently, posterior regions of the mandible including the rami are involved[37] (**Fig. 7**). In advanced cases, the condition may also involve anterior part of the mandible. If the condition involves the maxilla, sinus floors are elevated and maxillary tuberosities are enlarged. Marked displacement of teeth and delayed eruption are frequent findings.

Management

The diagnosis of cherubism is achieved by clinical and radiographic findings.[38] Histopathologic examinations are usually not needed. Although a disorder of early childhood, treatment of

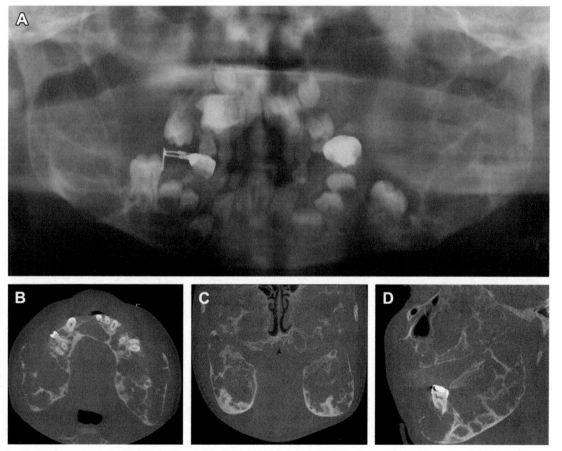

Fig. 7. (*A*) Panoramic radiograph of a child with cherubism shows bilateral, multilocular, expansile lesions in the posterior mandible and maxilla are evident and characteristic of the condition. Multiple teeth have been displaced largely in an anterior direction. (*B–D*) Axial, coronal, and sagittal cone-beam computed tomography sections demonstrate significant bony expansion bilaterally in both jaws. Note the multilocular appearance of the lesions.

cherubism can be safely delayed past puberty for the lesions to become static, when surgical recontouring of the jaws is done. Orthodontic treatment can be continued during active growth of the lesions to maintain dental occlusion.[39] There are reports of death owing to malnutrition secondary to cherubism.

Paget Disease of Bone

Paget disease or osteitis deformans is an autosomal-dominant condition that affects multiple bones. A discrepancy in the rate of resorption and apposition of the bone leads to the clinical condition where the affected bones are distorted and weakened.[40] Apart from hereditary causes, inflammatory and endocrine disturbances also play a role in contributing to the formation of Paget disease.

Patient demographics
Paget disease is mostly limited to middle or older age individuals. Rarely, it affects people under 40 years of age. There is a male predilection, with a ratio of 2:1 to females. There seems to be a geographic distribution, with higher incidence in Great Britain and Australia.[41] The incidence seems to be lower among Asians.[42]

Imaging features
Involvement of the jaws by Paget disease is infrequent compared with skull, pelvis, or femur. When jaws are affected, the maxilla is involved more frequently (**Fig. 8**). Usually, the whole jaw is

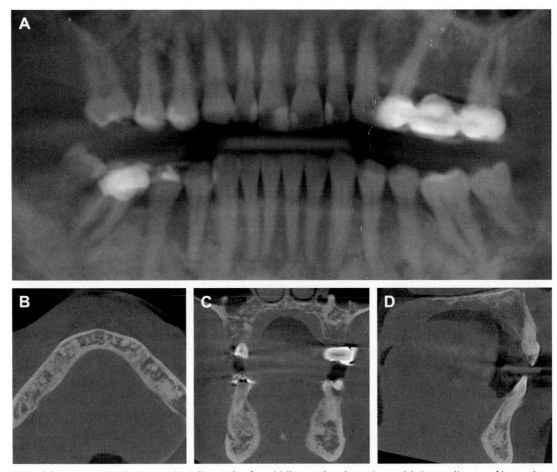

Fig. 8. (*A*) Reconstructed panoramic radiograph of a middle-aged male patient with Paget disease of bone shows irregular and heterogenous regions of calcification of the medullary bone is present in both jaws, bilaterally. Hypercementosis, an occasional associated finding, is noted on a lower left premolar tooth. (*B–D*) Axial, coronal, and sagittal cone-beam computed tomography sections demonstrate irregular regions of calcification with a high-density, homogenous appearance and other regions with a grainy, intermediate density. (*C*) The presence of multiple opaque, protrusive bony growths into the maxillary sinus is considered a finding possibly unique to this condition. (*Courtesy of* Heidi Kohltfarber, DDS, MS, Chapel Hill, NC.)

involved, but occasionally only a part of the jaw may be affected. Similar to other bony disorders, Paget disease may have 3 radiographic stages: (1) in the early stage, the involved bone is radiolucent, undergoing a resorptive process, (2) in the second stage, the bone assumes a granular pattern, and (3) finally, there is a more radiopaque appearance of the bone.[43] In the jaws, the final stage of radiopacity, mostly as irregular bone, is displayed. The radiographic features often mimic fibrous dysplasia, a condition, as mentioned, that is of the younger population. Therefore, there is little confusion between Paget disease and fibrous dysplasia. Tooth hypercementosis is a not uncommon associated finding.

Management

The mild form of Paget disease does not require any treatment. A surgical approach may have to be taken if the bony changes encroach into neurovascular canals. Most Paget disease patients are managed medically, to correct the serum calcium and alkaline phosphatase imbalance.[44,45] The risk of osteomyelitis after extraction is greater in these patients owing to reduced vascularity of the affected bone.

Idiopathic or Simple Bone Cavity

Idiopathic or simple bone cavity is included in this article as a bony condition that does not meet the histologic criteria of a cyst or a tumor. In the dental literature, this condition has been termed simple bone cyst, traumatic bone cyst, or hemorrhagic bone cyst. Such terms are misnomer, because the condition does not fulfill histologic diagnosis of a cyst. Because these cavities do not have epithelial linings, they are not true cysts. In addition, there is a minimal amount of fluid, if any, present in these cavities. The etiology of such cavities

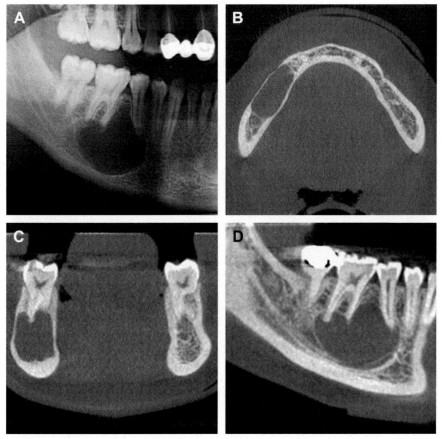

Fig. 9. (*A*) Cropped panoramic radiograph of a 17-year-old male patient with idiopathic or simple bone cavity formation in the right mandible. Inferiorly, the radiolucent lesion seems to be thinly corticated; it is noncorticated superiorly. The lesion is scalloping between the teeth roots with no tooth displacement are characteristic of the condition. (*B–C*) Axial and coronal cone-beam computed tomography (CBCT) sections demonstrates thinning of the buccal and lingual cortical plates of the mandible. (*D*) Sagittal CBCT section confirms thin cortication at the inferior aspect of the lesion, absent cortication superiorly, and characteristic scalloping between teeth roots.

is unknown, and there is no definite relationship with trauma.[46]

Patient demographics

Idiopathic bone cavity is a common condition found in first 2 decades of life. There is a definite male predominance. The mean age at the time of identification is 17 years of age. Patients are asymptomatic.

Imaging features

The most common location of idiopathic bone cavity is the mandible. In older patients, simple bone cavity is mostly limited to posterior mandible (**Fig. 9**). The defects are uniformly radiolucent, with occasional septa. The borders of these cavities are well-defined. Various widths of corticated margins are visible, including noncorticated margins. Between the roots of teeth, the defect takes up a scalloped appearance.[47] Cross-sectional imaging reveals scalloping of the buccal or lingual cortical plates of the mandible. A simple bone cavity, owing to lack of any tissue content, does not displace a tooth or the inferior alveolar canal. Root resorption is rare. However, thinning and perforation of the cortical plate is seen. Expansion of the cortical plates is not common, but does happen.

A variant of idiopathic bone cavity is seen in older female patients, accompanied by POD[48–50] (**Fig. 10**). Occasionally, simple bone cavity is also seen with fibrous dysplasia and, as discussed, florid osseous dysplasia.

Management

A simple bone cavity may spontaneously heal.[51] The current protocol involves a conservative surgical approach and careful curettage of the wall of

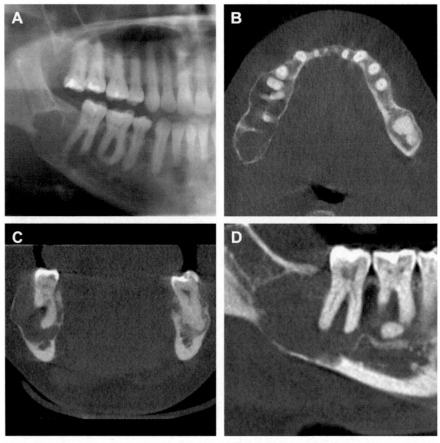

Fig. 10. (A) Cropped panoramic radiograph of a 40-year-old female patient of Somalian descent shows a mixed density lesion in the periapical regions of the mandibular first molars consistent with periapical osseous dysplasia. Formation of a larger radiolucency with thinly corticated borders in the right mandible indicates a secondary idiopathic or simple bone cavity formation. (B–D) Axial, coronal, and sagittal cone-beam computed tomography sections show thinning of the buccal, lingual, and inferior cortical plates and mild expansion associated with a secondary idiopathic or simple bone cavity formation. Mixed density periapical lesions are visible in the periapical region of the right and left mandible. (D) Thinly corticated borders of the secondary bone cavity lesions are clearly visible in the sagittal view.

the cavity to initiate bleeding and subsequent osseous resolution. Recurrence of these lesions is rare. Large, simple bone cavities may predispose the mandible to pathologic fracture.

SUMMARY

This article has described common fibro-osseous and other bony conditions encountered in the jaws and facial bones. An understanding of the varying lesion pathophysiologies and etiologies will hopefully inform radiographic findings. Most of the conditions described are diagnosed radiographically, without heavily relying on histologic examinations. In some of the conditions, for example, POD, cherubism, and simple bone cavity, histopathologic examination is not needed or may even be contraindicated, particularly with POD. In other conditions, for example, ABC, an aspirational biopsy helps in differentiating it from CGCG. In some conditions, for example, cherubism, clinical examination may be sufficient to arrive at a diagnosis. However, imaging is still needed in cherubism to identify the extent of the lesion and for treatment planning.[38] A proper diagnosis based on imaging findings can judiciously guide patients to curative surgical procedures when they need it, and noninvasive monitoring when they do not.

REFERENCES

1. Slootweg PJ. Maxillofacial fibro-osseous lesions: classification and differential diagnosis. Semin Diagn Pathol 1996;13(2):104–12.
2. Waldron CA. Fibro-osseous lesions of the jaws. J Oral Maxillofac Surg 1993;51(8):828–35.
3. Alsharif MJ, Sun ZJ, Chen XM, et al. Benign fibro-osseous lesions of the jaws: a study of 127 Chinese patients and review of the literature. Int J Surg Pathol 2009;17(2):122–34.
4. White SC, Pharoah MJ. Oral radiology: principles and interpretation. 7 edition. St Louis (MO): Elsevier; 2014.
5. Brannon RB, Fowler CB. Benign fibro-osseous lesions: a review of current concepts. Adv Anat Pathol 2001;8(3):126–43.
6. Mainville GN, Turgeon DP, Kauzman A. Diagnosis and management of benign fibro-osseous lesions of the jaws: a current review for the dental clinician. Oral Dis 2016;23(4):440–50.
7. Abramovitch K, Rice DD. Benign fibro-osseous lesions of the jaws. Dent Clin North Am 2016;60(1):167–93.
8. Alsufyani NA, Lam EW. Osseous (cemento-osseous) dysplasia of the jaws: clinical and radiographic analysis. J Can Dent Assoc 2011;77:b70.
9. Islam MN, Cohen DM, Kanter KG, et al. Florid cemento-osseous dysplasia mimicking multiple periapical pathology–an endodontic dilemma. Gen Dent 2008;56(6):559–62.
10. Fenerty S, Shaw W, Verma R, et al. Florid cemento-osseous dysplasia: review of an uncommon fibro-osseous lesion of the jaw with important clinical implications. Skeletal Radiol 2017;46(5):581–90.
11. MacDonald-Jankowski DS. Florid cemento-osseous dysplasia: a systematic review. Dentomaxillofac Radiol 2003;32(3):141–9.
12. Cavalcante MB, de Oliveira Lima AL, Junior MA, et al. Florid cemento-osseous dysplasia simultaneous the chronic suppurative osteomyelitis in mandible. J Craniofac Surg 2016;27(8):2173–6.
13. Kucukkurt S, Rzayev S, Baris E, et al. Familial florid osseous dysplasia: a report with review of the literature. BMJ Case Rep 2016;2016 [pii: bcr2015214162].
14. McCarthy EF. Fibro-osseous lesions of the maxillofacial bones. Head Neck Pathol 2013;7(1):5–10.
15. Ozek C, Gundogan H, Bilkay U, et al. Craniomaxillofacial fibrous dysplasia. J Craniofac Surg 2002;13(3):382–9.
16. Cohen MM Jr, Howell RE. Etiology of fibrous dysplasia and McCune-Albright syndrome. Int J Oral Maxillofac Surg 1999;28(5):366–71.
17. Abdelkarim A, Green R, Startzell J, et al. Craniofacial polyostotic fibrous dysplasia: a case report and review of the literature. Oral Surg Oral Med Oral Pathol Oral Radiol Endod 2008;106(1):e49–55.
18. MacDonald-Jankowski DS, Yeung R, Li TK, et al. Computed tomography of fibrous dysplasia. Dentomaxillofac Radiol 2004;33(2):114–8.
19. Petrikowski CG, Pharoah MJ, Lee L, et al. Radiographic differentiation of osteogenic sarcoma, osteomyelitis, and fibrous dysplasia of the jaws. Oral Surg Oral Med Oral Pathol Oral Radiol Endod 1995;80(6):744–50.
20. Larheim TA, Westesson PL. Maxillofacial imaging. New York: Springer; 2006.
21. El-Mofty SK. Fibro-osseous lesions of the craniofacial skeleton: an update. Head Neck Pathol 2014;8(4):432–44.
22. Eversole R, Su L, ElMofty S. Benign fibro-osseous lesions of the craniofacial complex. A review. Head Neck Pathol 2008;2(3):177–202.
23. Eversole LR, Merrell PW, Strub D. Radiographic characteristics of central ossifying fibroma. Oral Surg Oral Med Oral Pathol 1985;59(5):522–7.
24. El-Mofty S. Psammomatoid and trabecular juvenile ossifying fibroma of the craniofacial skeleton: two distinct clinicopathologic entities. Oral Surg Oral Med Oral Pathol Oral Radiol Endod 2002;93(3):296–304.

25. Engelbrecht V, Preis S, Hassler W, et al. CT and MRI of congenital sinonasal ossifying fibroma. Neuroradiology 1999;41(7):526–9.

26. Titinchi F, Morkel J. Ossifying Fibroma: analysis of treatment methods and recurrence patterns. J Oral Maxillofac Surg 2016;74(12):2409–19.

27. MacDonald-Jankowski DS, Li TK. Ossifying fibroma in a Hong Kong community: the clinical and radiological features and outcomes of treatment. Dentomaxillofac Radiol 2009;38(8):514–23.

28. Kaffe I, Ardekian L, Taicher S, et al. Radiologic features of central giant cell granuloma of the jaws. Oral Surg Oral Med Oral Pathol Oral Radiol Endod 1996;81(6):720–6.

29. De Lange J, Van den Akker HP. Clinical and radiological features of central giant-cell lesions of the jaw. Oral Surg Oral Med Oral Pathol Oral Radiol Endod 2005;99(4):464–70.

30. Bodner L, Bar-Ziv J. Radiographic features of central giant cell granuloma of the jaws in children. Pediatr Radiol 1996;26(2):148–51.

31. Kruse-Losler B, Diallo R, Gaertner C, et al. Central giant cell granuloma of the jaws: a clinical, radiologic, and histopathologic study of 26 cases. Oral Surg Oral Med Oral Pathol Oral Radiol Endod 2006;101(3):346–54.

32. Kaffe I, Naor H, Calderon S, et al. Radiological and clinical features of aneurysmal bone cyst of the jaws. Dentomaxillofac Radiol 1999;28(3):167–72.

33. Omami G, Mathew R, Gianoli D, et al. Enormous aneurysmal bone cyst of the mandible: case report and radiologic-pathologic correlation. Oral Surg Oral Med Oral Pathol Oral Radiol 2012;114(1):e75–9.

34. Asaumi J, Konouchi H, Hisatomi M, et al. MR features of aneurysmal bone cyst of the mandible and characteristics distinguishing it from other lesions. Eur J Radiol 2003;45(2):108–12.

35. Urs AB, Augustine J, Chawla H. Aneurysmal bone cyst of the jaws: clinicopathological study. J Maxillofac Oral Surg 2014;13(4):458–63.

36. Redfors M, Jensen JL, Storhaug K, et al. Cherubism: panoramic and CT features in adults. Dentomaxillofac Radiol 2013;42(10):20130034.

37. Jain V, Sharma R. Radiographic, CT and MRI features of cherubism. Pediatr Radiol 2006;36(10):1099–104.

38. Lima Gde M, Almeida JD, Cabral LA. Cherubism: clinicoradiographic features and treatment. J Oral Maxillofac Res 2010;1(2):e2.

39. Abela S, Cameron M, Bister D. Orthodontic treatment in cherubism: an overview and a case report. Aust Orthod J 2014;30(2):214–20.

40. Reddy SV. Etiology of Paget's disease and osteoclast abnormalities. J Cell Biochem 2004;93(4):688–96.

41. van Staa TP, Selby P, Leufkens HG, et al. Incidence and natural history of Paget's disease of bone in England and Wales. J Bone Miner Res 2002;17(3):465–71.

42. Merashli M, Jawad A. Paget's disease of bone among various ethnic groups. Sultan Qaboos Univ Med J 2015;15(1):e22–6.

43. Tillman HH. Paget's disease of bone. A clinical, radiographic, and histopathologic study of twenty-four cases involving the jaws. Oral Surg Oral Med Oral Pathol 1962;15:1225–34.

44. Lyles KW, Siris ES, Singer FR, et al. A clinical approach to diagnosis and management of Paget's disease of bone. J Bone Miner Res 2001;16(8):1379–87.

45. Selby PL, Davie MW, Ralston SH, et al. Guidelines on the management of Paget's disease of bone. Bone 2002;31(3):366–73.

46. Kaugars GE, Cale AE. Traumatic bone cyst. Oral Surg Oral Med Oral Pathol 1987;63(3):318–24.

47. Perdigao PF, Silva EC, Sakurai E, et al. Idiopathic bone cavity: a clinical, radiographic, and histological study. Br J Oral Maxillofac Surg 2003;41(6):407–9.

48. Peacock ME, Krishna R, Gustin JW, et al. Retrospective study on idiopathic bone cavity and its association with cementoosseous dysplasia. Oral Surg Oral Med Oral Pathol Oral Radiol 2015;119(4):e246–51.

49. Saito Y, Hoshina Y, Nagamine T, et al. Simple bone cyst. A clinical and histopathologic study of fifteen cases. Oral Surg Oral Med Oral Pathol 1992;74(4):487–91.

50. Mahomed F, Altini M, Meer S, et al. Cementoosseous dysplasia with associated simple bone cysts. J Oral Maxillofac Surg 2005;63(10):1549–54.

51. Sapp JP, Stark ML. Self-healing traumatic bone cysts. Oral Surg Oral Med Oral Pathol 1990;69(5):597–602.

Imaging of Dentoalveolar and Jaw Trauma

Reyhaneh Alimohammadi, DDS

KEYWORDS

- Dental fracture • Luxation • Root fracture • Alveolar bone fracture • Mandibular fracture
- Facial trauma

KEY POINTS

- Radiographic evaluation is an indispensable tool for diagnosing, assessing, and following-up fractures of the maxillofacial complex.
- Thorough knowledge of dentomaxillofacial plain film and 3-D radiographic anatomy leads to success in the diagnosis of fractures.
- Detailed clinical evaluation is essential prior to any radiographic evaluation/prescription in trauma and fracture cases.
- Radiographic presentation may vary between
  - One or 2 well-defined sharply demarcated line(s) limited to the anatomic structure (rule out artifact).
  - Increase in density/radiopacity within the structure caused by overlap of fragments.
  - Discontinuity of the outline of the osseous and dental structures when a radiolucent fracture line cannot be seen within the structure.
  - Irregularity of the contour and step formation in areas where the osseous or dental structure outline is supposed to be smooth and continuous.

INTRODUCTION

Radiographic evaluation is an indispensable tool for diagnosing fractures and traumatic injuries to the maxillofacial complex. The presence or absence of a fracture line; the direction, orientation, and space between fragments; and the involvement of surrounding anatomic structures as well as the location of the attached fragments can be determined on radiographic images. If foreign bodies are suspected, their presence, position, number, and shape within the hard and soft tissue structures can be detected radiographically, guiding accurate surgical intervention for removal while sparing the neighboring anatomic structures, such as arteries, veins, nerves, and sinuses. Radiographic evaluation provides an accurate estimation of the healing process providing the details of osseous fusion and post-traumatic remodeling. Fibrous healing defects can be easily detected in cases of failure of bone fusion. This article presents an overview of the patterns of dental and maxillofacial fractures to familiarize general radiologists with the appearance and significance of common dentoalveolar and jaw fractures.

RADIOGRAPHIC TECHNIQUES

Detailed clinical evaluation is essential prior to any radiographic prescription and subsequent evaluation in trauma and fracture cases. Variable presentation of fractures, however, even though occurring in the same area, dictates a

The author does not have any commercial or financial conflicts of interest and any funding sources.
Oral and Maxillofacial Radiology, University of Texas Health Science Center San Antonio, School of Dentistry, 7703 Floyd Curl Drive, San Antonio, TX 78229, USA
E-mail address: Alimohammadi@uthscsa.edu

Radiol Clin N Am 56 (2018) 105–124
http://dx.doi.org/10.1016/j.rcl.2017.08.008
0033-8389/18/Published by Elsevier Inc.

radiologic.theclinics.com

customization of the technique depending on the degree of patient discomfort, gravity of the trauma, and involvement of multiple structures.

When using plain film techniques, 1 projection is usually not enough to provide detailed information about the fracture line, displaced fragments, or involvement of surrounding structures. Two projections made perpendicular to one another are usually used as a minimal requirement, and the addition of the third technique is often required.

Gradually, 3-D imaging, such as CT or cone beam computed tomography (CBCT), is replacing plain film techniques; 3-D imaging provides detailed information of the oral and maxillofacial complex that is less technique sensitive and more comprehensive than that seen with plain film imaging.

For dental and dentoalveolar trauma cases and in the absence of 3-D imaging techniques, such as in a general dentist's office settings, periapical films provide high-resolution images, and the use of multiple projections is indispensable for the detection of a thin alveolar bone fracture. A panoramic radiograph associated with an occlusal projection can be helpful in detecting fractured teeth and direction of the displacement. A panoramic projection combined with posteroanterior (PA) head film can be helpful in detecting condylar process fractures and determining the direction of proximal fragment displacement. A PA coupled with a lateral projection is useful in assessing sinus walls fractures. More complicated trauma cases as well as midface fractures need CT evaluation due to the complexity of the anatomy in this area.[1]

RADIOGRAPHIC FEATURES OF FRACTURES

The key to success in diagnosis of fractures is a comprehensive knowledge of dentomaxillofacial anatomy as seen on different imaging acquisitions.

A fracture by definition is a separation between 2 fragments of the same anatomic structures, such as tooth or mandible. The separation can extend throughout the structure to reach the adjacent tissues. On plain film imaging, the x-ray beam has to pass through the fracture gap to be able to generate a radiolucent line that can be seen and diagnosed as a fracture line.

The following are the general features that are usually seen radiographically in fracture cases:

- Presence of 1 or 2 well-defined sharply marked lines situated and limited to the anatomic borders of the structure
- Presence of increase in density/radiopacity within the structure caused by the overlap of the separated fragments due to muscular activity
- Discontinuity of the outline in cases where a radiolucent line cannot be seen within the structure itself
- Irregularity of the contour of the structure with interruption and formation of a step in the areas where the outline is supposed to be smooth and continuous

DENTAL LUXATION
Definition

Dental luxation is a general term that covers multiple types of injuries; the common feature is absence of root fracture and absence of alveolar bone fracture. The structures that are mainly affected by luxation incidence are the periodontal ligament (PDL) space and lamina dura.[2]

Luxation injuries include concussion, subluxation, intrusive or extrusive luxation, lateral luxation, and avulsion.

Etiology

Predominant etiologic factors in the permanent dentition are bicycle injuries, falls, fights and sports injuries. In the primary dentition, falls dominate as the cause.

Clinical Presentation

The clinical presentation of luxation injuries differs according to the type of injury sustained.[3,4] These can be seen in **Table 1**.

Radiographic Appearance

The radiographic appearance of luxation injuries differs according to the type of injury sustained. These can be seen in **Table 1** and an example of lateral luxation can be seen in **Fig. 1**.

DENTAL FRACTURES
Definition

Dental injuries have been classified according to a variety of factors, such as etiology, anatomy, pathology, and therapeutic considerations. But in general, fractures are mostly divided as coronal fractures and root fractures with and without pulp involvement.

Crown Fractures

Etiology
Etiology is severe force to the teeth sufficient to disrupt the enamel, dentin, or both of a tooth. Predisposing factors include abnormal occlusion, maxillary protrusion, an overjet exceeding 4 mm,

Table 1
The clinical and radiographic presentation and treatment of the different luxation injuries

Type of Luxation Injury	Clinical Presentation	Radiographic Appearance	Treatment
Concussion	Marked reaction to percussion without abnormal loosening or displacement	Cannot be detected radiographically	Occlusal interferences should be relieved by selective grinding of opposing teeth. Splinting is needed if there is any severe loosening. Soft diet for 14 d is advised.
Subluxation	Abnormal loosening without clinically demonstrable displacement of the tooth	PDL space widening	Occlusal interferences should be relieved by selective grinding of opposing teeth. Splinting is needed if there is any severe loosening. Soft diet for 14 d is advised.
Intrusive luxation	Displacement of the tooth deeper into the alveolar bone accompanied by comminution or fracture of the alveolar socket	Severe periapical PDL space narrowing	Spontaneous eruption or orthodontic extrusion
Extrusive luxation	Partial displacement of the tooth out of its socket	Generalized PDL space widening	Repositioning and splinting
Lateral luxation	Eccentric displacement of the tooth accompanied by comminution of fracture of the alveolar crest	PDL space widening depending on the angulation of the central beam	Repositioning and splinting
Avulsion	Complete displacement of a tooth out of the alveolar socket	Empty socket	Replanting and splinting

a short upper lip, an incompetent lip, and mouth breathing.

Clinical presentation
Crown fractures are divided in 3 types:

- Fracture limited to the enamel: the fracture presents as a slight chip of the enamel; usually no clinical symptoms are noted but the patient feels the sharpness of the damaged tooth.
- Fracture involving the enamel and dentin but not the pulp: the dentin is clinically visible and the tooth is sensitive to thermal stimuli (**Fig. 2**).
- Fracture involving the enamel, dentin, and pulp; the tooth is very sensitive and the pulp is clinically exposed with some limited bleeding from the pulp chamber.

Radiographic appearance
Periapical images or limited volume with high-resolution CBCTs are the most used and the most useful in this situation; they provide detailed information about the level of fracture, the extension, and relationship with the pulp space. They also provide useful information regarding the degree of development of the apex. Assessment of the PDL space and lamina dura is also made on these images to detect any narrowing, widening, or interruption of the structures. Periapical images also are used as a baseline for future evaluation in cases of the apices not completely formed when the trauma was received or in presence of stabilization after intrusion/extrusion to detect the possibility of ankylosis in the long term (**Fig. 3**).

Root Fractures

Etiology
Two causes of the majority of dental fracture involving the roots are traumatic causes, especially sports activities, mainly seen in the anterior maxillary and mandibular teeth, and iatrogenic

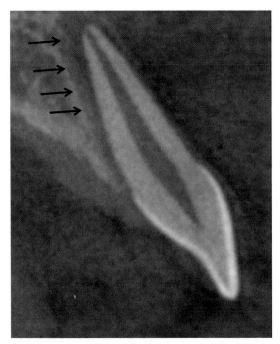

Fig. 1. CBCT sagittal cross-sectional view shows extrusive luxation with widening of the palatal PDL space (*arrows*).

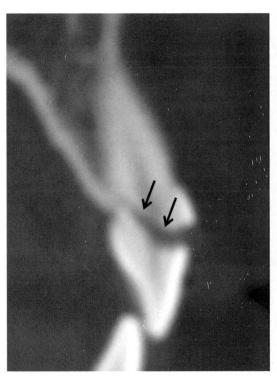

Fig. 3. CBCT sagittal cross-sectional view shows a horizontal-oblique fracture of the cervical third of the crown with subcrestal root involvement lingually (*arrows*).

causes, related to large restoration and posts placement in posterior teeth. Fractures due to traumatic incidents are mainly horizontal; they usually involve single-rooted teeth and the fracture line can be situated at any level of the root; however, a majority are seen at the level of the mid-height of the root. The line extends from side to side with displacement and reparation enough to be detected radiographically.

Fractures due to iatrogenic conditions are mainly vertical and the most common cause of these fractures is endodontic treatment with placement of a large post or some large coronal restoration; both types of restoration create a weak point in the structure of the root and sometimes limited trauma is enough to create a fracture. The trauma can cause a crack in the root that can progress with time to a radiographically visible fracture with fragment separation (**Fig. 4**).

Clinical findings

Clinical findings in vertical fractures are similar to other conditions, such as pulpal necrosis, failed root canal treatment, and/or periodontal disease,

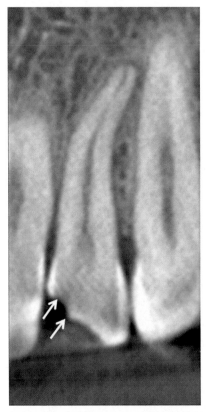

Fig. 2. CBCT coronal oblique cross-sectional view shows an oblique coronal fracture involving the enamel and dentin but without the pulp space (*arrows*).

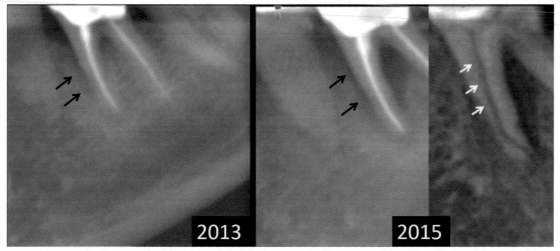

Fig. 4. CBCT panoramic reformation of a root canal treated molar shows the progression (from *left* to the *right*) of bone loss after vertical root fracture in an endodontically treated tooth (*arrows*).

and other conventional methods (eg, transillumination, projection radiography, bite testing, periodontal probing, sinus tract detection, and direct visual examination) were suggested to detect vertical fractures; however, they showed limited reliability and the results were not specific. Definitive diagnosis of vertical root fractures in posterior teeth is more challenging than anterior teeth due to the more complex dental and osseous anatomy. Fast identification of a root fracture prevents unnecessary treatment, extended patient discomfort, and severe adjacent bone resorption.

Radiographic appearance

The expected radiographic features indicating a fractured root include

- A radiolucent line between the fragments
- An alteration in the outline shape of the root
- Discontinuity of the PDL space

CBCT became the favored imaging modality for root fracture detection because it eliminates the superimposition and provides a multidirectional view for the area of interest. Beam hardening and streak artifacts, however, caused by high-density material placed within the canal pulp space pose a significant radiographic challenge for fracture detection, because these fractures are most commonly seen in endodontically treated teeth that are commonly filled with high-density material, such as gutta-percha, metallic restorations, and posts[5] (**Figs. 5–7**).

Definitive diagnosis of vertical root fractures in posterior teeth is more challenging than anterior teeth due to the more complex dental and osseous anatomy. Clinical findings in vertical fractures are similar to other conditions, such as pulp necrosis, failed root canal treatment, and/or periodontal disease; other

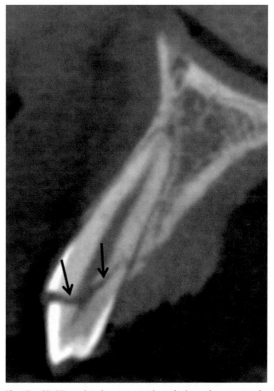

Fig. 5. CBCT sagittal cross-sectional view shows an oblique crown fracture with subcrestal involvement of the cervical third of the root (arrows).

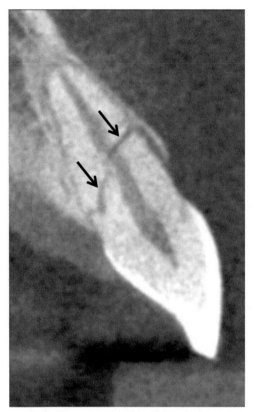

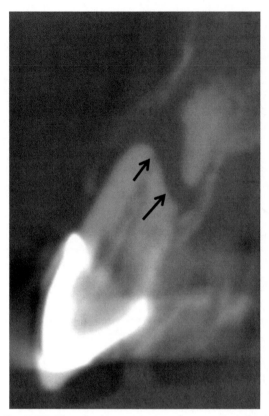

Fig. 6. CBCT sagittal cross-sectional view shows a horizontal-oblique fracture involving the middle third of the root facially and the cervical third of the root lingually. There is minimal tooth fragment displacement noted (*arrows*).

Fig. 7. CBCT sagittal cross-section shows apical third root fracture with severe fragments displacement (*arrows*).

conventional methods (eg, transillumination, projection radiography, bite testing, periodontal probing, sinus tract detection, and direct visual examination) were suggested to detect vertical fractures; however, they showed limited reliability and the results were not specific.

Fast identification of a root fracture prevents unnecessary treatment, extended patient discomfort, and severe adjacent bone resorption (**Figs. 8 and 9**).

CBCT became the favored imaging modality for root fracture detection because it eliminates the superimposition and provides a multidirectional view for the area of interest. Beam hardening and streak artifacts caused by high-density material placed within the canal pulp space, however, pose a significant radiographic challenge for fracture detection, because these fractures are most commonly seen in endodontically treated teeth that are commonly filled with high density material, such as gutta percha, metallic restorations, and posts[6] (**Figs. 10 and 11**).

DENTOALVEOLAR FRACTURES
Definition

Fracture of the alveolar process usually involves the facial or lingual plates or both; most of these fractures are accompanied by injuries to teeth; thus, they are referred to as dentoalveolar fractures.[7,8] In some cases, injuries to the alveolar process can occur independently. In cases of trauma involving multiple teeth, the possibility of an alveolar bone fracture increases; this possibility increases also in cases of dental intrusive and lateral luxation. Most of the fractures of the alveolar process are open with trauma to the gingiva and the alveolar mucosa.

Etiology

Motor vehicle accidents, sports activities, and falls are the main causes of these injuries.

Clinical Presentation

In fracture of the alveolar socket wall, the fracture is usually limited to the facial or lingual socket wall.

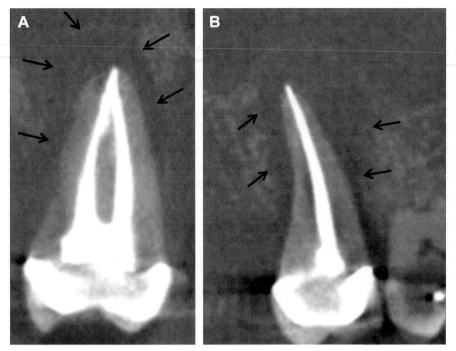

Fig. 8. CBCT coronal (*A*) and sagittal (*B*) cross-sections of a root canal treated maxillary molar shows the severe bone loss associated with a vertically fractured tooth (*arrows*).

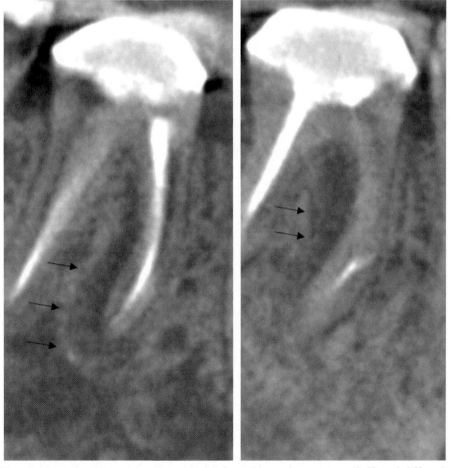

Fig. 9. CBCT sagittal cross-sections show the typical J-shaped bone loss pattern (*left*) and diffuse bone defect (*right*) in a vertically fractured tooth (*arrows*).

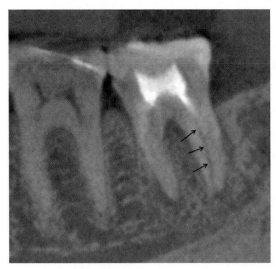

Fig. 10. CBCT sagittal cross-section shows a radicular vertical fracture with actual separation of the root fragments (*arrows*).

It affects multiple teeth and is mostly seen in anterior regions. In the maxillary arch, typically the dentoalveolar segment is displaced in a palatal and inferior direction, with the fracture occurring on the labial or buccal alveolar socket wall. In the mandible, especially in the anterior region, both labial and lingual alveolar socket wall fractures usually occur, with the displacement of the segment directed facially or lingually. They are associated with luxation. The facial osseous plate is usually mobile with associated contusion of the gingiva. In cases of dental intrusion, 1 plate is usually fractured (**Fig. 12**).

Fracture of the alveolar process: the fracture involves both facial and lingual cortical plates, which may or may not involve the alveolar socket and associated tooth. Due to the change in position of the involved fragment, the patient reports the occlusion change. It can accompany concomitant with extrusive and luxation and root fracture. These fractures are predominantly found in anterior teeth, canine, and premolar regions (**Fig. 13**).

In fracture of the mandible or maxilla, the fracture involves the base of the mandible or maxilla and the alveolar process. Clinical findings include displacement of the segment and disturbance of the occlusion, crepitus, and provoked pain.

Radiographic Appearance

Lateral extraoral radiographs can be used to detect the fracture site in fractures of the anterior alveolar socket wall if displaced. In fractures of mandible or maxilla, intraoral radiographs reveal relationship between involved tooth and fracture line and extraoral radiographs can show the position of the fracture line. Although intraoral and extraoral radiographs can help detecting these fractures, CBCT images can provide greater details about the extension of the fracture line, and the involvement of 1 or 2 cortical plates. It can also help in assessing the width of the fracture, the displacement of the fragments, and the continuity of the outline. The involvement of surrounding structures can be confirmed or ruled out using CBCT as well. Alveolar socket fracture associated with dental trauma is usually seen with small bone splinters always associated with an intrusive or lateral luxation of an associated tooth or teeth (**Fig. 14**). Detached bone fragments can be situated within the thickness of the gingival tissues or displaced and located within the oral mucosa or mainly the lips (**Fig. 15**). Cross-sectional images can show these fragments and are useful for treatment planning.[9]

MANDIBULAR AND TEMPOROMANDIBULAR JOINT FRACTURES

The mandible's prominence and its relative lack of support make it a commonly fractured

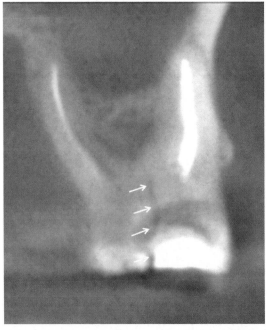

Fig. 11. CBCT coronal cross-section shows a coronal vertical fracture involving the root furcation area (*arrows*).

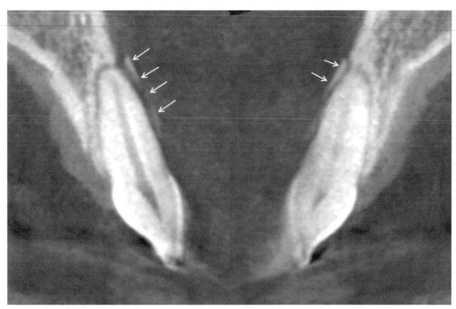

Fig. 12. CBCT sagittal cross-sections show tooth intrusion with fracture of buccal plates (*arrows*).

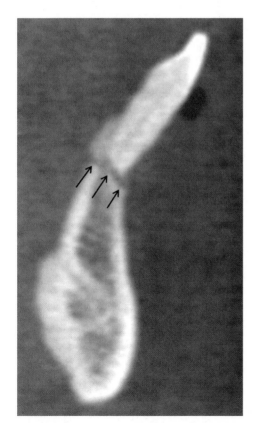

bone. Fractures of the mandible have been reported to account for 36% to 59% of all maxillofacial fractures. Mandibular fractures have been classified in several ways. The most common classification is based on the anatomic location of the fracture (ie, condyle, coronoid process, ramus, angle, body, symphysis, and alveolar crest).

Depending on the angulation of the fracture and the force of the muscle pull, proximal and distal to the fracture, fractures are divided as *favorable* and *unfavorable*, meaning when the fractures are

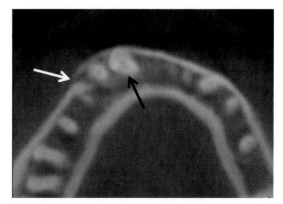

Fig. 13. CBCT sagittal cross-section of the anterior mandibular alveolus shows a horizontal fracture of the alveolar process involving the PDL space tooth apex (*arrows*).

Fig. 14. CBCT panoramic and axial views show intrusion of the mandibular lateral incisor (*black arrow*) with fracture of the facial plate of the alveolar process (*white arrow*).

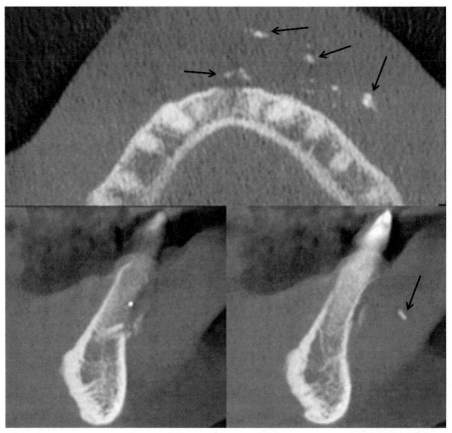

Fig. 15. CBCT axial and sagittal views show fracture of the mandibular alveolar facial plate of the alveolar process with multiple high density fragments (*upper* and *lower right*) suggestive of bone or foreign bodies within the soft tissues (*arrow*).

vertically and horizontally unfavorable, the fragments tend to be displaced.

Definition and Classification

Condylar fractures

The higher incidence of mandibular condylar process fracture is due to the binding of the wide and rigid mandibular ramus to the condyle through a thin and narrow condylar neck. Condylar process fractures can be classified according to their position of the condyle as follows: condylar fracture, condylar neck fracture, and subcondylar fracture. Fractures limited to the condyle are also called intracapsular fracture because the joint capsule extends usually inferiorly to the condylar neck. Condylar neck fractures occur inferior to the area where the joint capsule attaches to the bone; the neck of the condyle is narrower than the condyle. Condylar neck fractures are considered extracapsular fracture because it is not within in the joint capsule.[10] A subcondylar fracture is situated inferiorly to the condylar neck in the area between the mandibular sigmoid notch and posterior border of the mandibular ramus.

Five types of condylar fractures are described in order of increasing severity. These can be seen in **Figs. 16–19** and **Table 2**.

Angle fractures

Angle fractures occur in the triangular region bounded within the anterior and posterosuperior attachments of the masseter muscle (usually distal to the third molar). There are 2 main proposed reasons why the angle of the mandible is commonly associated with fractures; presence of a thinner cross-sectional area relative to the neighboring segments of the mandible and presence of third molars, in particular those that are impacted, which weakens the region. Angle fractures are usually unfavorable due to the actions of the masseter, temporalis, and medial pterygoid muscles, which pull the proximal segment superiorly and medially (**Fig. 20**).

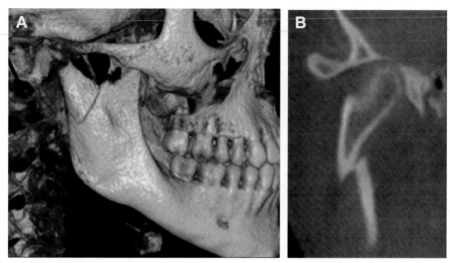

Fig. 16. CBCT surface rendering (A) and coronal view (B) show subcondylar fracture with lateral displacement and telescoping of the proximal fragment on the lateral aspect of the distal ramus segment.

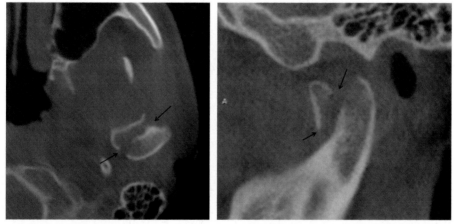

Fig. 17. CBCT axial (left) and sagittal oblique views (right) show intracapsular fracture of the condyle with anterior displacement of the fragment (arrows). This is due to the direction of action of the lateral pterygoid muscle that is attached to the pterygoid fovea.

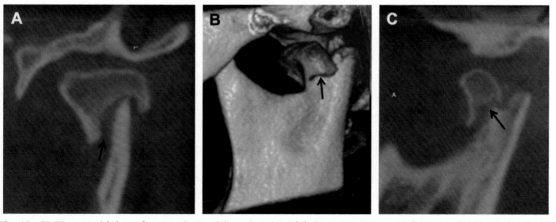

Fig. 18. CBCT coronal (A), surface rendering (B), and sagittal (C) show condylar neck fracture with limited anterior displacement due to the lodging of the fragment into the neck (arrows).

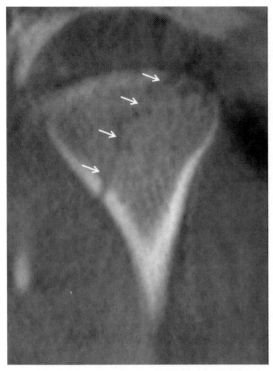

Fig. 19. CBCT coronal view shows intracapsular condyle fracture with minimal displacement of the fragments (*arrows*).

Table 2 A classification for severity of condylar fractures		
Condylar Fracture Type	Fracture Position	Condylar Position
Type I	Neck	Slight displacement of the condyle; angle between the condyle and the axis of the ramus between from 10° and 45°
Type II	Neck	Angle from 45° to 90°, resulting in tearing of the medial portion of the joint capsule
Type III	Neck/subcondylar	Fragments not in contact; displaced medially and forward
Type IV	Neck/subcondylar	Condyle articulates on or in a forward position with regard to the articular eminence
Type V	Vertical or oblique fractures through the head of the condyle	Fragment can be displaced or within the fossa.

Symphysis fractures

Symphysis fractures occur in the region of the central incisors and run from the alveolar process through the inferior border of the mandible. Fractures of the symphysis are unfavorable due to the presence of suprahyoid muscles that cause inferior rotation around the axis of the temporomandibular joint and the mylohyoid muscles that depress the mandible and raise the floor of the mouth during the beginning of deglutition (**Fig. 21**).

Body fractures

Body fractures happen between the distal symphysis and a line coinciding with the anterior border of the masseter muscle (usually including the third molar).

Body fractures are often unfavorable because of the actions of the masseter, temporalis, and medial pterygoid muscles, which distract the proximal segment superomedially. Additionally, the mylohyoid muscle and anterior belly of the digastric muscle may contribute to the unfavorable nature of this fracture by displacing the fractured segment posteriorly and inferiorly (**Fig. 22**).

Complex fractures

Studies on the number of fractures per mandible have shown remarkable consistency. In patients with mandible fractures, 53% of patients had unilateral fractures, 37% of the patients had 2 fractures, and 9% had 3 or more fractures. Because approximately 50% of patients with mandibular fracture have more than 1 fracture, a second fracture site or location should always be considered. When double fractures occur, they are usually on contralateral sides of the mandible. Common combinations include the angle or symphysis plus the contralateral body or condyle (**Fig. 23**). Triple fractures occasionally occur, and the most common type is fracture of both condyles and the symphysis (**Fig. 24**).

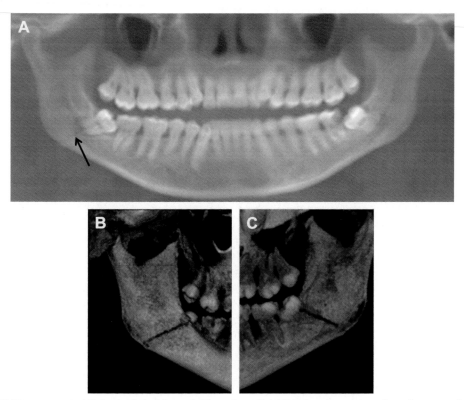

Fig. 20. CBCT panoramic (*A*) (*arrow*) and lateral (*B*) and medial (*C*) 3-D reformation show fracture of the right angle of the mandible in the area of the third molar. The presence of impacted third molars may weaken the bone in this area and make it more prone to fracture if subject to trauma.

Glenoid Fossa Fracture

The roof of the glenoid fossa is formed by a very thin bone; it separates the articular space of the joint from the floor of the middle cranial fossa.

Glenoid fossa fractures are rare and can be clinically confused with condylar fractures, due to multiple common clinical symptoms. After

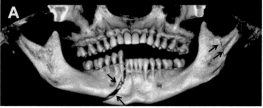

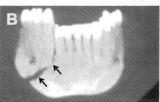

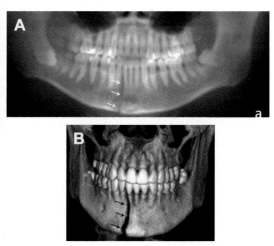

Fig. 21. CBCT panoramic (*A*) (*white arrows*) and 3-D reformation (*B*) (*black arrows*) show fracture of the mandibular symphysis.

Fig. 22. CBCT 3-D panoramic reformation (*A*) and maximum intensity projection (*B*) show fractures of the right parasymphyseal area and the left condyle (*arrows*). These fractures often occur together due to the distribution of the upwards and laterally directed force in the bone.

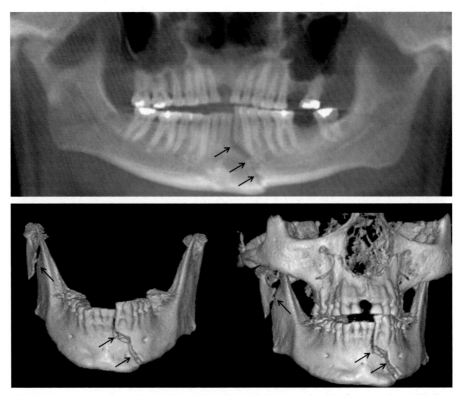

Fig. 23. CBCT panoramic (*upper*) and 3-D reformation (*lower*) shows a double fracture (mandibular parasymphysis and contralateral condyle) and displacement of the of the left body and right condyle (*arrows*).

trauma, an intracranial displacement of the condyle can cause the disruption of the roof of the glenoid fossa and intracranial structures, such as meningeal or cerebrospinal elements, could be affected (**Fig. 25**).

Etiology

Individual studies demonstrate that location of the fracture varies depending on the type of injury and direction and force of trauma. Studies show that assaults and fights lead to a higher percentage of angle fractures, whereas motor vehicle accidents result in more ramus fracture.

Clinical presentation

A typical feature of mandibular fracture is any change in occlusion. Premature posterior dental contact or an anterior open bite may result from bilateral fractures of the mandibular condyle or angle and from maxillary fractures with inferior displacement of the posterior maxilla. Anterior alveolar process or parasymphyseal fractures result in posterior open bite. Ipsilateral angle and

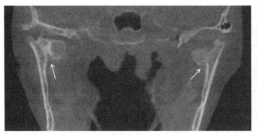
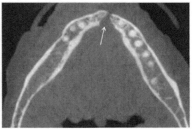

Fig. 24. CBCT coronal (*left*) and axial views (*right*) show triple fracture of both condyles and the symphysis. This pattern is also called guardsman fractures.

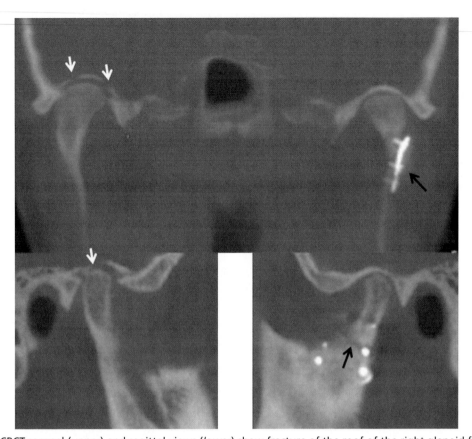

Fig. 25. CBCT coronal (*upper*) and sagittal views (*lower*) show fracture of the roof of the right glenoid fossa and repaired fracture of the left condylar neck (*arrows*).

parasymphyseal fractures are associated with unilateral open bite.

Abnormal mandibular movement, including trismus or limited opening, changes in sensation of the lower lip, loose teeth, and crepitation on palpation, and flattened appearance of the lateral aspect of the face are other signs and symptoms of mandibular fracture.

Radiographic appearance

Radiographic evaluation is indispensable in primary and follow-up assessments of fracture of the mandible and midface. Radiographs play a major role in detecting the presence or absence of a fracture and location and direction of fracture line(s); assessing the amount of fragment displacement and separation; detecting, if any, the involvement of teeth with the fracture line; and determining the location of associated foreign bodies in hard and soft tissues. Radiographic examination is also important in detecting the presence of a local or general condition that might contribute, complicate, or exaggerate the effect of a fracture.

In short-term and long-term follow-up, radiographic evaluation is needed to assess the alignment of the bone fragments and the healing or presence of complications, such as fibrous healing, nonunion, infection, and involvement of adjacent anatomic structures. Panoramic radiographs are the single most informative radiograph for the diagnosis of mandibular fractures due to simplicity of the technique and ability to visualize the entire mandible. The Caldwell PA view shows medial or lateral displacement of fractures of the ramus, angle, body, and symphysis. The lateral oblique view of the mandible is helpful in diagnosing ramus, angle, and posterior body fractures. The reverse Towne view is useful in evaluating medial displacement of the condyle and condylar neck fracture. With the advent of newer technology, multidetector CT (MDCT), CBCT, and MRI provide more accurate details if needed.

FRACTURES OF THE MAXILLA, MIDFACE, AND SURROUNDING STRUCTURES
Zygomaticomaxillary Complex

Definition
Zygomaticomaxillary complex fracture is called a tripod fracture because there are 3 fracture lines

through the 3 osseous connections of the zygomatic bone with the adjacent structures; the first through the lateral orbital wall, the second separating the zygoma from the maxilla, and the third seen through the zygomatic arch.

With a lesser force and dependent on the direction of the strike, the fracture can occur only in 1 site of the 3 sites.[11,12]

Etiology
Zygomaticomaxillary complex fractures are usually caused by a direct blow to the zygomatic bone. Fractures of the zygomatic arch are frequently seen during ski accident due to a hit on the face by the ski pole handle.

Clinical presentation
Mobilization of the zygomatic bone (displacement and/or rotation) is the common finding.

Radiographic appearance
Plain film evaluation for zygomaticomaxillary complex fractures include Waters, submentovertex, and Caldwell views. Waters view is the most useful view to evaluate for zygomatic injuries. CT and CBCT are the modalities of choice (**Fig. 26**).

Sinus Wall Fractures

Definition
Sinus wall fractures are considered as one of the major nondental source of maxillary sinusitis alongside allergic conditions and chemical irritation. Fractures due to facial trauma can involve 1 or multiple walls of the maxillary sinuses.[13,14]

Etiology
Maxillary sinus fractures can be isolated but they are systemically seen in all types of Le Fort

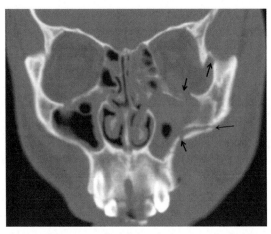

Fig. 26. CBCT coronal oblique shows zygomaticomaxillary, zygomaticofrontal, and orbital floor fractures (*arrows*).

fractures. They can also be associated with partial fractures of the maxilla that usually result from a hit delivered by a narrow object directly superior to the anterior aspect of the maxilla. A fracture sustained in this manner usually involves the anterolateral wall of the maxillary sinuses.

Fractures of the posterolateral wall of the sinus are most probably due to a transient increased pressure in the masticatory space, causing fracture and internal displacement of the fragments within the maxillary sinus.

Traumatic dental extractions can cause a fracture of the floor of the sinus that may lead to an oroantral communication. The possibility of intruding a tooth or a root tip during traumatic extraction can also cause an oroantral communication.

Clinical presentation
Fractures of the maxillary sinuses are usually associated with zygomatic bone fractures. In cases of isolated maxillary sinus fractures, presence of air under the skin of the cheek or bleeding during nose blowing is helpful in diagnosis. Isolated maxillary sinus fractures, however, can easily go undiagnosed, because few symptoms are associated with them.

Radiographic appearance
The radiographic manifestations of trauma to the sinuses vary from total opacification (cloudiness) of the sinus to mucosal thickening (hyperplastic mucosa) to presence of fluid level. The walls of the maxillary sinuses are remarkably thin; fragment displacement after fracture is easily detectable radiographically. Two major signs usually accompany fractures of the sinus walls: fluid in the sinus and air bubble collection within the soft tissues in the vicinity of the sinus. A direct impact of the coronoid process can also cause similar radiographic findings (**Figs. 27 and 28**).

Orbital Walls Fractures

Definition
Fractures of the orbits can be divided in 2 types: fracture of the orbital rim and fractures of the thin superior, lateral, and inferior walls of the orbit. The second type also is known as orbital blow-in or blow-out fractures, depending on the direction of the fracture and the displacement of the fragments.[13]

Etiology
Like so many other facial traumas, orbital wall fractures usually happen as a result of motor vehicle

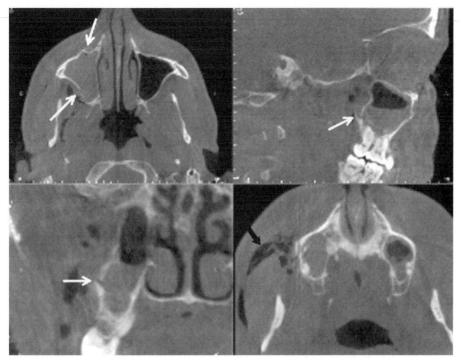

Fig. 27. CBCT multiplanar reformats show fractures of the anterior and lateral walls of the maxillary sinuses (*black arrow, lower right*) with air collection within the soft tissues (*white arrows, upper and lower left*).

accidents, industrial accidents, sports-related facial trauma, and assaults.

Clinical presentation
Black eyes, relative afferent pupil defect, diplopia, and significant periocular ecchymosis and edema are common findings.

Radiographic appearance
CT scans with coronal views are the most appropriate for specific evaluation of the orbit in cases

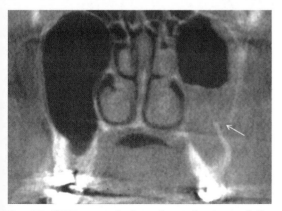

Fig. 28. CBCT coronal view shows fracture of the lateral wall of the left sinus with a fluid level noted (*arrow*).

of blow-out fractures. If the floor of orbit is fractured, the typical feature is inferior displacement of the fragments with periorbital fat herniation within the maxillary sinus. If the medial wall of the orbit, called also lamina papyracea, is fractured, the fragments are displaced within the ethmoid air cells and fluid material detected within these air cells; orbital soft tissues can be entrapped within the fracture. The possibility of muscle entrapment between the fragments needs to be always considered when diagnosing blow-out fractures; if the floor of the orbit is fractured, the inferior rectus muscle might be affected. When the medial wall is fractured, the mesial rectus muscle might become entrapped (Fig. 29).

Le Fort Fractures

Definition
Le Fort fractures are fractures of the midface with 1 major common feature: the separation of 2 or multiple portions of the midface from the skull base. The pterygoid plates of the sphenoid bone connect the midface to the skull base; involvement of pterygoid plates almost always indicates a fracture in one of the Le Fort planes.[15]

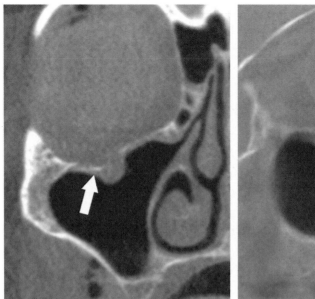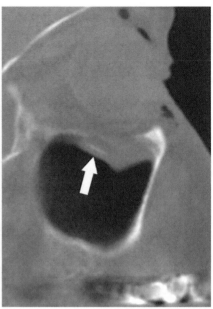

Fig. 29. CBCT coronal (*left*) and sagittal views (*right*) show a blow-out fracture of the floor of the orbit (*arrows*).

The Le Fort classification system attempts to categorize according to the plane of fracture and separation.

To classify the type of Le Fort fracture, radiologists need to assess the 3 bone structures that are unique to each type of Le Fort fracture.[16]

- Anterolateral margin of the nasal fossa for Le Fort I
- Inferior orbital rim for Le Fort II
- Zygomatic arch for Le Fort III

For a proper and efficient Le Fort fracture diagnosis, the radiologist and clinician should pause after identifying 1 Le Fort fracture because fractures may occur in more than 1 Le Fort plane on the same side. It should not be assumed that Le Fort fractures are perfectly symmetric, because they can occur in different planes on each side. Le Fort fractures are not always isolated; they may be associated with other types of fractures that do not fit the plane of the already diagnosed Le Fort–type fracture.

Le Fort I Le Fort I fracture involves the anterolateral margin of the nasal fossa, the walls of maxillary sinuses, the lower nasal septum, and the inferior part of the pterygoid plates (**Fig. 30**).

Maxillary teeth are movable relative to the remainder of face.

Le Fort II Le Fort II fracture involves the inferior orbital rim, root of the nose, posterior and lateral walls of maxillary sinuses, orbital floor, lamina papyracea, and nasofrontal suture. Posteriorly, the fracture extends inferiorly across the infratemporal surface of the maxilla and involves the lower pterygoid plates.

Teeth and nose as a unit are movable relative to the skull.

Le Fort III Le Fort III fracture involves the zygomatic arch, lateral orbital wall and rim, medial orbital wall, and nasofrontal suture. First fracture is situated near junction of frontal bone, and

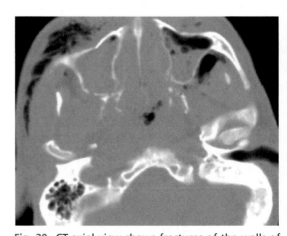

Fig. 30. CT axial view shows fractures of the walls of maxillary sinuses and the inferior part of the pterygoid plates. Air emphysema is noted in the left masticator space and in the right cheek.

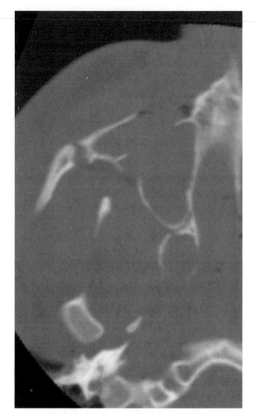

Fig. 31. Cropped axial CT shows fractures of the anterior and lateral walls of the sinus, zygomatic arch, and pterygoid plates.

greater wing of sphenoid. A second fracture line extends from the orbital floor down across the back of each maxilla to the lower portion of the pterygoid plates. The fracture of the zygomatic arches completes the separation of the facial skeleton from the skull base (**Figs. 31** and **32**).

Teeth, nose, and zygomatic bones are movable as a unit relative to the rest of skull.

Etiology

The Le Fort I fracture usually results from a direct horizontal blow to the face mostly from motor vehicle accidents.

Clinical appearance

Obstruction of the bony architecture with soft tissue swelling, ecchymoses, gross blood, and hematoma are some common findings. Periorbital swelling or dish-face or pan-face deformity may indicate Le Fort II or III fractures. Premature contact of the molar teeth, resulting in an anterior open bite deformity, is another clinical finding.

Radiographic appearance

CT and CBCT are the radiographic modalities of choice for the most comprehensive evaluation of the facial fractures; they are currently the reference standard for assessing maxillofacial injuries. The radiologist is normally the primary specialist evaluating these injuries. The most useful diagnostic information is obtained by examining multiplanar reconstructions because a single-plane sectional image does not provide sufficiently detailed information as examining the same area from 3 different perspectives. The ability of generating a multitude of customized sections, made possible with the latest acquisition and processing technology, provides the radiologist and surgeon with more advanced diagnostic and treatment planning tools.

MDCT and CBCT provide excellent 3-D reconstructions. Although some details might be compromised by the reconstruction software programs and the operating computer specifications, 3-D images serve as an excellent communication tool between the radiologists and surgeons; they can provide accurate interpretation and, potentially just as relevant, clear communication of the findings to facilitate appropriate care of these patients. 3-D images usually permit clinicians to

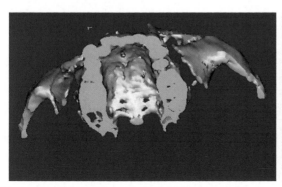
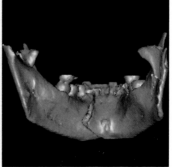

Fig. 32. This image shows the use of CBCT 3-D rendering for detection and evaluation fractures. This 3-D rendering of a patient's maxilla, zygoma (*left*), and mandible (*right*) after a motor vehicle accident showing a triple mandibular fracture and bilateral fracture of the zygomatic bones with complete separation.

envision the fragments and their relationship to one another better than plane 2-D scan images, especially if large surfaces are involved with displaced fragments. Currently, many institutions are using advanced technology, such as advanced 3-D image processing, rapid prototyping, and virtual surgical repair. 3-D reconstruction software programs occupy a larger place in the treatment planning for facial trauma cases than before, and clinicians can now manipulate the bone fragments on the screen to plan the appropriate treatment approach and predict the results. Improved surgical outcome has been seen in 33% of cases because of better diagnostic ability using CT.[17]

SUMMARY

Complexity of osseous maxillofacial anatomic structures and importance of the tissues they protect emphasize the importance of detection of any injury caused by a traumatic aggression. Plain film radiography, for a long time, has played a major role in detecting fractures of the maxillofacial complex and planning their treatment approach. Introduction of advanced imaging techniques with sectional abilities and high resolution have improved the sensitivity of radiographic examinations in detecting fine details and in providing a more comprehensive picture of complex fractures for better diagnosis. Addition of 3-D reconstruction, moreover, improved the treatment planning protocols mainly for large traumatic injuries with loss of structures.

REFERENCES

1. Noikura T, Shinoda K, Ando S. Image visibility of maxillo-facial fractures in conventional and panoramic radiography. Dentomaxillofac Radiol 1978; 7(1):35–42.
2. Andreasen JO, Borum MK, Jacobsen HL, et al. Replantation of 400 avulsed permanent incisors. 4. Factors related to periodontal ligament healing. Endod Dent Traumatol 1995;11:76–89.
3. Andersson L, Andreasen JO, Day P, et al. International association of dental traumatology guidelines for the management of traumatic dental injuries: 2. Avulsion of permanent teeth. Dent Traumatol 2012; 28:88–96.
4. Evans D. Splinting duration for replanted avulsed teeth. Evid Based Dent 2009;10(4):104.
5. Bornstein M, Wölner-Hanssen AB, Sendi P, et al. Comparison of intraoral radiography and limited cone beam computed tomography for the assessment of root-fractured permanent teeth. Dent Traumatol 2009;25(6):571–7.
6. Wang P, Yan XB, Lui DG, et al. Detection of dental root fractures by using cone-beam computed tomography. Dentomaxillofac Radiol 2011;40(5): 290–8.
7. Gassner R, Bosch R, Tuli T, et al. Prevalence of dental trauma in 6000 patients with facial injuries: implications for prevention. Oral Surg Oral Med Oral Pathol Oral Radiol Endod 1999;87:27–33.
8. Glendor U, Marcenes W, Andreasen JO. Classification, etiology and epidemiology of traumatic dental injuries. In: Andreasen JO, Andreasen FM, Andersson L, editors. Textbook and color atlas of traumatic injuries to the teeth. Oxford (England): Blackwell Munksgaard; 2007. p. 217–54.
9. Lechner K, Connert T, Kühl S, et al. Lip and tooth injuries at public swimming pools in Austria. Dent Traumatol 2017;33(3):214–20.
10. McDonnell DG, Masterson J, Barry HJ, et al. The use of two-dimensional CT reconstruction to demonstrate a vertical fracture of the condylar head. Dentomaxillofac Radiol 1990;19(1):34–6.
11. Birgfeld C, Mundinger G, Gruss J. Evidence-based medicine: evaluation and treatment of zygoma fractures. Plast Reconstr Surg 2017; 139(1):168e–80e.
12. Yamsani B, Gaddipati R, Vura N, et al. Zygomaticomaxillary complex fractures: a review of 101 cases. J Maxillofac Oral Surg 2016;15(4):417–24.
13. Fama F, Cicciu M, Sindoni A, et al. Maxillofacial and concomitant serious injuries: an eight-year single center experience. Chin J Traumatol 2017; 20:4–8.
14. Imai T, Sukegawa S, Kanno T, et al. Mandibular fracture patterns consistent with posterior maxillary fractures involving the posterior maxillary sinus, pterygoid plate or both: CT characteristics. Dentomaxillofac Radiol 2014;43(2):20130355.
15. Christensen J, Sawatari Y, Peleg M. High-energy traumatic maxillofacial injury. J Craniofac Surg 2015;26:1487–91.
16. Patterson R. The Le Fort fractures: René Le Fort and his work in anatomical pathology. Can J Surg 1991; 34:183–4.
17. Shah S, Uppal SK, Mittal RK, et al. Diagnostic tools in maxillofacial fractures: is there really a need of three-dimensional computed tomography? Indian J Plast Surg 2016;49(2):225–33.

Alterations in Tooth Structure and Associated Systemic Conditions

Farah Masood, BDS, DDS, MS[a],*, Erika Benavides, DDS, PhD[b]

KEYWORDS

• Dental • Anomalies • Tooth abnormalities • Systemic • Syndromes

KEY POINTS

• Tooth development is a complex process that involves precise and time-dependent orchestration of multiple genetic, molecular, and cell interactions.
• The cause of most dental anomalies is multifactorial, including genetic and environmental contributors.
• Some dental abnormalities are commonly seen with specific systemic diseases and syndromes.
• Dental abnormalities can be broadly categorized as anomalies affecting the tooth number, size, shape, structure, eruption pattern, and position in the dental arch.

INTRODUCTION

The development of a normal dentition occurs from the dental lamina, which originates from a string of epithelial cells in the oral ectoderm during the early months of embryonic development. A variety of factors can affect the normal development of tissues and may lead to variation in the normal compliment of teeth and development of alterations and defects in the shape and size of teeth. These dental anomalies can be congenital, developmental, or acquired. This article discusses some of these tooth alterations with associated systemic and genetic conditions.

TOOTH NUMBER ANOMALIES
Hyperdontia

Definition: the presence of extra or supernumerary teeth in the dental arches beyond the normal 32 teeth of the permanent dentition and 20 teeth of the primary dentition.

Cause: genetic predisposition as well as environmental factors may increase the activity of the dental lamina leading to formation of the extra tooth/teeth.[1,2]

Clinical presentation: clinical intraoral and radiographic examinations are key in accurate diagnosis. Supernumerary teeth may occur in variable numbers, size, and locations, and tend to have variable morphology. They can be found in the primary and permanent dentitions. Supernumerary teeth may develop in any region of the dental arches; however, the most common sites tend to be the anterior maxilla, maxillary molar, and mandibular premolar regions. The term mesiodens is used when a supernumerary tooth is located close to the maxillary midline, between the central incisors.

Radiographic appearance: often, extra teeth remain embedded in bone because they do not have enough space to erupt. If not seen clinically, the presence of more than the normal number of

[a] Department Oral Diagnosis and Radiology, The University of Oklahoma, College of Dentistry, Office 286-A, 1201 North Stonewall Avenue, Oklahoma City, OK 73117, USA; [b] Department of Periodontics and Oral Medicine, The University of Michigan, School of Dentistry, Office 2029F, 1011 North University Avenue, Ann Arbor, MI 48109, USA
* Corresponding author.
E-mail address: Farah-Masood@ouhsc.edu

Radiol Clin N Am 56 (2018) 125–140
http://dx.doi.org/10.1016/j.rcl.2017.08.009

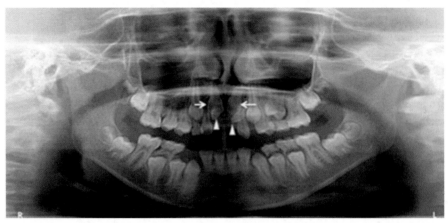

Fig. 1. Supernumerary teeth. Panoramic image shows 2 mesiodens (*arrowheads*) blocking the eruption of the permanent maxillary central incisors (*white arrows*). (*Courtesy of* Frederico Sampaio Neves, DDS, Brazil.)

teeth can be detected radiographically. The tooth may be inverted in position and located facial to, lingual to, or between the adjacent teeth (**Figs. 1–3**).

Clinical relevance: the effect of the supernumerary teeth on the surrounding teeth and bone may differ according to their relation to the adjacent teeth. Supernumerary teeth may cause impaction of adjacent teeth, varying degrees of root resorption, and thinning of the surrounding bone.

Associated conditions: supernumerary teeth can be an incidental finding or they may be associated with systemic or genetic disorders[3] (**Box 1**).

Hypodontia

Definition: the term hypodontia or oligodontia is used when the patient has less than the normal complement of teeth in the arches. This condition can be congenital or acquired. The term anodontia or agenesis is used for congenital absence of all teeth (failure of teeth to develop), which is a rare occurrence.

Cause: to date, the mutation spectra of nonsyndromic forms of familial and sporadic tooth agenesis in humans have revealed defects in various genes that encode transcription factors, Msh homeobox 1 gene (MSX1) and Paired box gene 9 (PAX9), or genes that code for a protein involved in canonical Wnt signaling (Axis inhibition protein 2 [AXIN2]), and a transmembrane receptor of fibroblast growth factor receptor 1 (FGFR1).[4]

Possible causes of acquired hypodontia include destruction of tooth buds and follicles caused by trauma or primary teeth infection affecting the developing permanent dentition, or extraction of teeth.

Clinical presentation: hypodontia can be partial or complete. The most commonly missing teeth are the third molars, followed by maxillary lateral incisors and mandibular second premolars. Hypodontia can be seen in primary and permanent dentition.

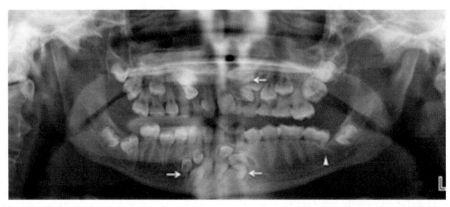

Fig. 2. Cleidocranial dysplasia. Panoramic image shows several supernumerary teeth in maxilla and mandible (*white arrows*). Arrowhead is showing root dilaceration. (*Courtesy of* Kevin Smith, DDS, Oklahoma City, OK.)

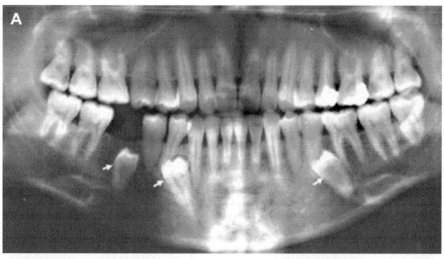

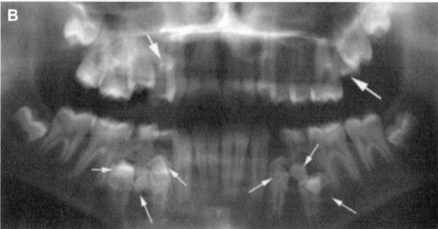

Fig. 3. Familial nonsyndromic supernumerary teeth. (*A*) Panoramic image of the mother. (*B*) Her 11-year-old son with 2 maxillary and 6 mandibular supernumerary teeth (*white arrows*). (*Data from* Orhan AI, Ozer L, Orhan K. Familial occurrence of nonsyndromal multiple supernumerary teeth. Angle Orthod 2006:76(5);891–7.)

Radiographic appearance: congenital or hereditary failure of teeth development shows single or multiple missing teeth (**Figs. 4** and **5**). Acquired hypodontia after tooth extraction may result in horizontal and vertical alveolar bone loss and malpositioning of teeth.

Clinical relevance: esthetic problems, or possible increased risk of sleep-disordered breathing caused by decreased development of the transverse dimension of the jaw arches, may be reported.

Associated conditions: conditions associated with hypodontia are listed in **Box 1**.

Solitary Median Maxillary Incisor

Definition: solitary median maxillary incisor (SMMI) is the presence of a single or solitary central incisor located in the midline of the maxillary arch.

Box 1
Hyperdontia and hypodontia: associated syndromes

Hyperdontia

Cleidocranial dysplasia

Gardner

Nance-Horan

Ehlers-Danlos

Hypodontia

Down

Ectodermal dysplasia

Axenfeld-Rieger

Leukemia

Hypophosphatasia

Radiation therapy

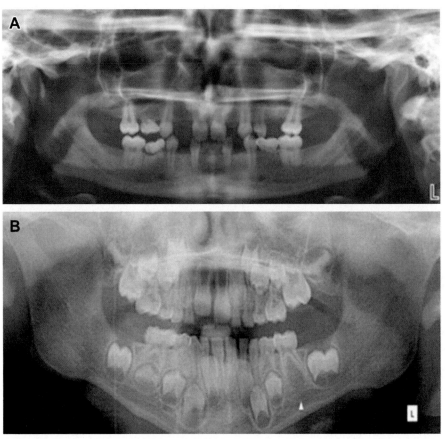

Fig. 4. Congenital hypodontia. (*A*) Multiple missing teeth noted in the dental arches. (*B*) Second left premolar is missing (*white arrowhead*). (*Courtesy of* Martha Garzon, DMD, MS, Edmond, OK.)

Cause: this is rare developmental anomaly and the cause is uncertain but may be associated with mutations in the sonic hedgehog (SHH) gene in chromosome 7q.

Clinical presentation: the single central incisor usually develops exactly along the midline, with the crown and root sizes the same as those of a normal central incisor (**Fig. 6**). The condition rarely presents as an isolated trait and is also known as SMMI syndrome when associated with other abnormalities. It occurs in 1 in 50,000 live births, with greater occurrence in girls.[5] It may affect

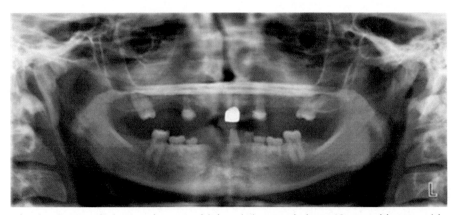

Fig. 5. Hypodontia. Panoramic image shows multiple missing teeth in a 19-year-old man with ectodermal dysplasia.

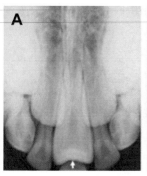
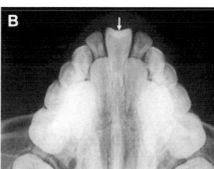

Fig. 6. Solitary median maxillary central incisor syndrome. Intraoral images (A, B) show the single central maxillary incisor (*white arrows*). *From* Machado E, Machado P, Grehs B, et al. Sindrome do incisive central superior solitário: relato de caso. Dental Press J Orthod 2010;15(4)55-61; with permission.

both the primary and permanent dentitions and it is commonly associated with defects of midline structures, including the craniofacial bones, nasal airways (choanal atresia, nasal pyriform aperture stenosis), and the brain (holoprosencephaly), along with an increased risk of pituitary malformation and malfunction.[6]

Radiographic appearance: radiographically, the single central incisor appears normal except for its position in the midline. It is superimposed over the intermaxillary suture on two-dimensional views but it usually forms buccal to it along the alveolar ridge (Fig. 7).

Clinical relevance: in contrast with a mesiodens, which is a conically shaped tooth, usually asymmetric in position and present in the permanent dentition between 2 normal central incisor teeth off the midline, an SMMI is commonly associated with developmental midline structural malformations such as short stature, congenital nasal abnormalities, microcephaly, scoliosis, heart disease, and growth deficiencies.

Associated conditions: SMMIs may be associated with growth hormone deficiency or other structural anomalies in the midline of the body; therefore, early diagnosis and follow-up are important, because it may be a sign of other severe congenital or developmental abnormalities.[7]

TOOTH SIZE ANOMALIES
Macrodontia (Megadontia)

Definition: teeth are larger than normal in size compared with the adjacent teeth.

Cause: localized occurrence may be caused by disturbance in morphodifferentiation, whereas generalized macrodontia may be attributed to hormonal imbalance.

Clinical presentation: a single tooth or multiple teeth may appear larger than normal compared with the adjacent teeth. The total number of teeth in the dentition is usually not affected, differentiating it from tooth gemination or fusion.

Radiographic appearance: the localized form of macrodontia is limited to single to few teeth. Proportional enlargement of the crown, pulp chamber, root canal, and root is noted. Hyperplasia of the jaw is also present in some cases.

Clinical relevance: oral complications include esthetic and periodontal issues, impaction of teeth, malocclusion, and crowding. Clinicians

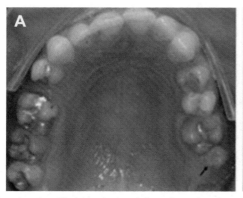
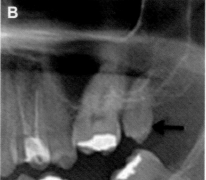

Fig. 7. Microdontia. Clinical picture (A) and cropped panoramic image (B) show a microdont (*black arrow*). (*Courtesy of* Frederico Sampaio Neves, DDS, Brazil.)

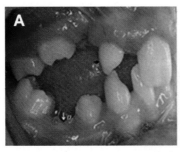 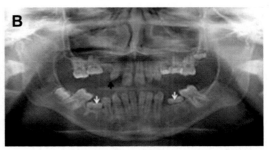

Fig. 8. Microdontia of maxillary right lateral incisor. (*A*) Clinical picture; (*B*) panoramic image (*black arrows*). White arrows are pointing towards retain primary mandibular molars. (*Courtesy of* David M. Sarver, DDS, Birmingham, AL.)

must differentiate this condition from fusion and gemination.

Associated conditions: systemic diseases such as pituitary gigantism and hemifacial hypertrophy may result in a more generalized form of macrodontia.[8]

Microdontia

Definition: teeth appear abnormally small compared with the surrounding teeth in the dental arches.

Cause: genetic and environmental factors play a role, although the initiating factors causing microdontia remain unknown.[9,10]

Clinical presentation: a single tooth or multiple teeth may be involved (**Fig. 8**). The maxillary lateral incisors and third molars are most commonly affected. When maxillary lateral incisors are smaller than normal, they are called peg laterals.

Radiographic appearance: abnormally small tooth or teeth are noted (see **Fig. 8**).

Clinical relevance: cosmetic concerns may arise caused by the size and shape of these teeth when present in the esthetic zone.

Associated conditions: syndromes associated with microdontia are listed in **Box 2**.

Abnormalities in tooth eruption
Primary failure eruption: primary failure eruption is idiopathic failure of the eruptive mechanism of the tooth. This condition is a rare anomaly of unknown cause that involves arrested eruption of teeth in the absence of a local or general contributory factors (**Fig. 9**).

GENETIC ALTERATION IN TOOTH STRUCTURE
Amelogenesis Imperfecta

Definition: amelogenesis imperfecta (AI) is a developmental condition that consists of a rare group of inherited abnormalities that involve an abnormal or defective enamel formation and/or calcification process that is not associated with defects in other parts of the body.

Cause: mutations in the Amelogenin, X isoform (AMELX), Enamelin (ENAM), Matrix metalloproteinase-20 (MMP20), and Uncharacterized protein FAM83H (FAM83H) genes can cause AI.[11]

Clinical presentation: teeth may be unusually small, discolored, pitted, grooved, and prone to rapid wear and breakage. Both primary and permanent dentitions may be involved. Enamel defects are present in the absence of a systemic condition. Researchers have described at least 14 forms of AI, which are distinguished by their specific dental abnormalities and by their pattern of inheritance; however, it can be classified into 4 main types: hypoplastic, hypomaturation, hypocalcified, and hypomaturation-hypocalcified.

Radiographic appearance: pitted teeth appear as radiolucent flecks on the crowns of the involved teeth. Dentin, pulp chambers, and roots appear normal. Crown height may appear vertically reduced because of wear (**Fig. 10**). Because of missing enamel in advanced cases, the coronal portion of the tooth may have homogeneous radiodensity.

Clinical relevance: the main concerns with AI are caries susceptibility, tooth wear, and esthetic issues.

Box 2
Macrodontia and microdontia: associated syndromes

Macrodontia

Pituitary gigantism

Hemifacial hypertrophy

Localized hemangioma and lymphangioma

Microdontia

Ectodermal dysplasia

Cleft lip and palate

Van der Woude

Down

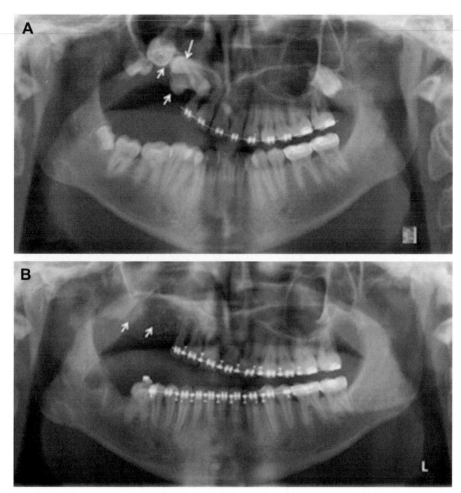

Fig. 9. Primary failure of eruption. (*A*) Panoramic image shows asymmetry and multiple unerupted malpositioned teeth (*white arrows*) in right posterior maxilla. (*B*) Follow-up panoramic image shows removal of unerupted teeth. (*Courtesy of* Kevin Smith, DDS, Oklahoma City, OK.)

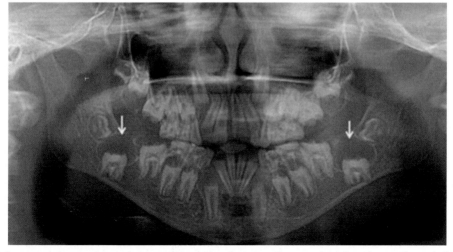

Fig. 10. AI. Panoramic image shows absence of enamel surfaces on all erupted teeth and several cysts (*white arrows*). (*Courtesy of* Frederico Sampaio Neves, DDS, Brazil.)

Associated conditions: the literature describes AI and AI-like changes associated with many syndromes. Some of these are listed in **Box 3**.

Box 3
Amelogenesis imperfecta: associated syndromes

AI

Tricho-dento-osseous syndrome, Kohlschutter syndrome, platyspondyly with AI

Nephrocalcinosis and AI

Cone rod dystrophy and AI

Data from Crawford PJM, Aldred M, Bloch-Zupan A. Amelogenesis imperfecta. Orphanet J Rare Dis 2007;2:17.

Dentinogenesis Imperfecta

Definition: dentinogenesis imperfecta (DI) is a rare inherited defect of the mesodermal portion of the developing teeth and is transmitted in an autosomal dominant or recessive mode.[8] Researchers have described 3 types of DI with similar dental abnormalities. Type I occurs in people who also have osteogenesis imperfecta, a genetic condition in which bones are brittle and easily broken. DI type II and type III usually occur in people without other inherited disorders.

Cause: it is a rare dentin genetic disease. Mutations in the dentin sialophosphoprotein gene have been identified in DI types II and III.

DI type I occurs as part of osteogenesis imperfecta, which is caused by mutations in one of several other genes (most often the collagen type 1 alpha 1 chain [COL1A1] or collagen type 1 alpha 2 chain [COL1A2] genes).

Clinical presentation: DI affects the 2 dentitions, with blue-amber opalescent teeth, bulbous crowns, and important attrition, but the major difference between the different types of DI comes from the pulpal aspect. Affected teeth are described as shell teeth because of an important pulp enlargement on dental radiographs. Pulp is apparent through occlusal dentin and exposures are frequent.

Radiographic appearance: the pulpal enlargement results in a reduction in dentin tissue. The radiographic appearance is pathognomonic. Images show reduced bulbous crowns caused by cervical constriction, short and thick roots, and pulp obliteration (**Fig. 11**).

Clinical relevance: because of the shape abnormality of teeth, periodontal disease may occur.

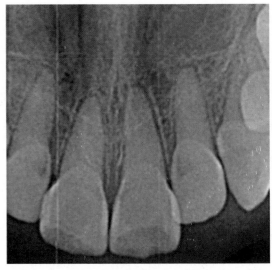

Fig. 11. DI. Intraoral image shows obliteration of the pulp chambers and canals. (*Courtesy of* Martha Garzon, DMD, MS, Edmond, OK.)

Enamel may fracture easily and teeth may wear down to the gingival level.

Associated conditions: type I DI is associated with osteogenesis imperfecta.

Dentin Dysplasia

Definition: dentin dysplasia (DD) is a condition is characterized by the presence of normal tooth enamel but atypical dentin with abnormal pulpal morphology.

Cause: DD is a genetic disorder of dentition with an autosomal dominant trait.

Clinical presentation: this dentinal defect is an extremely rare condition. Both primary and permanent dentitions may be involved. In the radicular type (type 1), the teeth may appear normal on clinical examination. However, tooth mobility may develop, leading to mobility and eventually premature exfoliation of teeth either spontaneously or after minor trauma.[12] In the coronal type (type 2), the teeth have a clinical appearance similar to that of DI.

Radiographic appearance: characteristic radiographic findings may include presence of shorter, abnormally shaped roots or absence of roots in severe cases (rootless teeth) (**Fig. 12**). Merged roots with an apical conical aspect with sharp construction have been reported.[13] Premature loss of teeth and short roots and/or length alterations help to distinguish this condition from hypophosphatasia. The pulp is replaced by a calcified/mineralized tissue that resembles pulp stones. Pulp chambers become completely or partially obliterated and crescent-shaped horizontal radiolucent lines may be observed on the radiographs. Rarefying osteitis

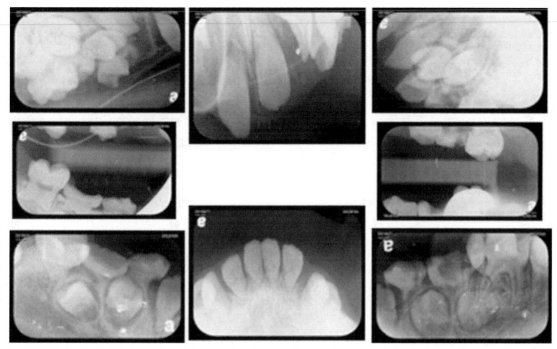

Fig. 12. DD. Periapical images show abnormal pulp chambers and short roots. (*Courtesy of* James R. Boynton, DDS, MS, Elizabeth A. Barber, DDS, MS, and Kristin K. Auer, DDS, MS, University of Michigan, School of Dentistry.)

has been also reported, caused by communication between the remaining pulp and the oral cavity.[8]

Clinical relevance: esthetic issues and tooth retention are the main concerns. Long-term prognosis of teeth is questionable because of very short roots.

Associated conditions: DD is closely associated with DI type II and III.

Regional Odontodysplasia

Definition: this rare developmental anomaly of the dental hard tissues affects ectodermal and mesodermal dental components. It has characteristic clinical and radiographic findings that include localized occurrence within a particular segment in either or both dentitions; hypocalcification and hypoplasia of the enamel and dentin; discolored, small, and distorted affected teeth with various surface markings; and delayed or failed eruption caused by arrested root formation.[14]

Cause: unknown. Contributing factors may include genetic mutations, vascular abnormalities, or viral causes.

Clinical presentation: only a few isolated cases have been reported. Primary teeth are most commonly involved. Single or multiple quadrants may be affected. Most often the maxilla is involved. Patients report delay or failure in tooth eruption. Clinically, teeth show malformed, rough, grooved, hypoplastic, and discolored coronal surfaces. Gingival tissue can be hyperemic and usually presents a

fistula. In the permanent dentition, teeth are usually not erupted or can be partially erupted with fibrous gingival tissue coverage.[15] The condition often presents in other members of the patient's family.

Radiographic appearance: radiographic features of the involved teeth include thin and defective layers of enamel and dentin, resulting in faint, fuzzy outline, creating a ghostlike appearance caused by dental enamel hypoplasia and hypomineralization (**Fig. 13**).

Clinical relevance: significant functional and esthetic problems may occur. Some clinicians advocate early extraction of the affected teeth because many of them are not restorable and could develop dental abscesses soon after eruption. In contrast, retaining noninfected teeth helps maintain the height of alveolar bone, avoids the need for a removable prosthesis, and eliminates the psychological effects of premature tooth loss.

Associated conditions: regional odontodysplasia may be associated with hypophosphatasia, hypocalcemia, hyperpyrexia, as well as local trauma and irradiation.

CHANGES ASSOCIATED WITH CROWN MORPHOLOGY
Fusion

Definition: fusion is a rare developmental disorder characterized by the union of 2 adjacent teeth at

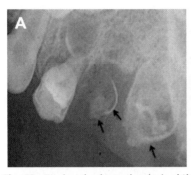

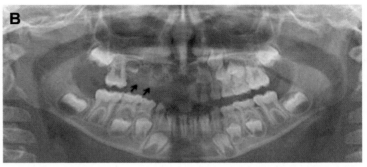

Fig. 13. Regional odontodysplasia. (*A*) Periapical radiograph shows ghostlike teeth (*black arrows*). (*B*) Panoramic image shows thin shell of hypoplastic enamel and dentin (*black arrows*). (*Courtesy of* [*A*] David Lewis, DDS, MS, University of Oklahoma College of Dentistry, Oklahoma City, OK; and [*B*] Jae Hyun Park, DMD, MSD, MS, PhD, AT Still University, Arizona School of Dentistry and Oral Health.)

the crown level (enamel and dentin), causing the formation of a tooth with an enlarged clinical crown.

Cause: involvement of epithelial and mesenchymal germ layers results in irregular tooth morphology. The cause of the condition is unknown, but the influence of surrounding physical forces causing close contact between 2 developing tooth buds and genetic predisposition are often suggested as possible causative factors.[16]

Clinical presentation: fusion may be partial or total, depending on the stage of tooth development at the time of union. It can occur in any phase of dental development, and is characterized most commonly by the appearance of a clinically large and wide tooth. Fused teeth are more prevalent in the primary dentition than in the permanent dentition. Fusion usually involves the incisors and canines, and the occurrence of fusion is rare in permanent posterior teeth. When the fusion or union occurs, pulp chambers and canals may be joined or remain separated, depending on the developmental stage of dentition.

Radiographic appearance: fused teeth may have a single large crown combined with dentin. The pulp canals may be joined as 1 or the fused tooth may have a divided pulp chamber. Both of the conjoint buds may be normal, or 1 may be supernumerary.

Clinical relevance: esthetic, spacing, periodontal, eruption, and caries issues may arise because of unusual and irregular tooth morphology.

Associated conditions: dental fusion may be associated with the otodental syndrome, which is an inherited autosomal dominant condition characterized by a striking dental phenotype known as globodontia, associated with sensorineural high-frequency hearing loss and eye coloboma, which has been described in at least 9 families.[12] Globodontia refers to the enlarged, bulbous,

fused, malformed posterior teeth with no discernible cusps or grooves and occurs in both primary and permanent dentitions, affecting canine and molar teeth.

Gemination

Definition: gemination or dental twinning is a phenomenon in which a single tooth bud attempts to divide into 2 teeth. There may be a partial or complete division.

Cause: local metabolic interferences, which occur during morphodifferentiation of the tooth germ, may be the cause and there could be a relationship between gemination, twinning, and odontoma.[17]

Clinical presentation: gemination most frequently affects the primary teeth, but it may occur in the permanent dentition, usually in the incisor region. Geminated teeth are typically disfigured or bifid because of irregularities of the enamel. The total number of teeth in the arch is normal.[8]

Radiographic appearance: teeth affected by gemination have a single root. The crown appears abnormally large and the root may or may not be of normal size (**Fig. 14**).

Clinical relevance: the area of hypoplasia may be prone to caries and may present esthetic issues.

Associated conditions: dental fusion and gemination have been reported in some cases of Kabuki make-up syndrome (KMS). KMS is a rare, multisystem disorder characterized by multiple abnormalities, including distinctive facial features, growth delays, varying degrees of intellectual disability, skeletal abnormalities, and short stature. Oral manifestations are commonly observed in KMS (68% of the cases) and may comprise micrognathia; retrognathia; high-arched palate; posterior crossbite; cleft lip/palate; bifid tongue and

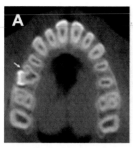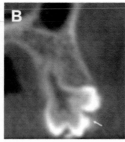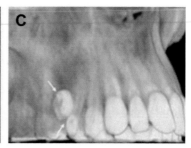

Fig. 14. Gemination of posterior maxillary premolar (*white arrows*) shown on the Cone beam computed tomographic images. (*A*) axial, (*B*) cross-section, (*C*) 3-D.

uvula; widely spaced teeth; ectopic permanent first molars; delayed tooth eruption pattern; external root resorption of the permanent upper incisors and molars; impacted teeth; and dental anomalies such as hypodontia, conical teeth, neonatal teeth, and teeth with large pulp chambers.[18]

Talon Cusp

Definition: talon cusp is development of an extra (supernumerary) cusp on a tooth and is also referred to as eagle's talon, dens evaginatus, and supernumerary cusp.[19]

Cause: the cause of the formation of the talon cusp is unknown.

Clinical presentation: clinically it is seen as a prominent accessory hornlike structure that projects from the cingulum or cementoenamel junction of the maxillary or mandibular teeth. It can occur in primary and permanent dentition and can lead to occlusal interference, irritation of the tongue, pulpal necrosis, caries, and periodontal problems. Talon cusps occur most often on the palatal surface of permanent maxillary incisors. Deep developmental groves may be present. The classification of talon cusps is shown in **Box 4**.

Radiographic appearance: radiopaque smooth outline of the talon cusp is superimposed over the crown of the affected tooth (**Fig. 15**).

Clinical relevance: talon cups may interfere with normal occlusion. Also, the deep developmental groves may be prone to dental caries, which may not be detected until pulp inflammation occurs.

Box 4
Classification of talon cusps according to degree of cusp formation and extension

Type I (talon)

Morphologically well-delineated additional cusp that projects from the palatal surface to at least half the distance between CEJ and incisal edge.

Type II (semitalon)

Additional cusp (≤1 mm) that may blend with the palatal surface or stand away from the rest of crown. It extends less than halfway between CEJ and incisal edge

Type III (trace talon)

Enlarged cingula that may have a conical, bifid, or tuberclelike appearance

Abbreviation: CEJ, cemento-enamel junction.

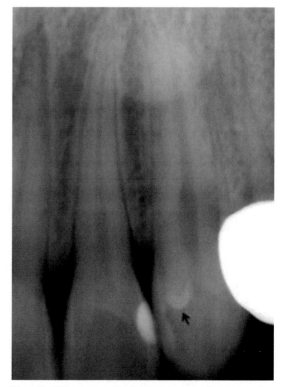

Fig. 15. Talon cusp. Periapical image shows a talon cusp on maxillary left canine (*black arrow*).

Associated conditions: patients with Rubinstein-Taybi syndrome may have hypodontia, hyperdontia, natal teeth, and talon cusps.[20]

Turner Hypoplasia

Definition: hypoplasia is defined as a visual quantitative defect in the enamel surface or reduction in the normal thickness of enamel layer of a tooth.[7] Clinically, Turner hypoplasia appears as an external deformity involving the surface of the enamel. The enamel may be partially or completely missing. Enamel is reduced in thickness locally compared with adjacent areas.

Cause: Turner hypoplasia is usually caused by either trauma or infection to a primary tooth that affects the developing permanent tooth underneath.

Clinical presentation: Turner hypoplasia usually manifests as a portion of missing or diminished enamel, generally affecting 1 or more permanent teeth. If it involves anterior teeth, the most likely cause is traumatic injury leading to primary incisors being knocked out or driven into the alveolus and affecting the permanent tooth bud.

Developmental defects of the permanent successor tooth range from mild changes in enamel mineralization in the form of simple white or yellow-brown discoloration to crown malformations. The characteristics of clinical enamel hypoplasia include unfavorable esthetics, higher dentin sensitivity, malocclusion, and dental caries susceptibility.[8] The types of Turner hypoplasia are shown in **Box 5**.

Radiographic appearance: altered contour of the coronal surface of the tooth and irregularity are noted (**Fig. 16**).

Clinical relevance: Turner hypoplasia can cause unfavorable esthetics, higher dentin sensitivity, malocclusion, and increased caries susceptibility.

Associated conditions: enamel hypoplasia may occur during radiation therapy and multiple teeth may be involved.

Dens Evaginatus

Definition: dens evaginatus is an uncommon condition characterized by out-pouching of the enamel organ and there is formation of an extra cusp or tubercle on the occlusal surface of a posterior tooth or lingual aspect of the anterior tooth.

Cause: the cause of dens evaginatus remains unknown.

Clinical presentation: dens evaginatus has been described as a hard polyplike protuberance predominantly located in the central groove or lingual ridge of a buccal cusp of posterior teeth and in the cingulum fossa of anterior teeth. Rarely it may occur on the facial aspect of a tooth. Enamel covers a dentinal core that usually contains pulp tissue. Premolars are most likely to be affected by dens evaginatus and the condition is sometimes called the Leong premolar.

Radiographic appearance: radiographs may show the extension of the tooth's pulp horn into the tubercle of the dens evaginatus. The dentin

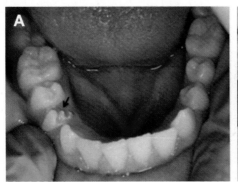 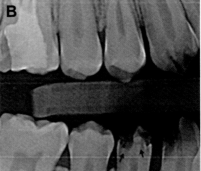

Fig. 16. Turner hypoplasia. (*A*) Clinically defective enamel on the first mandibular premolar (*black arrow*). (*B*) Bitewing radiograph shows the radiolucent defect (*black arrows*). (*Courtesy of* Martha Garzon, DMD, MS, Edmond, OK.)

core is usually covered with a radiopaque enamel layer (**Fig. 17**).

Clinical relevance: because of excessive occlusal trauma over time this tubercle tends to fracture leading to pulpal exposure of the involved tooth and the tooth may need root canal treatment. This condition may be discovered incidentally in asymptomatic patients.

Associated conditions: most cases reported in the literature indicate that dens evaginatus is an isolated anomaly rather than an integral part of any disorder. It has not been reported as an integral part of any specific syndrome, although it seems to be more prevalent in patients with Rubinstein-Taybi syndrome, Mohr syndrome (orofacial-digital II syndrome), and Ellis-van Creveld syndrome.[21]

Dens Invaginatus

Definition: dens invaginatus is also known as dens in dente or tooth within a tooth. There is invagination or the infolding of the enamel surface into the interior aspect of the tooth.

Cause: the cause of this malformation is still unclear.

Clinical presentation: classification of invaginated teeth is described in **Box 6**.

Radiographic appearance: this condition may affect the normal morphology of a tooth and the root canal system may be involved in larger anomalies. The defect may vary in size and shape from a

---

Box 6
Forms of dens invaginatus

Type I

Enamel-lined minor form within the crown, not extending beyond the CEJ

Type II

Enamel-lined form invading the root but confined as a bind sac, which may or may not communicate with the dental pulp

Type IIIA

Penetrates through the root and communicates laterally with the periodontal ligament space through a pseudoforamen. Usually no communication with the pulp

Type IIIB

Penetrates through the root and perforates at the apical area through a pseudoforamen

Rare radicular form

Arises secondary to a proliferation of the Hertwig root sheath and, radiographically, the affected tooth shows an enlargement of the root

---

looplike, pear-shaped, or slightly radiolucent structure to a severe form resembling a tooth within a tooth (**Fig. 18**). The outline of the invagination is generally well defined, with an opaque layer of enamel.[22]

Clinical relevance: this invagination on the tooth acts as niche for bacterial growth and food impaction, leading to dental caries in many cases. Early detection and sealing of its opening with restorative materials can effectively prevent those complications, as well as infection.

Associated conditions: there are multiple case reports in the dental literature of invaginated teeth coincident with other dental anomalies and syndromes, including microdontia, macrodontia, hypodontia, oligodontia, taurodontism, germination, fusion, supernumerary teeth, AI, invagination in an odontome, multiple odontomes, coronal agenesis, William syndrome, mesiodens, talon cusp, dens evaginatus, Crouzon syndrome, and Apert syndrome.[23]

CHANGES ASSOCIATED WITH PULP CHAMBER AND ROOT MORPHOLOGY
Taurodontism

Definition: also called bull teeth, taurodontism is a morphologic abnormality of teeth with large pulp chambers and short roots. This condition

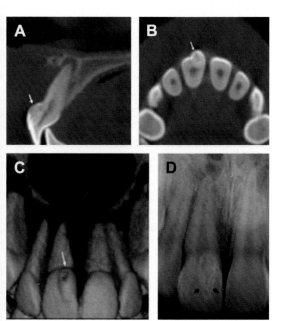

Fig. 17. Dens evaginatus (*arrows*) shown on CBCT (*A–C*) and periapical image (*D*).

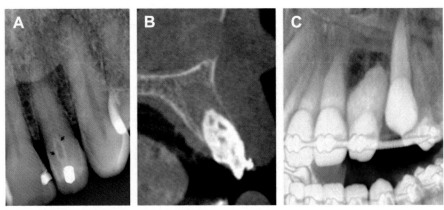

Fig. 18. Dens invaginatus. (A) Periapical image shows dens invaginatus on maxillary left lateral incisor (arrows). (B, C) CBCT images shows the anomaly dilating the root of the tooth and periapical infection caused by caries in the enamel defect in the crown.

can be described as a change in the shape of a tooth caused by failure of the Hertwig epithelial sheath diaphragm to invaginate at the proper horizontal level most frequently observed in molar teeth.

Cause: it has been suggested that this anomaly represents a primitive pattern, a mutation, a specialized or retrograde character, an atavistic feature, an X-linked trait, and a familial or autosomal dominant trait.[24]

Clinical presentation: teeth appear normal clinically.

Radiographic appearance: characteristic radiographic features of a taurodont tooth include vertical enlargement, apical displacement of the pulpal chamber, and no constriction at the level of the cementoenamel junction (Fig. 19). Radiographically, the distance from the roof of the pulp chamber to the root bifurcation is greatly increased.

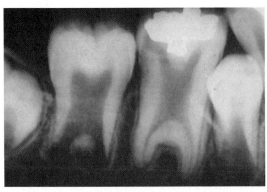

Fig. 19. Taurodontism. Periapical image shows the anomaly in first and second mandibular molars. Pulp chambers are vertically elongated. (Courtesy of David Lewis, DDS, MS, University of Oklahoma College of Dentistry, Oklahoma City, OK.)

Clinical relevance: endodontic treatment may become difficult as roots are apically displaced and the root canal orifices are apically located.

Associated conditions: it may exist as an isolated trait (autosomal dominant) or as part of several syndromes, including Down syndrome, tricho-dento-osseous syndrome, otodental dysplasia, ectodermal dysplasia, tooth and nail syndrome, AI, Mohr syndrome, and Klinefelter syndrome.

External Root Resorption

Definition: external root resorption refers to the loss of the outer aspect of the root caused by osteoclastic activity.

Cause: the definite cause of external root resorption is unknown but several factors, including impacted teeth, localized inflammation, trauma, and occlusal stresses and disorders, may contribute to its initiation and progression.

Clinical presentation: cervical invasive external root resorption is the only type of external root resorption that is clinical apparent as it starts at the cementoenamel junction level and extends coronally, apically, and toward the pulp, causing a pink discoloration of the crown where the resorptive defect is present. Single or multiple teeth may be involved. Advanced cases of external root resorption may present with pain, mobility, or even tooth fracture.

Radiographic appearance: it is most common at the apex and cervical aspect of the root. Radiographic features in an asymptomatic tooth may include blunting of root apex, normal surrounding bone, and intact lamina dura around the resorbed root (Fig. 20). The apical foramen also becomes prominent in some cases. The mesial and distal

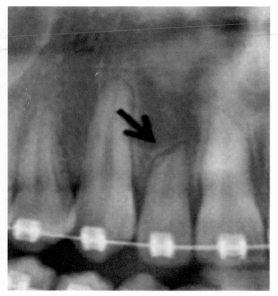

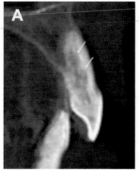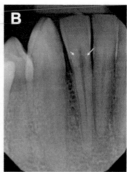

Fig. 21. Internal tooth resorption (*white arrows*). (*A*) CBCT cross-sectional image of maxillary lateral incisor shows large internal resorption. This pattern is consistent with a subtype called invasive cervical resorption. (*B*) Periapical radiograph of the anterior mandibular teeth shows a similar but milder presentation of the lesion.

Fig. 20. External root resorption noted on right maxillary lateral incisor (*black arrow*).

aspects of the root may be resorbed because of the pressure from an adjacent impacted tooth or a nearby lesion.

Clinical relevance: the resorptive defect may extend to the pulp, causing complications like inflammation, infection, and tooth loss.

Associated conditions: external root resorption may be associated with benign and malignant lesions. Benign lesions usually cause a decrease in root length, whereas malignant lesions cause a decrease in root width (spiky-looking roots).

It may also be associated with orthodontic tooth movement.

Internal Resorption

Definition: internal resorption is progressive loss of tooth structure that originates internally within a tooth and may involve the pulp chamber or root canal.

Cause: unknown, but possible causes include pulpal trauma and inflammation. Odontoclasts act to initiate the process.

Clinical presentation: internal root resorption is usually an incidental finding. In advanced resorption of the pulp chamber, the crown may show a dark pinkish shadow. Both primary and permanent dentitions may be involved. Central incisors and second molars are most commonly affected.

Radiographic appearance: enlargement of the pulp chamber or root canal is noted with the resorptive process (**Fig. 21**). The lesion appears radiolucent, round to oblong, and the borders are well demarcated. The pulp chamber and root

canal may appear irregular or abnormal in shape. On conventional radiographic images, resorptive defects within the pulp chamber may be confused with dental caries on the buccal or lingual surfaces of the tooth.

Clinical relevance: there is a risk of tooth perforation and fracture as the resorption expands.

Associated conditions: internal root resorption may be associated with chronic apical periodontitis.

Hypercementosis

Definition: hypercementosis is the excessive deposition of cementum on the external surfaces of the roots.

Cause: the exact cause is unknown but possible contributing factors include periapical chronic inflammation, supraeruption, and occlusal trauma.

Clinical presentation: hypercementosis is an idiopathic condition with no clinical finding. Clinical signs and symptoms may be present when the condition is associated with other entities, such as rarefying osteitis.

Radiographic appearance: hypercementosis is a radiographic finding. The root outline of the involved tooth may appear smooth but large and bulbous because of formation of extra cementum (**Fig. 22**). It may occur on the apex of the tooth only or may involve other parts of the root.

Clinical relevance: hypercementosis may complicate the extraction procedure because the diameter of the roots is increased relative to the cervical aspect of the alveolus.

Associated conditions: Paget disease, acromegaly, and vitamin A deficiency have been associated with hypercementosis.

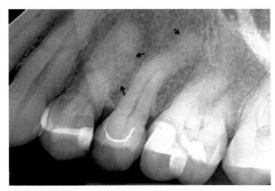

Fig. 22. Hypercementosis. Periapical image shows hypercementosis (*black arrows*) on left maxillary premolars.

SUMMARY

It is important that both dentists and physicians understand the link between dental anomalies and systemic conditions. Early identification of various dental anomalies may also help diagnose the underlying condition. Interdisciplinary management assists in formulating a better treatment plan and may improve the overall quality of life for patients.

REFERENCES

1. Barale SD, Kiran SDP. Non-syndromic occurrence of true generalized microdontia with mandibular mesiodens - a rare case. Head Face Med 2011;7:19.

2. Langlais RP, Langland OE, Nortje CJ. Diagnostic imaging of jaws. Baltimore (MD): Williams and Wilkins; 1995.

3. Lubinsky M, Kantaputra PN. Syndromes with supernumerary teeth. Am J Med Genet A 2016; 170:2611–6.

4. Chhabra N, Goswami M, Chhabra A. Genetic basis of dental agenesis–molecular genetics patterning clinical dentistry. Med Oral Patol Oral Cir Bucal 2014;19(2):e112–9.

5. Machado E, Machado P, Grehs B, et al. Solitary median maxillary central incisor syndrome: case report. Dental Press J Orthod 2010;15(4):55–61.

6. Hall RK. Solitary median maxillary central incisor (SMMCI) syndrome. Orphanet J Rare Dis 2006;1:12.

7. Utreja A, Zahid SN, Gupta R. Solitary median maxillary central incisor in association with hemifacial microsomia: a rare case report and review of literature. Contemp Clin Dent 2011;2(4):385–9.

8. White SC, Pharoah MJ. Oral radiology: the principles and interpretation. Chapter 31. St Louis (MO): Mosby; 2014. p. 582–611.

9. Thesleff I. The genetic basis of tooth development and dental defects. Am J Med Genet A 2006; 140(23):2530–5.

10. Elhaq S, Abdulghani A. Primary failure of eruption combined with bilateral transmigration of mandibular canines, transposition, torus palatinus, and class III incisor relationship: A rare case report. Eur J Dent 2015;9(4):594–8.

11. Aldred MJ, Savarirayan R, Crawford PJ. Amelogenesis imperfecta: a classification and catalogue for the 21st century [review]. Oral Dis 2003;9(1):19–23.

12. Bloch-Zupan A, Goodman JR. Otodental syndrome. Orphanet J Rare Dis 2006;1:5.

13. O'Carroll MK, Duncan WK, Perkins TM. Dentin dysplasia: review of the literature and a proposed subclassification based on radiographic findings. Oral Surg Oral Med Oral Pathol 1991;72(1):119–25.

14. Farman AG, Nortje CJ, Wood RE. Oral and maxillofacial diagnostic imaging. St Louis (MO): Mosby; 1993. p. 65–101.

15. Volpato L, Botelho G, Casela L, et al. Regional odontodysplasia: report of a case in the mandible crossing the midline. J Contemp Dent Pract 2008;9:142–8.

16. Rao BD, Sapna HS. A talon cusp on fused teeth associated with hypodontia: report of a unique case. Eur J Dent 2010;4(1):75–80.

17. Chipashvili N, Vadachkoria D, Beshkenadze E. Gemination or fusion? - challenge for dental practitioners (case study). Georgian Med News 2011;(194):28–33.

18. dos Santos BM, Ribeiro RR, Stuani AS, et al. Kabuki make-up (Niikawa-Kuroki) syndrome: dental and craniofacial findings in a Brazilian child. Braz Dent J 2006;17(3):249–54.

19. Praveen P, Anantharaj A, Venkataraghavan K, et al. Talon cusp in a primary tooth. J Dental Sci Res 2011;2(1):35–40.

20. Hennekam RC, Van Doorne JM. Oral aspects of Rubinstein-Taybi syndrome. Am J Med Genet Suppl 1990;6:42–7.

21. Hattab FN, Yassin OM, Sassa IS. Oral manifestations of Ellis-van Creveld syndrome (chondroectodermal dysplasia): report of two siblings with unusual dental anomalies. J Clin Pediatr Dent 1998;22(2):159–63.

22. Munir B, Tirmazi SM, Majeed HA, et al. Dens invaginatus: etiology, classification, prevalence, diagnosis and treatment considerations. Pakistan Oral Dental J 2011;31(1):191–8.

23. Oehlers FAC. Dens invaginatus. Part I: variations of the invagination process and association with anterior crown forms. Oral Surg Oral Med Oral Pathol 1957;10:1204–18.

24. Manjunatha BS, Kovvuru SK. Taurodontism - a review on its etiology, prevalence and clinical considerations. J Clin Exp Dent 2010;2(4):e187–90.

Radiology of Implant Dentistry

Asma'a Abdurrahman Al-Ekrish, MDS, Cert Diag Sci (OMFR)

KEYWORDS

- Dental implants • Multidetector computed tomography • Algorithms • Image processing
- Computer-assisted • Radiation dosage

KEY POINTS

- Multidetector computed tomography is useful in treatment planning, but has limited use during implant surgery and follow-up of cases.
- Low-dose protocols should be applied without compromising the diagnostic quality of images.
- Radiographic stents are necessary in multiple-implant and esthetically challenging cases.
- Proper image reformatting is necessary with sectional images being parallel and perpendicular to the jaws.
- Implant simulations are preferable to linear measurements of implant sites.

INTRODUCTION

Dental implant therapy is rapidly becoming more widespread in the management of missing teeth, and is considered the standard of care in the prosthetic treatment of completely edentulous cases.[1] Implant therapeutics begins with the treatment-planning phase, during which the oral and occlusal conditions are assessed clinically and the prosthetic needs are evaluated. A radiographic examination is then performed to evaluate the bone and the teeth associated with the edentulous area. A prosthetic treatment plan is then formulated that includes the type of prosthesis that will replace the missing tooth/teeth and the number, size, and position of the implants that will support the prosthesis (the implant treatment plan). The next phase in implant therapeutics is the surgical phase, during which the implants are placed. The postoperative phase is then entered, which includes the follow-up and prosthetic stages. In the follow-up stage, sufficient time is allowed for bone healing and osseointegration of the implant(s) to take place. After bone healing, the prosthetic stage is entered, in which the implant-supported prosthesis is fabricated. After insertion of the prosthesis, long-term follow-up is continued to monitor the overall oral condition. In cases of immediate implant loading, a prefabricated prosthesis is attached to the implants during the surgical phase.

With proper case selection and treatment planning, implant therapy has shown high success rates. Imaging is an important part of implant diagnostics, on which case selection and treatment planning are based. Imaging is also an important tool during the surgical and postoperative phases. Various imaging modalities are of use in this regard, the most commonly used being panoramic and periapical radiographs, which are 2-dimensional (2-D) imaging modalities, cone-beam computed tomography (CBCT), and multidetector CT (MDCT). **Fig. 1** demonstrates the sectional planes in which MDCT images may be viewed. This article presents an overview of the goal of imaging at each stage of implant

The author declares no conflict of interest and has not received any funding for this article.
Department of Oral Medicine and Diagnostic Sciences, Division of Oral and Maxillofacial Radiology, College of Dentistry, King Saud University, PO Box 56810, Riyadh 11564, Saudi Arabia
E-mail addresses: asma.alekrish@gmail.com; aalekrish@ksu.edu.sa

Radiol Clin N Am 56 (2018) 141–156
http://dx.doi.org/10.1016/j.rcl.2017.08.010

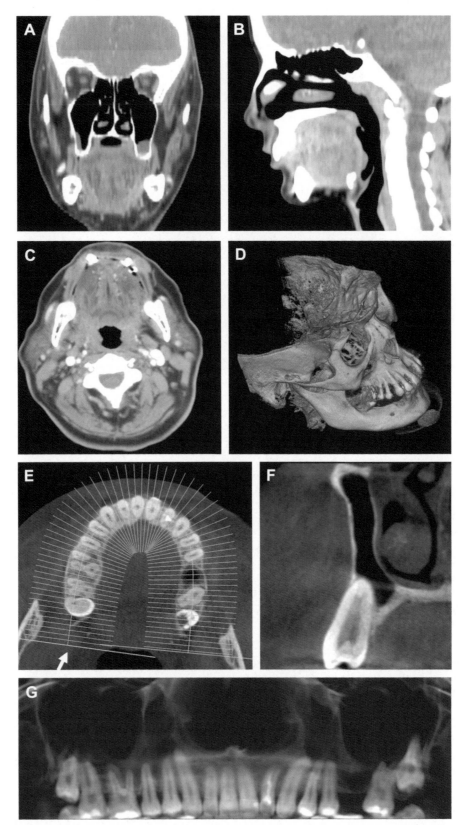

Fig. 1. The MDCT data set may be viewed as sectional images in the orthogonal planes, coronal (*A*), sagittal (*B*), and axial (*C*), or as a volumetric image (*D*). For dental implant imaging, use of specialized reformatting software allows drawing a curvilinear plane parallel to the curve of the arch in axial section (*arrow in E*) to produce sectional images perpendicular (*F*) and parallel (*G*) to the jaws.

therapy and the usefulness of MDCT in achieving those goals. The various CT protocols of use in implant imaging also are presented, as well as the options for viewing and analysis of CT images and issues related to image interpretation, interactive treatment planning, and transfer of information from the images to the surgical field during implant surgery. Due to space limitations, panoramic and periapical radiography and CBCT are not discussed in this article, but readers may find detailed information regarding these modalities in relation to dental implantology elsewhere.[1]

GOALS OF IMAGING IN IMPLANT THERAPEUTICS

The goals of imaging in implant therapeutics depend on the phase of the implant therapy.[2–4]

Treatment Planning (Preoperative) Phase

The aims of imaging during this phase are to determine, based on a prosthetically driven treatment plan, the optimum implant location, size, and angulation, and to determine if the residual ridge (the jaw bone after tooth removal) requires augmentation or reduction procedures. The information needed at this phase includes the following:

1. Presence or absence of disease in implant sites (and jaws in general)
2. Morphology of bone at proposed implant sites, including the following:
   a. Ridge dimensions
   b. Ridge angulation
   c. Presence of undercuts
   d. Thickness of cortical bone
3. Relationship of critical structures (neurovascular canals, nasal cavity, and maxillary sinus) to proposed implant sites
4. Quality of trabecular bone (the importance of this point is questionable with the new machined surface implants)
5. Reference information for transfer of treatment plan from the images to the surgical field (computer-guided surgery).

MDCT is useful in achieving all the aims of the treatment-planning phase (**Fig. 2**).

Surgical (Intraoperative) Phase

The aims of imaging during this phase are to verify and assist in optimal positioning and orientation of the implants as determined during the treatment-planning phase. MDCT is not generally useful during this phase, except in complex cases, and only when placement of the implants is carried out in a facility in which MDCT is available.

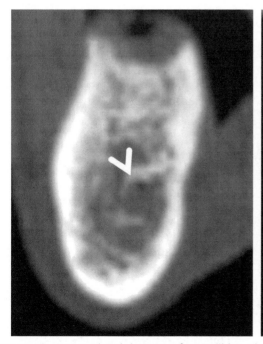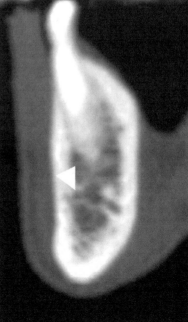

Fig. 2. Transverse cross-sectional images of mandibles obtained using MDCT. The voxel size is 0.39 × 0.39 × 0.625 mm. The images clearly demonstrate the bone margins and IAC (*open arrowheads*) and the narrower mandibular incisive canal (*closed arrowheads*).

Follow-up (Postoperative) Phase

The aims of imaging during this phase are to evaluate the relationship between the implant and the adjacent bone, the position and relationships of the prosthetic components to the implant and surrounding bone, and to evaluate the long-term prognosis of the implant therapy. Generally, MDCT is not of use during this phase due to presence of artifacts. However, it may be beneficial in evaluation of the relationship of implants to anatomic structures or grafts if abnormal symptoms develop.

COMPUTED TOMOGRAPHY IMPLANTOLOGY IMAGING PROTOCOLS
Standard Dose Protocols

Diagnostic reference levels (DRLs) for CT of the face and sinuses in medical imaging have been established as a volume CT Dose Index (CTDIvol) of 35 mGy.[5] The standard recommended exposure parameters for MDCT imaging for implantology (**Table 1**) impart a CTDI lower than a DRL of 35 mGy.[13,16]

Ultra-Low-Dose Protocols

Dose optimization in dental implantology imaging (determination of the minimum dose that will provide the required diagnostic quality) allows dose reduction to levels much lower than those required for other medical and dental tasks, and should always be pursued.[3,17] Although CBCT is considered a lower-dose alternative to MDCT, considerable reductions in radiation dose with MDCT have been shown to impart effective doses comparable to, or lower than, those of CBCT.[13,18,19] Although such ultra-low-dose protocols have produced images with reduced spatial and contrast resolution and increased image noise levels,[16] the images were found to be diagnostically acceptable.[13,19]

The suitable level of dose reduction depends on the diagnostic task involved. Use of 10 mA/80 kV and a pitch factor of 0.53 (CTDIvol: 0.53 mGy), a 98% reduction in MDCT dose compared with a standard protocol, allowed linear measurements of bone dimensions at prospective implant sites comparable to those obtained with standard doses.[13] The same dose reductions also did not adversely affect suitability of the images for surgical planning.[19] Images of a maxillary ridge with thin cortical outlines obtained with ultra-low doses is depicted in **Fig. 3**. However, for visualization of the inferior alveolar canal, more modest dose reductions are possible. The lowest dose at which the inferior alveolar canal was identified in all test samples was

---

Table 1
Recommended exposure parameters for MDCT standard-dose and low-dose examinations

MDCT Dose Protocol	Recommended Exposure Parameters
Standard	• Scan length should include regions of interest only. • The mA and kV depend on CT system being used, but low mA (70–80) recommended.[6,7] • Slice thickness should be smallest slice thickness permitted by MDCT device.[6,8,9] • Slice spacing should be equal to, or less than, slice thickness to produce contiguous or overlapping slices.[6] • Helical pitch should not exceed 0.75, 0.9375, and 0.9844 for 4-row, 16-row, and 64-row scanners, respectively, to avoid helical interpolation artifacts.[10] • Scan field of view: H-Head. • DFOV: 16.5 cm (may range between 15 and 20 cm according to size of jaw).[7] • Matrix size: 512 × 512.[7]

Low- dose	The most practical way to reduce dose while maintaining small voxel sizes:
	• Limit the scan length to include only the regions of interest.
	• Reduce the mA through manual adjustment or AEC.[11,12]
	  ○ If manual reduction of mA performed:
	    ■ Reduction should be aimed at lowest level that does not adversely affect visibility of the anatomic boundaries.
	    ■ mA of 40 with 80 kV imparts effective doses comparable to CBCT, with no detectable adverse effect on subjective MDCT image quality.[13,14]
	  ○ If AEC is used:
	    ■ The "noise index" setting (or other image quality setting) should be increased to permit the maximum level of noise that does not adversely affect visibility of the anatomic boundaries.[11]
	    ■ Care must be taken to position the head at the center of the gantry.[15]

Abbreviations: AEC, automatic exposure control; CBCT, cone-beam computed tomography; DFOV, display field of view; MDCT, multidetector computed tomography.

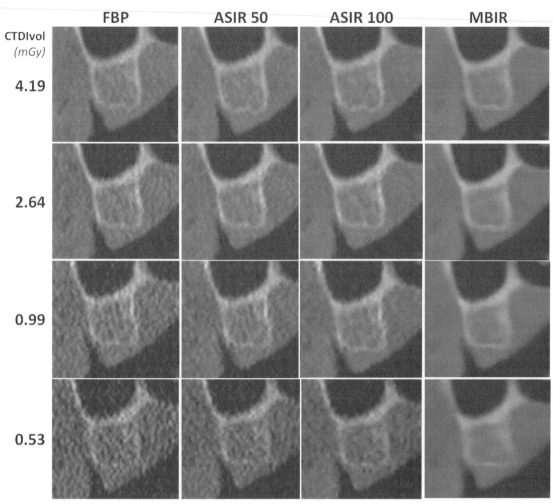

Fig. 3. Cross-sectional MDCT images of a cadaveric maxilla obtained with progressively lower dose protocols and reconstructed with 4 different reconstruction techniques, FBP, and the IRTs of ASIR and MBIR. The lowest dose (*bottom row*) is 2% of the standard dose used to produce the image in **Fig. 2**. For all the images, window width/window level is 4500/650. Although MBIR and ASIR show less noise than FBP, even the lowest-dose FBP protocol allows the identification of the bone–soft tissue interface. The oversmoothening of MBIR images also does not appear to adversely affect identification of ridge boundaries.

found to be CTDIvol: 2.64 mGy, using 40 mA/80 kV and a pitch factor of 0.53 (Al-Ekrish and colleagues, personal communication, 2017) (**Fig. 4**). For production of computer-aided design (CAD) models of the jaws, a precursor to computer-aided manufacture (CAM) of surgical guides for dental implant surgery, an 86% reduction in dose by use of 35 mA/100 kV and a pitch factor of 0.53 (CTDIvol: 4.19 mGy) was found to produce subjectively acceptable model quality (Al-Ekrish and colleagues, personal communication, 2017).

Therefore, imaging protocols used should impart minimal doses, but the dose reductions applied should not be so extreme as to affect image quality and diagnostic accuracy. The effect of planned dose reductions on visibility of

anatomic structures may be assessed by the use of computer-simulated dose reduction software programs that add noise to an image to simulate the effects of lowered radiation. Use of such tools may aid in estimation of the optimum parameters before their use in patient examinations. **Table 1** outlines recommended parameters for dose optimization based on the currently available data.

Ultra-Low-Dose Multidetector Computed Tomography Combined with Iterative Reconstruction Techniques

Use of iterative reconstruction techniques (IRTs) produces images with less noise than with the traditionally used filtered backprojection (FBP) reconstruction algorithms.[16] As such, IRTs have the potential to allow even further dose reductions compared with FBP. The IRTs of adaptive statistical iterative reconstruction (ASIR) and model-based iterative reconstruction (MBIR) have been investigated for use in maxillofacial imaging with mixed results, depending on the diagnostic task.

Sectional and volumetric images obtained with ultra-low doses (as low as CTDIvol of 0.22 mGy) and FBP and ASIR and MBIR were subjectively assessed for their usefulness in craniofacial navigation surgery; and the highest subjective image quality scores were recorded for MBIR, followed by ASIR 100, then by ASIR 50 and FBP, which obtained comparable scores. However, all the images were found to be suitable for surgical planning.[19] For identification of dental implant site outer bony margins, ASIR 50, ASIR 100, and MBIR did not demonstrate an advantage over FBP at various ultra-low doses, even at the lowest dose tested (CTDIvol of 0.53 mGy)[13] (see **Fig. 3**).

Use of ASIR and MBIR for production of CAD models of the jaws demonstrated subjectively acceptable CAD model quality at lower doses when IRTs were used compared with FBP. Compared with the low dose achievable by FBP (CTDIvol of 4.19 mGy), ASIR 50 allowed a further 37% dose reduction (CTDIvol: 2.64), and ASIR 100 allowed a 76% dose reduction (CTDIvol: 0.99). The accuracy of the CAD models produced by MBIR was found to be questionable, but potential dose savings of 93% (CTDIvol: 0.29) compared with FBP were found (Al-Ekrish and colleagues, personal communication, 2017). Research into dose optimization using FBP and various IRTs for numerous other diagnostic tasks involved in dental implantology is also currently being performed by the author's research group. The use of IRTs has not been found to offer an advantage over FBP in depiction of the inferior alveolar canal (Al-Ekrish and colleagues, personal communication, 2017). The appearance of the inferior alveolar canal (IAC) on ultra-low-dose images combined with FBP, ASIR, or MBIR is depicted in **Fig. 4**.

Special Protocols

When CT data are to be used for CAD/CAM production of surgical guides for implant surgery, the protocols recommended by the surgical guide company must be followed to limit the potential errors in position of the implant osteotomies.[20] Such protocols may necessitate that the patient wear a radiographic stent during the CT scan and/or obtain a digital scan of the patient's teeth and jaw, which is fused to the CT scan. The digital scan may be obtained by 3-D laser scanning, CT scanning, or stereophotogrammetry of a stone cast of the jaw, or by direct intraoral dental scanning.

A dual-scan module involves 2 CT scans, one of the patient wearing a prosthesis, which guides in treatment planning of the implants, and another CT scan of the prosthesis itself; these scans are merged in planning software. Such special scanning protocols allow accurate manufacture of the surgical guides by providing higher-resolution images of teeth and mucosal surfaces, compared with those obtained by direct CT scanning of the jaw, and by eliminating artifacts caused by dental restorations.

Table 2 outlines MDCT imaging parameters and image features with clinical considerations for implant site imaging.

RADIOGRAPHIC STENTS

The restorative dentist evaluates the occlusion and determines where the ideal position and angulation of the implant would be in relation to the occlusion. The radiographic stent relays that information to the radiologist. Radiographic stents are removable devices worn by the patient during CT scanning; they are made of low-radiodensity materials and contain high radiodensity markers that indicate the relation of the proposed implants to the underlying bone (**Fig. 5**). They are especially useful in multiple-implant and esthetically challenging cases, and should be fabricated based on the intended prosthetic plan.[34]

The radiopaque markers in the stent should demonstrate the position and tilt of the proposed implants and the vertical distance between the proposed occlusal edge of the teeth and crest of bone. The stent must be well-fitting and stable during the CT exposure; mobility of the stent may invalidate the position and orientation of the markers seen in the images (see **Fig. 5E**). Therefore, to stabilize the stent during imaging, if a radiographic stent is required for one jaw only and there are an insufficient number of teeth in the other jaw, the denture for the other jaw should be worn to occlude against, and stabilize, the stent.

VIEWING AND ANALYSIS OF COMPUTED TOMOGRAPHY IMAGES
Factors Affecting the Diagnostic Quality of Computed Tomography Images

The diagnostic quality of CT images is influenced by certain factors, of which the effect on implant site imaging must be considered for appropriate imaging, reformatting, and image interpretation.

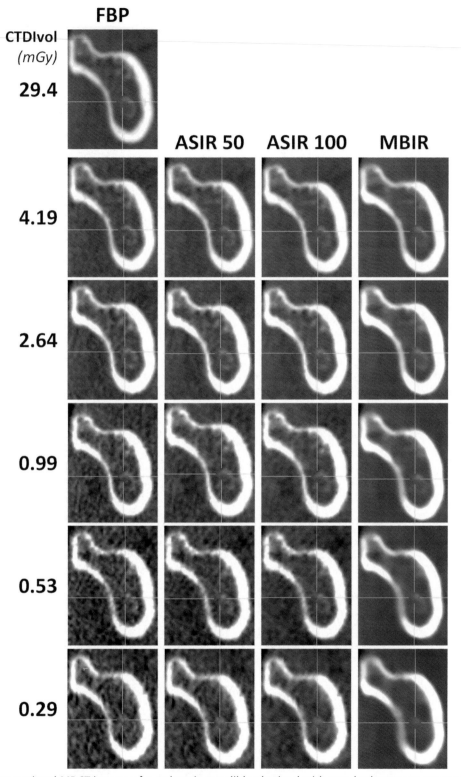

Fig. 4. Cross-sectional MDCT images of a cadaveric mandible obtained with standard exposure parameters (*top row*) and progressively lower dose protocols and reconstructed with 4 different reconstruction techniques, FBP, and the IRTs of ASIR and MBIR. The kV/mA used and volume CTDIvol imparted for each of the progressively lower dose protocols were 120/100 (29.4 mGy), 100/35 (4.19 mGy), 80/40 (2.64 mGy), 80/15 (0.99 mGy), 80/10 (0.53 mGy), and 80/10 (0.29 mGy). All the dose protocols used a pitch of 0.53, except the lowest dose (*bottom row*), which used a pitch of 0.97. With all the reconstruction techniques, the thin roof of the IAC (*at the intersection of the blue lines*) is still visible even at a CTDIvol of 0.53 mGy, which is less than 2% that of the reference dose. However, canals with an elusive roof may require higher doses.

Table 2
MDCT parameters and image features with clinical considerations for implant site imaging

	Technical Considerations	Clinical Considerations
Exposure parameters	• mA and kV depend on CT system being used, but low mA (70–80) recommended.[6,7] • Ultra-low-dose protocols (with FBP or IRTs) have demonstrated implant site measurements comparable to standard doses and comparable visibility of the roof of the IAC)[13,21–23] (see **Figs. 4** and **5**).	• With any combination of MDCT device and reconstruction algorithm, the lowest dose that produces diagnostic images of the implant sites should be pursued.[17]
Pitch factor	• Maximum acceptable pitch depends on the number of MDCT detector rows. • Maximum acceptable pitch values for 4-row, 16-row, and 64-row scanners are 0.75, 0.9375, and 0.9844, respectively.[10] • Pitch values larger than 1 increase helical interpolation artifacts that may lead to loss of image detail in the z-axis.	• Increasing pitch may reduce radiation dose to patient, but should not be increased to levels that adversely affect the diagnostic quality of the images.[17] • High pitch values may adversely affect visibility of the roof of the IAC (see **Fig. 4**).
Size of FOV	• Determined by scan length and DFOV. • Scan length in the craniocaudal dimension can be limited to one or both jaws. • The DFOV is the area reconstructed into an image. It can be smaller than or equal to the scan FOV. • The scan FOV is the area exposed to the radiation. It should encompass the entire circumference of the anatomy. The "Head" setting should be selected.	• Shortest scan length that covers field of interest should be used to avoid unnecessary exposure of tissues. • In general, 5-cm scan length is adequate for imaging of 1 jaw, and 10 cm for imaging of two jaws. Smallest DFOV that covers field of interest should be used.
Voxel size and spatial resolution	• Anisotropic (ie, unequal voxel dimensions in the 3 planes). • In-plane voxel size (ie, size of pixel in the originally acquired axial sections in the x-y dimensions) depends on DFOV and matrix size. • The size of the voxel in the z plane (along the cranio-caudal dimension) depends on the slice thickness of the originally acquired scan. • Smaller voxel sizes lead to reduced effect of partial-volume artifacts,[8] and permit higher spatial resolution of images. • Smaller voxels may be obtained by use of larger matrix size, smaller DFOV, and thinner slice thickness. • Reformatted images have lower spatial resolution compared with the originally acquired sectional images.[24,25]	• Smallest DFOV that covers region of interest should be used. • Smallest slice thickness permitted by MDCT device should be used.[6] • Small voxel size (0.25–0.3 mm) useful for evaluation of fine details. • Voxel sizes up to 0.4 mm have been demonstrated to allow accurate measurements of ridge dimensions.[26] • If MDCT acquired with slice thickness of 0.65 mm, spatial resolution is generally adequate for implant site imaging. • However, images may not display bone that is thinner than the voxel dimensions (ie, walls of neurovascular canals, crest of ridge, or covering roots of teeth).
Accuracy of density measurements	• Accurate density assessment possible using HU with individual CT scanner if kilovoltage peak is consistent.[27,28]	• Objective, accurate, and stable assessment of bone density possible. • The HU has been correlated with primary implant stability, but there is still no reference standard to relate specific HU values to the determinants of implant site treatment planning and/or success.[29–33]

Abbreviations: CT, computed tomography; DFOV, display field of view; FOV, field of view; HU, hounsfield units; IAC, inferior alveolar canal; IRT, iterative recon...

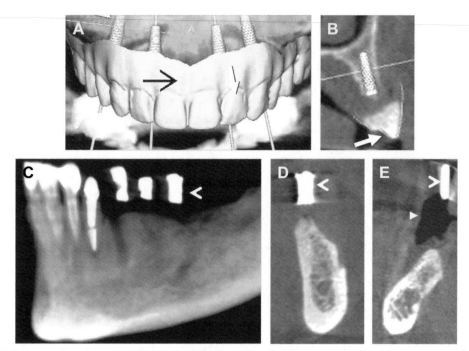

Fig. 5. CT images of patients wearing radiographic stents of different types. (*A, B*) Denture made of low-radiodensity flange (*black arrow*) and teeth of high radiodensity material (*white arrows*). (*C–E*) Low-radiodensity acrylic stent with radiodense markers (*open arrowheads*) along the long axis of the prosthetic teeth. Volume-rendered (VR) images of maxilla (*A*) and mandible (*C*) and transverse cross sections (*B, D*) display relation of radiodense teeth and linear markers to the bone, allowing the planning of implants based on the position and angulation of the proposed tooth. (*E*) Transverse cross section of mandible with patient wearing a stent that was not completely seated, as evidenced by the large gap (*closed arrowhead*) between the radiodense marker (*open arrowhead*) and the ridge. (*Adapted from* Tamimi D, editor. Specialty imaging—dental implants. Altona (Australia): Amirsys Inc.-Elsevier; 2014; with permission.)

Contrast resolution

Contrast resolution of an image is its ability to demonstrate subtle differences in radiodensity. Contrast resolution decreases with reduced radiation doses. However, identifying bone–soft tissue interfaces, which is the main task in implant site analysis, does not require high contrast resolution. Therefore, the higher levels of noise produced by low-dose exposure protocols have not been shown to adversely affect implant site measurements in MDCT.[13,21]

Spatial resolution

High spatial resolution leads to the production of sharply delineated interfaces between gray shades in a CT image. Most MDCT devices can produce images with adequate spatial resolution for measurement of implant site dimensions with submillimeter accuracy (see **Figs. 2, 3,** and **4**).

Voxel size is a primary, but not the only, determinant of spatial resolution. Smaller voxel sizes lead to increased spatial resolution if image noise remains constant. Conversely, increasing voxel size leads to increasing partial-volume averaging artifacts, which are of concern in implant site imaging when they occur at the bone–soft tissue interface. Their presence at such interfaces may result in reduced sharpness of the anatomic boundaries, which may compromise localization of anatomic borders.[8] To produce MDCT images with adequately small voxel size, the images should be acquired with the thinnest slice thickness, largest matrix size possible, and the smallest display field of view (DFOV), which includes the entire region of interest.

Artifacts

An artifact is a systematic discrepancy between the CT numbers in the reconstructed image and the true attenuation coefficients of the object. The artifacts of most concern in CT imaging for implantology are streaking and beam-hardening/missing data artifacts.[35,36]

High-density materials, such as amalgam restorations, dental implants, reconstruction plates and screws, and cast metals of prosthodontic appliances, may cause beam-hardening and/or streak artifacts, which may limit visualization of the anatomy adjacent to such materials (**Fig. 6**). Metallic jewelry or thyroid collars may also cause streaking

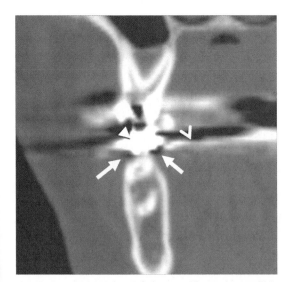

Fig. 6. Coronal section of the maxilla and mandible at the level of the molar teeth demonstrating amalgam restoration (*closed arrowhead*) causing beam-hardening (*arrows*) and streak (*open arrowhead*) artifacts. The effect of the artifacts is mostly in the horizontal plane, with minimum image degradation of the bone.

if situated at the horizontal level of the CT examination. The bone and tooth structures adjacent to such materials may appear missing to variable degrees. The effect of beam-hardening and streaking is mainly at the horizontal level; therefore, artifacts caused by objects crestal to the bone (eg, amalgam restorations and crowns) degrade visibility of only the crest of the bone, with minimal impact on accuracy of linear measurements of the jaws.[36] On the other hand, dental implants, metallic posts within the roots of the teeth, and reconstruction plates may degrade visibility of the adjacent bone. Beam-hardening artifacts around titanium implants may obscure subtle changes in marginal and peri-implant bone.[35]

Depending on the severity and position of such metallic artifacts, they may cause image degradation so severe as to render the images nondiagnostic. Various IRTs have been shown to reduce metallic artifacts caused by dental restorations, but their clinical impact needs further investigation.[37] Therefore, in the presence of metallic objects near the region of interest, it must be considered whether artifacts are likely to compromise the intended diagnostic task for which CT will be used.

Image-Reformatting Considerations

Figs. 7 and 8 provide a visual description of the optimum images used for implant site analysis and considerations for curvilinear reformatting for implant site assessment. The generated cross

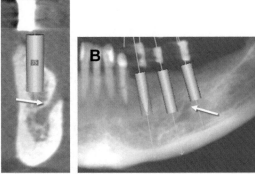

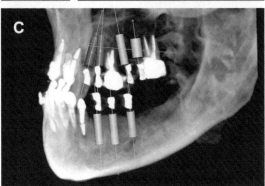

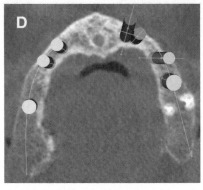

Fig. 7. Transverse (*A*) and parasagittal (*B*) sections, the optimum images used for visualizing the implant site area on CT images, demonstrating relationship of proposed implants to anatomic boundaries and critical structures clearly (*arrows*). VR image (*C*) and axial section (*D*) are also useful to demonstrate relationship of the proposed implants to each other and to the entire dental arch. Thin bone may not be visible in VR images; therefore, they should not be used to assess thin bone (eg, at crest of ridge).

sections should be aligned with the intended trajectory of the planned implant.

Ridge Measurement Considerations

1. Assessment of the adequacy of the available bone for the proposed implant treatment plan

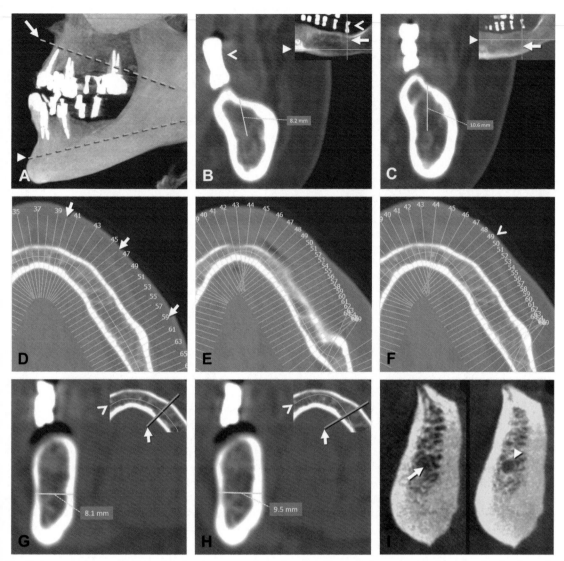

Fig. 8. Images demonstrating step-by-step procedures for curvilinear reformatting of images for implant site assessment. (*A*) Axial section on which curvilinear reformatting is performed must be properly angled. Maxillary section should be parallel to hard palate (*arrow*); mandibular sections should be parallel to long axis of mandible (*arrowhead*). (*B*) Cropped panoramic section produced by curvilinear reformatting (*top right insert*) on properly angled axial section (*arrowhead*), and the resultant orientation of the transverse cross sections supero-inferiorly (*arrow*). The transverse cross-sectional image is perpendicular to the bone and along the long axis of the proposed implant (as determined by the direction of the radiodense marker in the radiographic stent [*open arrowheads*]), thus demonstrating accurate ridge height above the IAC (*yellow line*). (*C*) Transverse cross-sectional image of the same site as in (*B*), but obtained by curvilinear reformatting on incorrectly angled axial section (*arrowhead*). The resultant transverse cross section is obliquely oriented supero-inferiorly (*arrow*), causing the ridge to appear longer with a false increase in the measured height of the ridge above the IAC. However, if the direction of the proposed implant is not perpendicular to the bone, then the transverse cross section should be angled to be parallel to the direction of the implant. (*D*) Cropped axial CT section of mandible at correct superio-inferior position for curvilinear reformatting. The axial section should correspond to the level of the mid-roots of the teeth (if present). The curvilinear plane parallel to the arch at this level produces transverse cross sections, which are properly oriented faciolingually (*arrows*). Drawing the reformatting curve on an axial section near the crest of the ridge (*E*) sometimes leads to the curve not being parallel to the jaw at the level of the roots/implants (*F*), which may cause the transverse cross sections to be obliquely oriented to the ridge faciolingually (*open arrowhead*). (*G*) Cropped axial section (*top right insert*) demonstrating proper shape of reformatting curve (*arrowhead*), and the resultant orientation of the transverse cross sections faciolingually (*arrow*). The

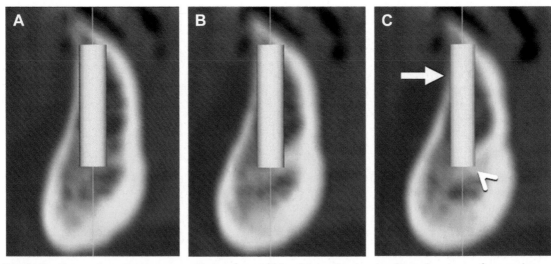

Fig. 9. Contiguous transverse cross sections of mandible obtained using implant planning software demonstrating the importance of analyzing all sectional images of the ridge along the mesiodistal extent of proposed implant site. Although sections (*A*) and (*B*) indicate implant would be covered by bone, (*C*) demonstrates insufficient amount of bone (*arrow*) and presence of lingual foramen (*open arrowhead*). (*Adapted from* Tamimi D, editor. Specialty imaging—dental implants. Altona (Australia): Amirsys Inc.-Elsevier; 2014; with permission.)

must take into consideration the bone morphology and position and angulation of the proposed implants.[2,3]

a. The position and angulation of the proposed implants may be determined by using a radiographic stent (see section entitled "Radiographic stents").

b. The position (point of insertion) of the proposed implant must be evaluated regarding the amount of mesiodistal space available and the faciolingual dimension and position of the bone.

c. The angulation (path of insertion) of the proposed implant must be evaluated relative to the faciolingual inclination of the bone and the mesiodistal inclination of the roots of the adjacent teeth.

d. All sectional images along the extent of the proposed implant site must be analyzed to verify that no aspect of the implant would encroach on a pathologic entity or vital structure (neurovascular canal, nasal cavity, maxillary sinus, adjacent tooth, external cortical boundaries, and especially lingual depressions of the mandible), or any accessory canals or anomalies (**Fig. 9**).

e. If the position of a neurovascular canal in the region of a proposed implant is not clear in a particular image section, identification of the canal may be improved by cross-referencing the image of the canal in perpendicular planes (the cross-sectional and parasagittal sections) (**Fig. 10**).

2. Placement of virtual implants (implant simulations) allows clear visualization of the previously mentioned morphology of the bone and anatomy relative to the proposed implants in all 3 dimensions (see **Figs. 7** and **9**), and is preferable to linear measurements of the bone. This is usually performed by the dentist or the implant planning specialist.

transverse cross-sectional image is perpendicular to the bone, thus demonstrating accurate ridge width (IAC) (*yellow line*). (*H*) Transverse cross-sectional image of the same site as in (*G*), but obtained by improper shape of curvilinear reformatting (*open arrowhead*). The resultant transverse cross section is obliquely oriented faciolingually (*arrow*), causing the ridge to appear wider with a false increase in the measured width of the ridge (*yellow line*). Small tilt in angle of section (below 20°) may not lead to significant changes in ridge dimensions.[8,38] (*I*) Transverse cross sections of an implant site demonstrating how identification of the neurovascular canals may be improved by changes in reformatting parameters. A 2-mm-thick cross-sectional image viewed in maximum-intensity projection mode (*right*), shows improved visibility of canal (*arrowhead*) compared with a 0.09-mm-thick section (*arrow*). (*Adapted from* Tamimi D, editor. Specialty imaging—dental implants. Altona (Australia): Amirsys Inc.-Elsevier; 2014; with permission.)

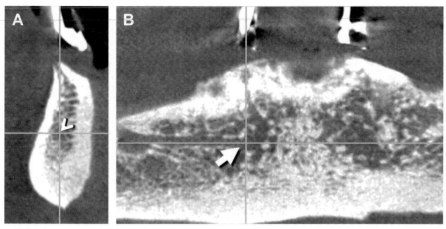

Fig. 10. Transverse cross section (*A*) of mandible demonstrating technique for localizing neurovascular canals at implant sites where the canal is not clearly visible. Canal localization may be improved by cross-referencing image with panoramic section (*B*). Canal is identified on panoramic section (*arrow*), and crosshairs of reformatting lines are placed at canal; intersection of lines on cross-sectional image (*open arrowhead*) indicates canal position. (*Adapted from* Tamimi D, editor. Specialty imaging—dental implants. Altona (Australia): Amirsys Inc.-Elsevier; 2014; with permission.)

3. Single linear measurements of the height and width of the bone at the implant site do not provide information regarding the spatial relationship of the proposed implant to the surrounding anatomy. In the absence of an implant simulation tool, an alternative, but less preferable, method of analysis is use of a rectangular measurement tool or linear measurements of the ridge performed in a rectangular shape (**Fig. 11**). Such measurements must be performed on all images along the extent of the proposed implant site.

4. Linear measurement errors with MDCT are mostly within 1 mm[8,21]; therefore, when

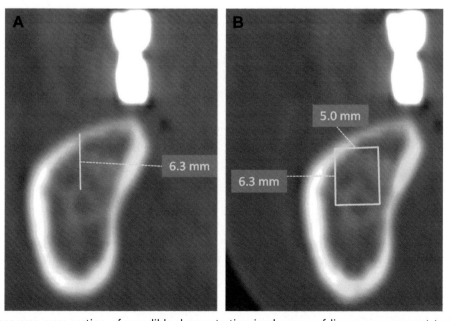

Fig. 11. Transverse cross section of mandible demonstrating inadequacy of linear measurement tool to assess availability of bone for implant placement. (*A*) Measurement of ridge height crestal to the roof of the IAC using linear measurement tool indicates 6.3 mm of bone is present crestal to IAC, but on the same cross-sectional image (*B*) the rectangular measurement indicates that an implant 6.3 mm in length and 4.0 mm in diameter would penetrate the roof of IAC if it was embedded within the bone. (*Adapted from* Tamimi D, editor. Specialty imaging—dental implants. Altona (Australia): Amirsys Inc.-Elsevier; 2014; with permission.)

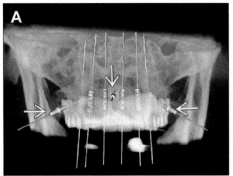
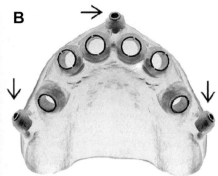

Fig. 12. (*A*) VR CT image shows the planning of a CAD/CAM surgical guide for the placement of 6 maxillary implants. (*B*) Photograph shows the corresponding surgical guide. The anchor pin sites (*arrows*) will guide the anchor pins into the underlying bone and help with the retention of this maxillary guide and its stability during the surgery. (*Adapted from* Tamimi D, editor. Specialty imaging—dental implants. Altona (Australia): Amirsys Inc.-Elsevier; 2014; with permission.)

planning implants, a safety margin of 1 mm is recommended,[39] with an additional 2 mm if surgical guides are used.[34]

5. Objective radiographic measurements of bone density not clinically useful in predicting implant stability.[29,40]

Interactive Treatment Planning

1. Virtual placement of implants (see **Figs. 7** and **9**) allows the following:
   a. Placement of simulated implants in optimum position to receive the planned crown prosthesis and analyzing their relationship to the surrounding anatomy in all 3 dimensions.
   b. Better evaluation of appropriate size and position of implant.
   c. Better assessment of need for sinus-lifting, bone-grafting, or bone-reduction procedures.
2. Virtual planning of prosthesis on virtual implants allows more advanced prosthetic treatment planning, which may be especially useful in complex cases.
3. Fusion of digital casts to CT images allows the following:
   a. Reduced artifacts from dental restorations.
   b. Creation of accurate surgical guides.
   c. Virtual wax-up of prosthesis.

TRANSFER OF INFORMATION FROM IMAGES TO THE SURGICAL FIELD

After optimum position of the implants has been determined within the CT images, the treatment plan must be transferred to surgical field. Precise determination of the intended implant sites and angulations during the surgery may be challenging. Such determination may be aided by manually constructed surgical guides or improved by computer-aided implant surgery

(CAS).[20,34,41,42] The potential benefits of CAS are more pronounced when minimally invasive (flapless) surgery is planned, and in complex and/or esthetically demanding cases. CAS is of the following 2 types.

Passive (or Semi-active): Computer-Aided Design/Computer-Aided Manufacture–Generated Surgical Guides

Passive CAS may be defined as the use of a static surgical template that reproduces virtual implant position directly from computerized tomographic data and does not allow intraoperative modification of implant position[20,34,43] (**Fig. 12**). Surgical guides can be classified, based on the type of tissue support, as tooth-supported, bone-supported, mucosa-supported, or mini-implant supported.[34] The type of support used depends on the number of teeth remaining and whether or not flapless surgery is planned. Surgical guides are difficult to use in cases of atrophied jaw bone or limited mouth opening.

Active: Computer-Guided Navigation

Computer-guided navigation, also known as CT-guided navigation or bur tracking, involves importing presurgical CT images into specialized surgical navigation software that interfaces with an optical tracking system to provide real-time tracking of the surgical drill within the CT images during surgery.[20]

ACKNOWLEDGMENTS

The author thanks Dr Gerlig Widmann, Department of Radiology, Medical University of Innsbruck, for providing the ultra-low-dose MDCT datasets used to extract the images for **Figs. 3** and **4**.

REFERENCES

1. Tamimi D, Koenig L, Al-Ekrish A, et al. Specialty imaging. Dental implants. Altona (Australia): Amirsys Inc.-Elsevier; 2014.
2. Harris D, Horner K, Gröndahl K, et al. EAO guidelines for the use of diagnostic imaging in implant dentistry 2011. A consensus workshop organized by the European Association for Osseointegration at the Medical University of Warsaw. Clin Oral Implants Res 2012;23(11):1243–53.
3. Tyndall DA, Price JB, Tetradis S, et al. Position statement of the American Academy of Oral and Maxillofacial Radiology on selection criteria for the use of radiology in dental implantology with emphasis on cone beam computed tomography. Oral Surg Oral Med Oral Pathol Oral Radiol 2012;113(6):817–26.
4. Gaetti-Jardim EC, Santiago-Junior JF, Goiato MC, et al. Dental implants in patients with osteoporosis: a clinical reality? J Craniofac Surg 2011;22(3):1111–3.
5. Bongartz G, Golding S, Jurik A, et al. EUR 16262: European guidelines on quality criteria for computed tomography. Luxembourg: Office for Official Publications of the European Communities; 2000.
6. GE medical systems. Advantage dentascan operator manual 2182400-100. Vol Revision 4: General Electric Company; 2010.
7. Au-Yeung K, Ahuja A, Ching A, et al. Dentascan in oral imaging. Clin Radiol 2001;56(9):700–13.
8. Al-Ekrish A, Ekram M. A comparative study of the accuracy and reliability of multidetector computed tomography and cone beam computed tomography in the assessment of dental implant site dimensions. Dentomaxillofac Radiol 2011;40:67–75.
9. Ruppin J, Popovic A, Strauss M, et al. Evaluation of the accuracy of three different computer-aided surgery systems in dental implantology: optical tracking vs. stereolithographic splint systems. Clin Oral Implants Res 2008;19(7):709–16.
10. Goldman LW. Principles of CT: multislice CT. J Nucl Med Technol 2008;36(2):57–68 [quiz: 75–6].
11. McCollough CH, Primak AN, Braun N, et al. Strategies for reducing radiation dose in CT. Radiol Clin North Am 2009;47(1):27–40.
12. Flohr T. Multi-detector row CT–recent developments, radiation dose and dose reduction technologies. In: Tack D, Kalra M, Gevenois P, editors. Radiation dose from multidetector CT. Berlin: Springer-Verlag; 2012. p. 3–20.
13. Al-Ekrish A, Al-Shawaf R, Schullian P, et al. Validity of linear measurements of the jaws using ultralow-dose MDCT and the iterative techniques of ASIR and MBIR. Int J Comput Assist Radiol Surg 2016;11(10):1791–801.
14. Widmann G, Fasser M, Schullian P, et al. Substantial dose reduction in modern multi-slice spiral computed tomography (MSCT)-guided craniofacial and skull base surgery. Rofo 2012;184(2):136.
15. Li J, Udayasankar UK, Toth TL, et al. Automatic patient centering for MDCT: effect on radiation dose. Am J Roentgenol 2007;188(2):547–52.
16. Widmann G, Al-Shawaf R, Schullian P, et al. Effect of ultra-low doses, ASIR and MBIR on density and noise levels of MDCT images of dental implant sites. Eur Radiol 2017;27(5):2225–34.
17. National Council on Radiation Protection (NCRP). Achievements of the past 50 years and addressing the needs of the future. Fiftieth annual meeting of the National Council on Radiation Protection and Measurements (NCRP). 2014. Available at: http://www.ncrponline.org/Annual_Mtgs/2014_Ann_Mtg/PROGRAM_2-10.pdf. Accessed March 10–11, 2014.
18. Ludlow J, Timothy R, Walker C, et al. Effective dose of dental CBCT—a meta-analysis of published data and additional data for nine CBCT units. Dentomaxillofac Radiol 2014;44(1):20140197.
19. Widmann G, Schullian P, Gassner E-M, et al. Ultra-low-dose CT of the craniofacial bone for navigated surgery using adaptive statistical iterative reconstruction and model-based iterative reconstruction: 2D and 3D image quality. Am J Roentgenol 2015;204(3):563–9.
20. Vercruyssen M, Fortin T, Widmann G, et al. Different techniques of static/dynamic guided implant surgery: modalities and indications. Periodontol 2000 2014;66(1):214–27.
21. Suomalainen A, Vehmas T, Kortesniemi M, et al. Accuracy of linear measurements using dental cone beam and conventional multislice computed tomography. Dentomaxillofac Radiol 2008;37(1):10–7.
22. Loubele M, Jacobs R, Maes F, et al. Radiation dose vs. image quality for low-dose CT protocols of the head for maxillofacial surgery and oral implant planning. Radiat Prot Dosimetry 2005;117(1–3):211–6.
23. Rustemeyer P, Streubühr U, Suttmoeller J. Low-dose dental computed tomography: significant dose reduction without loss of image quality. Acta Radiol 2004;45(8):847–53.
24. Ekestubbe A, Grondahl K, Ekholm S, et al. Low-dose tomographic techniques for dental implant planning. Int J Oral Maxillofac Implants 1996;11(5):650–9.
25. Lindh C, Petersson A, Klinge B. Visualization of the mandibular canal by different radiographic techniques. Clin Oral Implants Res 1992;3:90–7.
26. Waltrick KB, de Abreu Junior MJN, Corrêa M, et al. Accuracy of linear measurements and visibility of the mandibular canal of cone-beam computed tomography images with different voxel sizes: an in vitro study. J Periodontol 2013;84(1):68–77.
27. Nackaerts O, Maes F, Yan H, et al. Analysis of intensity variability in multislice and cone beam

computed tomography. Clin Oral Implants Res 2011; 22(8):873–9.

28. Norton MR, Gamble C. Bone classification: an objective scale of bone density using the computerized tomography scan. Clin Oral Implants Res 2001; 12(1):79–84.

29. Al-Ekrish A. Bone quality for implants. In: Tamimi D, editor. Specialty imaging—dental implants. Altona (Australia): Amirsys Inc.-Elsevier; 2014. p. 340–5.

30. Merheb J, Van Assche N, Coucke W, et al. Relationship between cortical bone thickness or computerized tomography-derived bone density values and implant stability. Clin Oral Implants Res 2010;21(6): 612–7.

31. Turkyilmaz I, McGlumphy EA. Is there a lower threshold value of bone density for early loading protocols of dental implants? J Oral Rehabil 2008; 35(10):775–81.

32. Turkyilmaz I, McGlumphy EA. Influence of bone density on implant stability parameters and implant success: a retrospective clinical study. BMC Oral Health 2008;8:32.

33. Ikumi N, Tsutsumi S. Assessment of correlation between computerized tomography values of the bone and cutting torque values at implant placement: a clinical study. Int J Oral Maxillofac Implants 2005;20(2):253–60.

34. Bornstein M, Al-Nawas B, Kuchler U, et al. Consensus statements and recommended clinical procedures regarding contemporary surgical and radiographic techniques in implant dentistry. Int J Oral Maxillofac Implants 2014;29:78.

35. Sirin Y, Horasan S, Yaman D, et al. Detection of crestal radiolucencies around dental implants: an in vitro experimental study. J Oral Maxillofac Surg 2012;70(7):1540–50.

36. Cremonini C, Dumas M, Pannuti C, et al. Assessment of linear measurements of bone for implant sites in the presence of metallic artefacts using cone beam computed tomography and multislice computed tomography. Int J Oral Maxillofac Surg 2011;40(8):845–50.

37. De Crop A, Casselman J, Van Hoof T, et al. Analysis of metal artifact reduction tools for dental hardware in CT scans of the oral cavity: kVp, iterative reconstruction, dual-energy CT, metal artifact reduction software: does it make a difference? Neuroradiology 2015;57(8):841–9.

38. Dantas J, Montebello FA, Campos P. Computed tomography for dental implants: the influence of the gantry angle and mandibular positioning on the bone height and width. Dentomaxillofac Radiol 2005;34(1):9.

39. Horner K. Cone-beam computed tomography: time for an evidence-based approach. Prim Dent J 2013;2(1):22–31.

40. Mathieu V, Vayron R, Richard G, et al. Biomechanical determinants of the stability of dental implants: influence of the bone–implant interface properties. J Biomech 2014;47(1):3–13.

41. Schneider D, Marquardt P, Zwahlen M, et al. A systematic review on the accuracy and the clinical outcome of computer-guided template-based implant dentistry. Clin Oral Implants Res 2009;20(s4):73–86.

42. Vercruyssen M, Jacobs R, Van Assche N, et al. The use of CT scan based planning for oral rehabilitation by means of implants and its transfer to the surgical field: a critical review on accuracy. J Oral Rehabil 2008;35(6):454–74.

43. Turbush SK, Turkyilmaz I. Accuracy of three different types of stereolithographic surgical guides in implant placement: an in vitro study. J Prosthet Dent 2012;108(3):181–8.

Temporomandibular Joint Imaging

Dania Tamimi, BDS, DMSc[a],*, Elnaz Jalali, DDS, MDSc[b], David Hatcher, DDS, MSc[c]

KEYWORDS

- TMJ imaging • Degenerative joint disease • Mandibular growth and morphology • TMJ Disc
- MR imaging analysis of TMJ

KEY POINTS

- Growth and development of the craniofacial complex are linked to temporomandibular joint (TMJ) growth and development.
- Changes in TMJ growth and development can change the appearance of the craniofacial complex.
- Changes include developmental (hemifacial microsomia, hypoplasia, hyperplasia), degenerative (juvenile or adult), inflammatory (juvenile idiopathic arthritis, rheumatoid arthritis, pigmented villonodular synovitis), and traumatic (subcondylar fracture/neonatal fracture) etiologies.

INTRODUCTION

The temporomandibular joint (TMJ) is an anatomically and biomechanically complex structure whose growth and development affects that of the mandible and subsequently the craniofacial complex. The mandible articulates with the temporal bone through the TMJ but also (and less acknowledged) through the interdigitation of the mandibular teeth with their maxillary counterparts. The TMJ can affect the position of the teeth and their occlusion if the mandibular growth is changed.[1] Understanding how the TMJ grows and functions and how it breaks down if its biomechanical threshold is exceeded remove is essential to accurate radiographic evaluation, because the radiographic appearance is usually a representation of the TMJ at one point in time along a continuum of disease or dysfunction. Knowing this continuum allows radiologists to give the referring clinician a clue to what factors preceded and precipitated the findings at the current time point as well as a prediction of what may be the future craniofacial manifestations of the disease.[2] Other entities affecting the TMJs and their radiographic appearance are discussed in this context as well. For reasons of space, plain film imaging and imaging modalities that were used in the past are not covered in this article.

Growth/Development of the Temporomandibular Joint

The TMJ condyle is capped with fibrocartilage and is one of the most important growth sites of the mandible.[3] Unilateral interruption of condylar growth through destruction or alteration of the fibrocartilage during the active growth phase leads to alteration of growth of the mandible, resulting in mandibular asymmetry[4] or a small mandible in cases of bilateral condylar growth disruption. Similarly, if there is a developmental change in the amount of fibrocartilage present (such as in condylar hypoplasia, hyperplasia, or hemifacial microsomia) mandibular asymmetry may occur. Benign condylar tumors have a similar effect on mandibular symmetry, but because they tend to occur after the growth phase is complete, the asymmetry is mostly caused by mandibular/condylar displacement and not actual size changes in the mandible.[5]

Imaging Protocols and Postprocessing

Patient mandibular posturing

For both osseous and soft tissue imaging, when evaluating the TMJs it is essential to view them while the mouth is in the closed position and the teeth are in maximum intercuspation. If the teeth

[a] Oral and Maxillofacial Radiology, Private Practice, Orlando, FL, USA; [b] Private Practice, Miami, FL, USA; [c] Private Practice, Diagnostic Digital Imaging, 99 Scripps road, Suite 101, Sacramento, CA 95825, USA
* Corresponding author.
E-mail address: daniatamimi2005@gmail.com

Radiol Clin N Am 56 (2018) 157–175
http://dx.doi.org/10.1016/j.rcl.2017.08.011
0033-8389/18/© 2017 Elsevier Inc. All rights reserved.

are not in maximum intercuspation, the spatial relationships of the TMJ components cannot be reliably evaluated and the diagnosis may not be accurate.[6] Images in the open mouth position give information about the position of the condyle and (in MR imaging) the disc. In patients who are not able to keep their mouths open and stable for the duration of the scan, a prefabricated mouth prop designed to replicate and maintain the patient's maximum opening can be used, which accurately stabilizes the mouth in maximum opening. Sometimes, a third scan is requested with a splint placed between the teeth. This device is fabricated by the dentist and changes the relationship of the condyle with the fossa to evaluate the effect of the splint on the condylar position and the soft tissues.

Soft tissue imaging (MR imaging)

TMJ coils are ideal for MR imaging of the TMJ. TMJ images should be obtained in the axially corrected sagittal oblique and coronal oblique planes through the TMJ (**Fig. 1**). This approach ensures that the images capture the correct spatial relationship of the disc to the condyle and fossa and helps to determine the presence of variations in the direction of displacement (rotational or sideways), which can be undetected or misdiagnosed if true (anatomic) sagittals or coronals images are obtained and evaluated. The most common protocols used for MR imaging evaluation of the TMJs are T1-weighted imaging (T1WI) or proton-density (PD) in the closed and open mouth positions, and T2-weighted imaging (T2WI) in the closed and open mouth positions. T1WI and PD show the structural and positional morphology of the TMJ components, whereas T2WI adds the ability to detect abnormal fluid, such as in joint effusion or bone marrow edema. Intravenous contrast may be used in suspected inflammatory disorders (such as juvenile

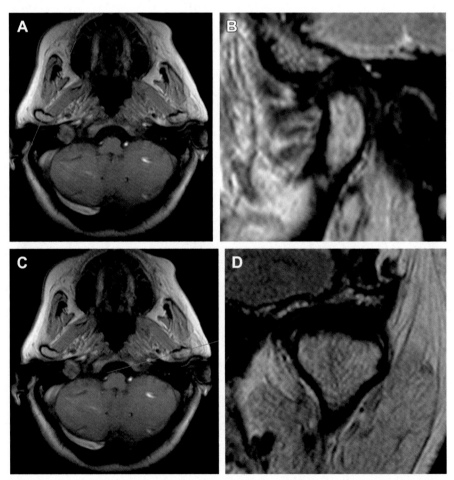

Fig. 1. MR images show the orientation and creation of axially corrected cross sections. (*A*) Axial MR imaging at the level of the condyles with a green indicator line shows the orientation and level of (*B*) the sagittal oblique cross section. (*C*) Axial MR imaging at the level of the condyles with an indicator line shows the orientation and level of (*D*) the coronal oblique cross section.

idiopathic arthritis) or in suspected malignancy. Other protocols may be requested or used by certain institutions, but those discussed earlier generally suffice for most TMJ imaging, especially for internal derangement.[2] Cine and dynamic MR imaging can also be used.

Osseous imaging (cone beam computed tomography or computed tomography)

For bone computed tomography (CT), a TMJ protocol that involves axially corrected images along and perpendicular to the long axis of the mandibular condyle is recommended. Cone beam CT (CBCT) images are acquired as a volume and can be manipulated at the workstation using DICOM-viewing software to create the corrected image reformations in the sagittal oblique and coronal oblique planes (**Fig. 2**).

Postprocessing reformations

As mentioned earlier, a thorough evaluation of the TMJs includes evaluation of the structures that are developmentally and functionally linked to it. In order to visualize the mandible and the occlusion, curvilinear reconstruction along the curve of the mandible (panoramic reformation) and three-dimensional (3D) surface renderings in the frontal and lateral views should be performed (**Fig. 3**). This approach aids in the visualization of the maxillofacial complex as a unit as well as the effect that alterations in form and function of the TMJ have on the mandible and the teeth.

Imaging Evaluation

Normal anatomy

Osseous structures of the temporomandibular joint When viewing the condyles and the fossa in the axially corrected sagittal oblique and coronal oblique views, there are a few key points to review:

Condylar contours The examiner should evaluate the position of the heights of contour of the condyle in relation to the fossa and to each other (**Fig. 4**). In the sagittal oblique view, when evaluating the posterior cortex of the condylar neck, it can be observed that it tapers to a point into a height of

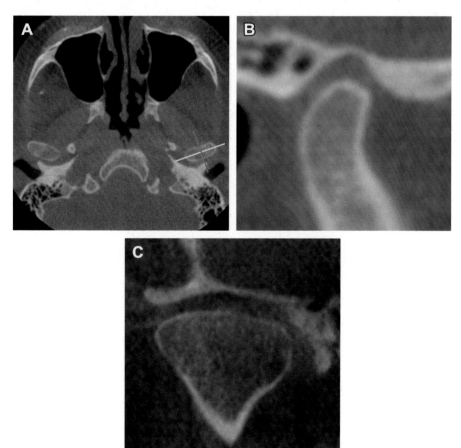

Fig. 2. (A) CBCT axial view with schematic plane lines to show the orientation of the axially corrected (B) sagittal oblique and (C) coronal oblique. These cross sections are correct and appropriate for the evaluation of the spatial relationships of the osseous structures.

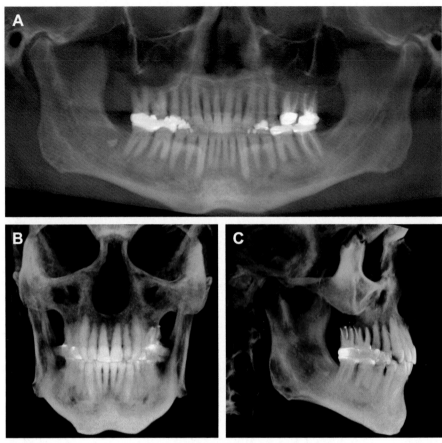

Fig. 3. CBCT (*A*) panoramic, (*B*) frontal 3D, and (*C*) lateral 3D reformats allow the evaluation of the effect of TMJ disorders on the facial skeleton and dental occlusion.

maximum curvature on the posterior surface (posterior height of contour). The cortex superior to this point becomes very thin and remains thin on the articular surface until the anterior height of contour just above the pterygoid fovea, where the cortex starts to flare down into the anterior aspect of the condylar neck. In a normal condyle, the posterior height of contour is more inferiorly positioned

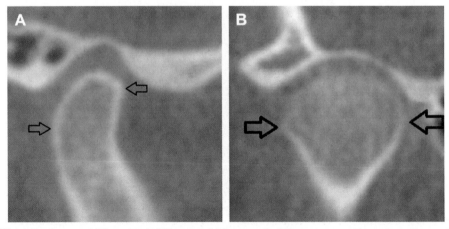

Fig. 4. CBCT axially corrected (*A*) sagittal oblique and (*B*) coronal oblique cross sections show the position of the condylar heights of contour (*arrows*) in relation to one another and to the fossa.

than the anterior height of contour and this distance becomes greater as the condyle grows to full adult size. In the coronal oblique view, the medial and lateral heights of contour can be visually connected with a line that passes through them and the posterior and anterior heights of contour and can be imagined to be the equator of the condyle. There should be fairly even condylar bone mass superior to this equator. A loss of bone on the articular surfaces may indicate degenerative or inflammatory changes and results in a superior migration of the heights of contours of the condyle in relation to the fossa, which can be a key distinguishing feature between condylar hypoplasia and stable degenerative joint disease.[2]

Condylar and fossa morphology The normal articular surfaces of the condyle and the fossa are incongruent, and the heights of maximum curvature of the anterior aspect of the condyle and the posterior slope of the eminence are opposite each other. This point is where the intermediate zone of the disc sits and acts as a cushion between these two surfaces. Rounded articular surfaces indicate a healthy joint, whereas flattened ones (ie, the formation of congruent articulation) indicate that the cushion of the disc is either no longer between these surfaces or has broken down to the point at which it can no longer perform its function.[2]

Cortical integrity and thickness On osseous imaging, the articular surface cortex of a normal adult condyle should be eggshell thin and continuous. Children have a thinner or nonvisible cortex but rounded contours. Growing individuals do not have a cortex on this surface because bone is forming through the process of endochondral

bone formation and rapidly turning over. On MR imaging, the articular cortex appears thicker because of the presence of a low-signal fibrocartilaginous cap that is indistinguishable from the underlying low-signal bony cortex. Thickening of the cortex on CT/CBCT indicates that the biomechanical threshold of the articular surfaces has been met or exceeded. Loss of integrity (erosion) indicates active degenerative joint disease.[2]

Trabecular bone density The trabecular bone should have homogeneous trabecular architecture and marrow spaces. Increased bone density on CT or CBCT and low signal intensity on T1WI and T2WI indicate sclerosis, and well-defined low density on CT and CBCT and a low signal on T1WI and a high signal on T2WI indicate the presence of a subchondral bone cyst.[7]

Homogeneity of the joint space attenuation A normal joint space should be isodense to soft tissue and homogeneous in density. The presence of calcifications within the joint space is not normal.

Spatial relationships of the condyle and the fossa In osseous imaging (CT or CBCT) in which the position and condition of the discs cannot be evaluated, the location of the condyle in the fossa in the closed and open mouth positions gives clues to the presence of soft tissue abnormality when no soft tissue imaging is available.[5] Clinicians must imagine the present of a normal biconcave disk between the osseous surfaces (**Fig. 5A**). In the sagittal oblique view with the anterior aspect being on the observer's left, the posterior band of the disc (the thickest part) should sit at the at the 12 or 11 o'clock position.[8] A thin intermediate

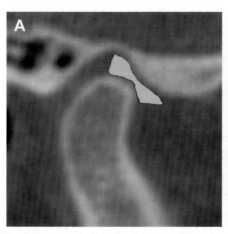
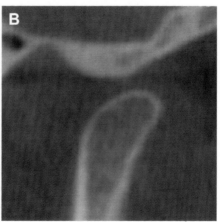

Fig. 5. CBCT axially corrected sagittal cross sections in the (*A*) closed and (*B*) open mouth positions show the normal spatial relationships of the osseous structures. (*A*) A normal-shaped biconcave disc can be imagined in the joint space by the examiner, indicating that the spatial relationships are within normal limits. (*B*) The condyle translates to a point inferior and slightly anterior to the crest of the eminence.

zone is interposed between the maximum heights of convexity of the articular surfaces. In the coronal oblique view, a crescent-shaped posterior band must be imagined sitting uniformly on top of the condyle and tapering out to the condylar poles. In the open mouth position, the normal condyle should translate to a point inferior to the crest of the eminence, with 1 to 3 mm of leeway anteriorly and posteriorly but still remaining below the eminence, and there should be enough space for the intermediate zone of the disc between the articular surfaces[9] (see **Fig. 5**B).

Soft tissue structures of the temporomandibular joint These structures can readily be shown on MR imaging but not on CT or CBCT. The disc and posterior attachment have low to intermediate signal intensity on both T1 and T2. In the sagittal oblique view, a normal TMJ disc is biconcave, and in the closed position the posterior band sits at the 11 to 12 o'clock position in relation to the condyle (**Fig. 6**A). The posterior band is generally the thickest part of the disc, followed by the anterior band and the thin intermediate zone. The intermediate zone is interposed between the convex articular surfaces and the anterior band appears to sit on the superior head of lateral pterygoid muscle fibers where they insert in the pterygoid fovea. The posterior attachment is made up of the temporal posterior attachment (superior lamina), the condylar posterior attachment (inferior lamina), and the area where they interweave and attach to the posterior band of the disc (intermediate posterior attachment). In the open mouth

position, the condyle and disc translate forward and, at this point, the part of the disc between the articular surfaces is the junction of the anterior band and the intermediate zone[8] (see **Fig. 6**B). A small amount of joint fluid can sometimes be seen on T2WI and is considered to be within normal limits.[10]

IMAGING OF TEMPOROMANDIBULAR JOINT DISORDERS
Imaging of Internal Derangement and Degenerative Joint Disease

Understanding the temporomandibular joint degenerative joint disease process
Soft tissue changes The TMJ is designed to withstand high multidirectional biomechanical forces. When the biomechanical demands exceed the biomechanical threshold of the disc, a loss of structural integrity of the disc and attachments occurs.[2] This loss of integrity leads to a gradual slipping (displacement) of the posterior band of the disc from the normal 11 to 12 o'clock position. If the biomechanical insult continues and increases, further damage can occur to these soft tissues and further displacement can occur. If the normal disc-condyle relationship is restored in the open mouth position, this is called disc displacement with reduction; if it does not, then this is called disc displacement without reduction[2,11–13] (**Fig. 7**). TMJ discs can become displaced in multiple directions, such as the anterior, anteromedial and anterolateral rotational, and sideways (pure medial or lateral) directions (**Fig. 8**). Some investigators

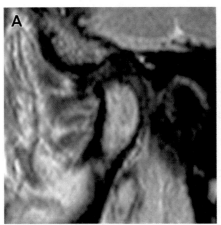 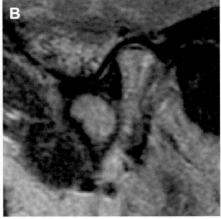

Fig. 6. MR PD sagittal oblique cross sections show the normal disc/condyle relationship in the (*A*) closed and (*B*) open positions. In the closed position, the posterior band of the disc should sit at the 11 to 12 o'clock position to the condyle. The thin intermediate zone should be positioned between the curvatures of the posterior slope of the eminence and the anterior aspect of the condyle. In the open position, the portion of the disc interposed between the articular surfaces of the osseous components should be the junction between the anterior band and the intermediate zone.

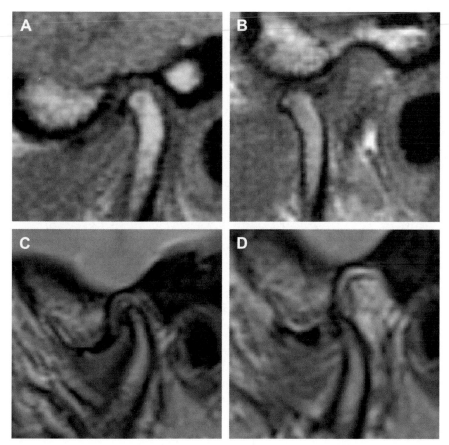

Fig. 7. MR images show (*A, B*) disc displacement with reduction and (*C, D*) disc displacement without reduction. (*A*) T1WI shows a biconcave disc that has maintained its anteroposterior dimension positioned anterior to the condyle. (*B*) T1WI in the same patient shows recapture of the disc by the condyle and translation of the condyle to normal range of motion. (*C*) T2WI shows a disc that is anteriorly displaced and appears morphologically altered. (*D*) T2WI in the same patient show lack of recapture of the disc by the condyle and limitation of condylar range of motion.

advocate the presence of posterior disc displacement, but it is the authors' opinion that this is most likely a false-positive appearance created by the formation of a pseudodisc; a thickening and fibrosis of the posterior attachment area that give a morphologically thick low signal similar to that of the disc.[8] Obtaining axially corrected sagittal oblique and coronal oblique cross sections is crucial for the correct evaluation and diagnosis of the direction of a disc displacement.

Osseous changes The soft tissue changes described earlier precede the osseous changes seen in degenerative joint disease (DJD) in both adults (called DJD) and children (called progressive condylar resorption [PCR] or idiopathic condylar resorption [ICR]). The morphology of the condyles and the effect of the degenerative process on the facial skeleton at the end stage of the degenerative change is different for adults and children, but the

process of destruction is similar. When the biomechanical threshold of the fibrocartilage and the articular surfaces is met, morphologic changes occur to the articular surfaces to adapt and to distribute these forces over a large surface area. These changes include thickening and sclerosis of the articular cortex and flattening of the articular surfaces (formation of congruent articulations). When the biomechanical threshold is exceeded, cortical breakdown (erosion) occurs (**Fig. 9**). The erosions destroy the articular surface and reduce its volume, and, when the forces are alleviated or when the body adapts to their presence, the articular surfaces start to repair and recorticate. However, the lost bone cannot be rebuilt, resulting in reduction of condylar height and volume with corticated surfaces and condylar heights of contour that have changed in relation to the fossa while the repair process was being completed. In adult DJD, it is common to see osteophytes as a method of increasing surface area for load

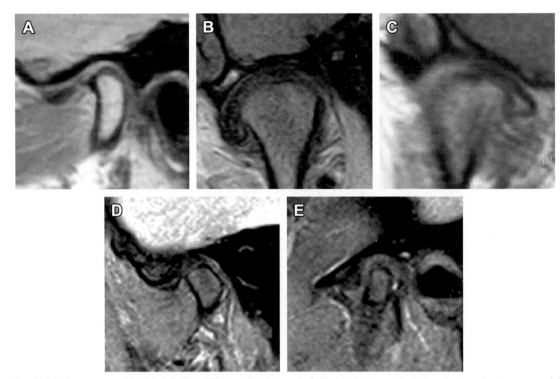

Fig. 8. MR images show some of the different directions of disc displacement: (*A*) anterior displacement, (*B*) lateral displacement, (*C*) medial displacement, and (*D, E*) anterior rotational displacement, where in the same TMJ (*D*) the disc is in the correct position in the center of the condyle and (*E*) it is displaced anteriorly off the lateral aspect of the condyle.

distribution (**Fig. 10**). Subchondral bone cysts can also be seen in adult DJD.[14]

Range of motion Condylar hypermobility is characterized by a condyle that moves more than 2 mm anterior and superior to the crest of the eminence. This hypermobility occurs when there is elongation of the posterior attachments and the sphenomandibular and stylomandibular ligaments. This condition may be seen in some early cases of internal derangement of the joint, or in Ehlers-Danlos syndrome.[15] It can manifest as subluxation of the condyle, in which the condyle can return to the closed position, or dislocation, in

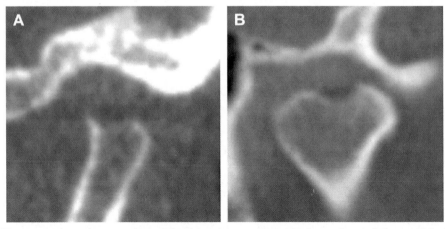

Fig. 9. CBCT cross sections show erosion and volume loss on the articular surface of the condyle in both the sagittal (*A*) and coronal (*B*) planes indicating active degenerative changes.

A

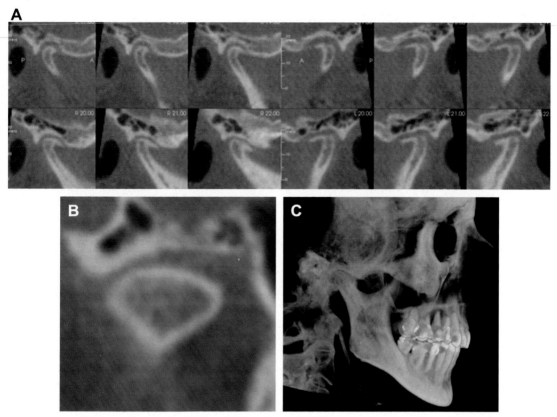

B

C

Fig. 10. CBCT reformations show the effect of end-stage degenerative changes on the condylar dimensions and the facial skeleton. (*A*) Serial sagittal cross sections show reduction of condylar height and the formation of an osteophyte anteriorly on each condyle. (*B*) The coronal view shows a reduction of the condylar height. (*C*) Lateral 3D rendering shows the effect of the reduction of condylar height bilaterally on the mandible: posterior rotation of the mandible, small mandible, and a steep mandibular plane, which can result in a convex facial profile.

which the condyle cannot return and the patient is in an open lock (**Fig. 11**). Condylar restriction is characterized by a condyle that remains posterior and superior to the crest of the eminence. It can occur with internal derangement. Disc displacement with reduction usually has a normal range of motion, but an acute closed lock is usually experienced in the acute phase of disc displacement without reduction. As the condition becomes more chronic, range of motion may be restored. Disc adhesions can be caused by trauma or by disc displacement (**Fig. 12**). Synovitis can lead to fibrin deposition and hence the decrease in lubrication that results in the stiction effect (2 solid objects pressed against each other but not sliding), reduced disc mobility, and further increase in fibrin depositions and formation of fibrous adhesions. This condition most commonly occurs in the superior joint compartment (where the translation motion of the TMJ occurs) but can occur in the inferior compartment (where the rotation motion of the condyle occurs). Thus, adhesions of the superior compartment manifest as more limitation

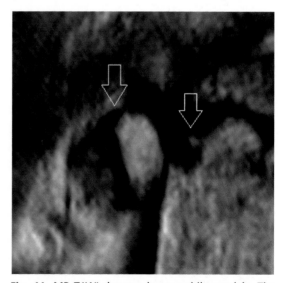

Fig. 11. MR T1WI shows a hypermobile condyle. The condyle (*yellow arrow*) is positioned anterior and superior to the crest of the eminence (*white arrow*). The portion of the disc between the condyle and fossa is the anterior band. This condyle is anterior to the normal position in relation to the disc indicated in **Fig. 6**.

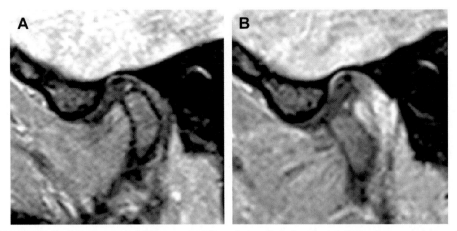

Fig. 12. MR T2WI in the (*A*) closed and (*B*) open positions shows that the disc position does not change in relation to the fossa, indicating a fibrous adhesion in the superior compartment.

of opening than those of the inferior compartment.[11–13] When investigating limited oral opening, coronoid hyperplasia should be ruled out as a causative factor.

Imaging of Inflammatory Disorders

Rheumatoid arthritis

Definition Rheumatoid arthritis is a chronic inflammatory disease that manifests as synovial membrane inflammation in many joints and can affect the TMJs. The inflammation of the synovial lining of the TMJ capsule in its chronic stage forms a granulomatous pannus that erodes the articular surface fibrocartilage and underlying bone.

Imaging findings The process mentioned earlier results in irregular resorption of the articular surfaces with subsequent flattening of the anterior and posterior aspects of the condyle, giving the sharpened-pencil appearance. In some late-stage cases, fibrous or bony ankylosis of the joint may occur. On T1WI and T2WI, the pannus has an intermediate signal intensity that can displace the temporal posterior attachment inferiorly and the condylar posterior attachment posteriorly (**Fig. 13**). Because the condition often occurs bilaterally, the condylar height is often reduced, which leads to posterior rotation of the mandible around a second molar fulcrum and results in an anterior open bite. This condition can occur unilaterally as well, or be more severe in one TMJ, resulting in mandibular asymmetry.[2,4]

Juvenile idiopathic arthritis

Definition Juvenile idiopathic arthritis is an autoimmune musculoskeletal inflammatory disease of childhood. It occurs primarily in large joints, but can affect the TMJs.

Imaging findings The inflammatory process usually destroys the condyle, resulting in a condylar-stump appearance and a wide and flat glenoid

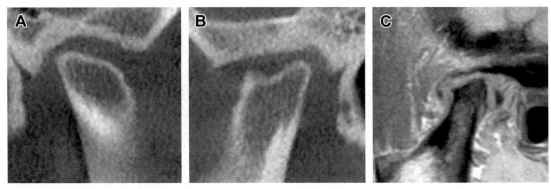

Fig. 13. (*A, B*) CBCT sagittal oblique cross sections show flattening of the condyles with a sharpened pencil appearance often seen with rheumatoid arthritis. (*C*) MR T1WI in another patient shows an intermediate-signal mass in the joint space representing pannus formation. (*From* Tamimi D, Hatcher DC. Specialty imaging: temporomandibular joint. Salt Lake City (UT): Elsevier; 2016; with permission.)

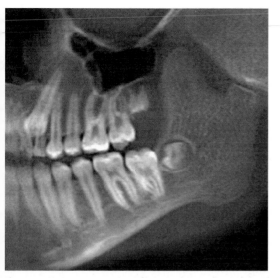

Fig. 14. CBCT panoramic reformat shows the left half of the mandible of a 15-year-old girl with bilateral juvenile idiopathic arthritis. The coronoid process is elongated and the condylar process is stumplike. The antegonial notch is deepened. (*From* Tamimi D, Hatcher DC. Specialty imaging: temporomandibular joint. Salt Lake City (UT): Elsevier; 2016; with permission.)

fossa (**Fig. 14**). The condyle may reposition anteriorly and superiorly because of the flattening of the eminence. On contrast-enhanced T2WI there is enhancement of the joint compartments, which allows the diagnosis to be made before the bone surface destruction is radiographically visible. Seventy-percent of patients with a positive diagnosis are asymptomatic.[16]

Pigmented villonodular synovitis

Definition Pigmented villonodular synovitis (PVNS), also called tenosynovitis and tenosynovial giant cell tumor, is a benign locally aggressive tumefactive disease of the synovium. It is rare in the TMJ.

Imaging findings PVNS has the radiographic appearance of an aggressive lesion destroying the condyle and invading into the middle cranial fossa. Bone CT shows erosion of the condyle and glenoid fossa. On T1WI and T2WI, low to intermediate signal with a peripheral rim of low signal can be seen. With contrast enhancement, some portions of the mass mildly enhance[17] (**Fig. 15**).

Imaging of Traumatic Changes

Neonatal fractures

Definition This specific type of fracture occurs perinatally with forceps delivery.

Imaging findings The condylar neck fractures and the fragment becomes anteriorly dislocated. Remodeling occurs and the result is an acute mandibular notch that projects radiographically as the characteristic pair-of-scissors appearance (**Fig. 16**). The anteriorly dislocated condyle does not function against the fibrocartilage of the eminence during feeding and mastication, resulting in an eminence that is flat because of the lack of stimulation of the fibrocartilage that is supposed to form it. Mild to moderate mandibular asymmetry is also noted, because the condyle is not functioning in its intended position, thus its growth and the growth of the mandible are affected.[2]

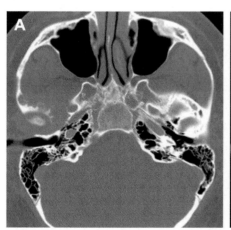
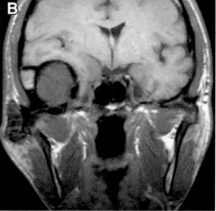

Fig. 15. (*A*) Axial bone CT shows widening of the right TMJ space and multiple rounded erosions of the adjacent skull base. (*B*) Coronal MR T1WI shows a hypointense right TMJ mass with peripheral lower signal intensity. There is a contiguous middle cranial fossa extra-axial mass with a similar markedly low-signal-intensity peripheral rim. This finding is consistent with pigmented villonodular synovitis. (*From* Tamimi D, Hatcher DC. Specialty imaging: temporomandibular joint. Salt Lake City (UT): Elsevier; 2016; with permission.)

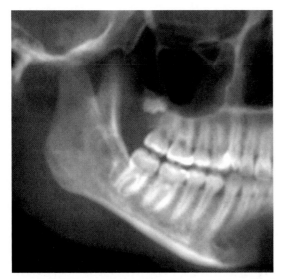

Fig. 16. CBCT panoramic reformat of the right half of the mandible shows anterior positioning of the condylar process. The condylar cortex traverses the ramus. There is an acute angle between the condylar process and the co-ronoid process. (*From* Tamimi D, Hatcher DC. Specialty imaging: temporomandibular joint. Salt Lake City (UT): Elsevier; 2016; with permission.)

Subcondylar and condylar fractures

Subcondylar and condylar fractures can occur in childhood or in adulthood. These types of fractures are discussed in Reyhaneh Alimohammadi's article, "Imaging of Dentoalveolar and Jaw Trauma," in this issue.

Bifid condyle

Definition Bifid condyle is a rare entity characterized by partial division of the mandibular condyle. It can have a congenital, developmental, or acquired cause and can be secondary to early trauma.[2]

Imaging findings Imaging findings range from a heart-shaped condyle, a vertical depression in the superior surface of the condyle best visualized on the coronal oblique view, to a duplication of the condyle (one condyle in front of the other) in the sagittal oblique view (**Fig. 17**).

Ankylosis

Definition Ankylosis of the TMJ can be fibrous or bony and is usually secondary to an insult to the joint. Trauma (hemarthrosis) is the most common cause, followed by inflammatory arthritides and previous joint surgery and infection. Fibrous ankylosis shows severely limited interincisal mouth opening and condylar translation.

Imaging findings On bone CT, there is maintenance of a low-density joint space in fibrous ankylosis, but the articular surfaces may be irregular. Bony ankylosis presents as complete immobility of the joint caused by fusion of the bony components of the joint (**Fig. 18**). Axially corrected coronal oblique bone CT shows a bony bridge of varying size extending medially and laterally beyond the confines of the capsule. It usually occurs on the lateral aspect of the joint, especially in cases of medial displacement of a fractured condyle.[2]

IMAGING OF TEMPOROMANDIBULAR JOINT NEOPLASIA
Benign

Osteochondroma

Definition Osteochondroma is a benign, cartilage-capped, exophytic lesion arising from bone. It can arise from the condyle and from the coronoid process.[18]

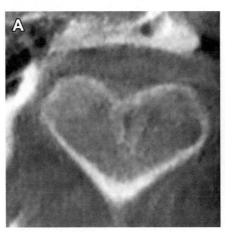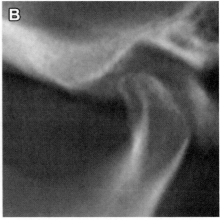

Fig. 17. CBCT (*A*) coronal oblique and (*B*) sagittal oblique cross sections show a bifid condyle. (*A*) The typical appearance of a deep groove in the superior aspect of the condyle. (*B*) The radiographic appearance of one condyle in front of the other that can be seen on panoramic plain film imaging and CBCT reformations. (*From* Tamimi D, Hatcher DC. Specialty imaging: temporomandibular joint. Salt Lake City (UT): Elsevier; 2016; with permission.)

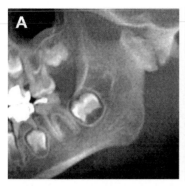
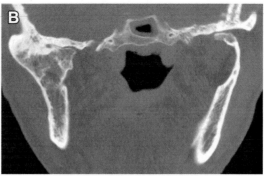

Fig. 18. (A) CBCT sagittal oblique view shows abnormal remodeling of the left condyle and fossa following trauma. There is maintenance of a thin low-density band between the temporal and mandibular components, suggestive of a fibrous union, not a bony one. (B) Coronal bone CT shows gross enlargement of the right condyle and bony fusion with the temporal bone. (*From* Tamimi D, Hatcher DC. Specialty imaging: temporomandibular joint. Salt Lake City (UT): Elsevier; 2016; with permission.)

Imaging findings Osteochondroma may appear as a pedunculated mass of mixed density attached to the condyle that often extends from the anterior or anteromedial surface of the condyle at the attachment of the lateral pterygoid muscle and can grow in the direction of the muscle fibers (**Fig. 19**). When small, it is difficult to differentiate this entity from osteophytes caused by degenerative changes.[2,19] When large, it can displace the condyle inferiorly in the fossa and displace the mandible contralaterally, resulting in an ipsilateral posterior open bite and a contralateral posterior crossbite.[4] Large osteochondromas may show secondary degenerative changes, making the diagnosis more difficult.[20]

Osteoma
Definition Osteoma is a benign, slow-growing, bone-forming tumor characterized by proliferation of either compact or cancellous bone. It usually originates from the surfaces of the condyle

that are covered with periosteum (nonarticular surfaces).

Imaging findings Osteoma appears as a pedunculated, homogeneous, well-defined, bone-based, high-density mass. It may be compact or cancellous and the bone pattern is normal (**Fig. 20**). This condition can also cause displacement of the condyle and the mandible if large enough.[2]

Malignant

Chondrosarcoma
Definition Chondrosarcoma is malignant tumor of cartilage that can arise centrally within the condylar or temporal bone, parosteally, or in the soft tissues of the TMJ.

Imaging findings On bone CT, a nonenhancing mass with flocculent calcifications around the condyle and in the joint space that may or may not destroy the bone is observed. The joint space is widened, and the condyle may appear enlarged

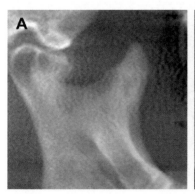
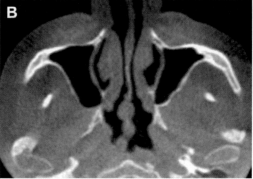

Fig. 19. (A) CBCT panoramic reformat shows how an osteochondroma can mimic an osteophyte. The normal condylar outline is seen but it is inferiorly displaced by the lesion. The fossa contours are within normal limits. (B) Axial view shows orientation of the lesion with fibers of the lateral pterygoid muscle fibers. (*From* Tamimi D, Hatcher DC. Specialty imaging: temporomandibular joint. Salt Lake City (UT): Elsevier; 2016; with permission.)

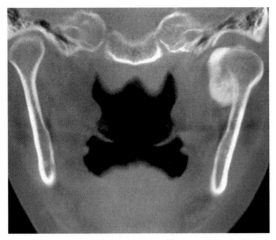

Fig. 20. Coronal CBCT shows a large, pedunculated, high-density mass arising from the neck of the condyle, suggestive of an osteoma. (*From* Tamimi D, Hatcher DC. Specialty imaging: temporomandibular joint. Salt Lake City (UT): Elsevier; 2016; with permission.)

or lengthened. There can be a ringlet pattern of calcification in and around the condyle. Periosteal reaction may or may not be present. It is of high signal intensity on T2WI, and the hypointense foci signifying calcifications may not be as prominent as the calcified appearance on CT. With contrast, a heterogeneously enhancing mass with whorls of intensifying lines within the tumor is often seen (**Fig. 21**). Other malignancies, such as osteosarcomas and metastases, can also affect the TMJs, the appearance of which has been covered in Susan M. White's article, "Malignant Lesions in the Dento-Maxillofacial Complex," in this issue.[21]

Imaging of Developmental Changes

Hemifacial microsomia

Definition Hemifacial microsomia is an anomaly of unknown origin. It affects structures developing from the first and second branchial arch, such as the ear, the TMJ and mandible, the orbit, the

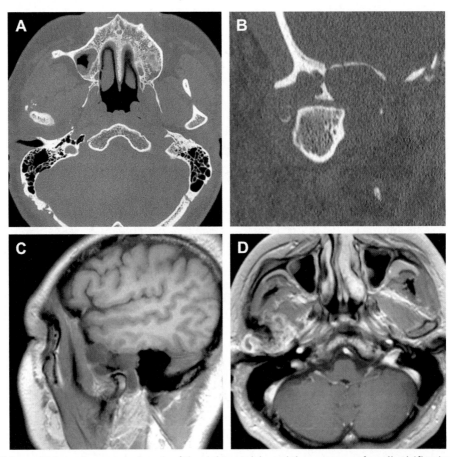

Fig. 21. (*A*) Bone CT shows increased sclerosis of the right condyle and the presence of small calcifications lateral to the condyle. (*B*) Coronal view shows ringlike calcifications lateral to the condyle and destruction of the glenoid fossa. (*C*) Sagittal MR T1WI shows a lobulated mass extending into the middle cranial fossa. (*D*) Axial contrast-enhanced T1WI shows extensive solid enhancement of the lesion, indicating that it is not inflammatory. (*From* Tamimi D, Hatcher DC. Specialty imaging: temporomandibular joint. Salt Lake City (UT): Elsevier; 2016; with permission.)

zygomatic arch, the facial nerve, and the facial soft tissues, including the muscles of mastication.

Imaging findings The degree of severity of mandibular asymmetry depends on the thickness of the fibrocartilaginous cap on the condyle, and the size of the condyle can range from condylar aplasia to a small condyle, with reduced development of the ipsilateral half of the mandible. The orbital floor is depressed and the zygomatic arch is often discontinuous. External ear canal atresia and lack of development of the middle ear structures can be seen, and an otic tag usually replaces the pinna[2,4] (**Fig. 22**).

Condylar hypoplasia
Definition Condylar hypoplasia is a developmental abnormality in which the condyle is smaller than the contralateral side because of a thinner

layer of, or insult to, the undifferentiated mesenchymal cells in the fibrocartilage cap of the condyle.

Imaging findings When reviewing the position of the condylar contours, the outlines and morphology of the condyle are within normal limits, but it may appear smaller overall, or it may be shorter than the other side, resulting in a smaller mandible ipsilaterally and mandibular asymmetry. An occlusal cant (tilt) in the coronal plane is noted, caused by this asymmetry, with the teeth on the affected side being more elevated. The osseous midline of the mandible may be shifted to the affected side[2,4] (**Fig. 23**).

Condylar hyperplasia
Definition Condylar hyperplasia is a slowly developing unilateral overgrowth of the condyle caused

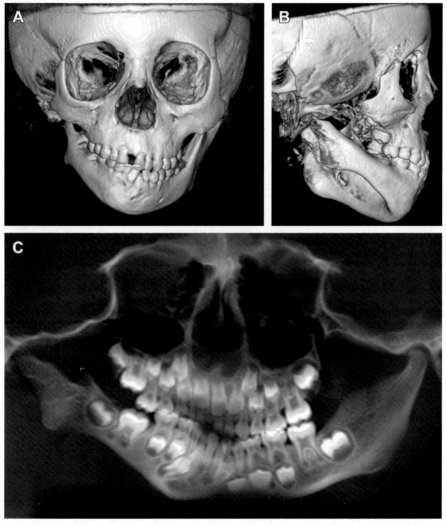

Fig. 22. CBCT reformats of a patient with hemifacial microsomia show (*A*) mandibular asymmetry and occlusal elevation on the affected side, (*B*) missing coronoid process and a zygomatic arch defect, and (*C*) decreased vertical height of the mandibular body and a flat undeveloped TMJ fossa and eminence. (*From* Tamimi D, Hatcher DC. Specialty imaging: temporomandibular joint. Salt Lake City (UT): Elsevier; 2016; with permission.)

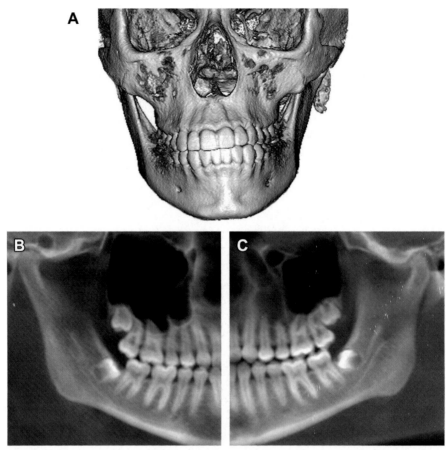

Fig. 23. (*A*) CBCT 3D frontal reformation shows mandibular asymmetry, deviation of the mandibular osseous midline to the left, and medial bowing of the left ramus, indicating a small left condyle. (*B, C*) Panoramic reformats of the right and left sides of the mandible show that the left side of the mandible is smaller than the right. The left condyle maintains the position of its posterior and anterior heights of contour, indicating left condylar hypoplasia. (*From* Tamimi D, Hatcher DC. Specialty imaging: temporomandibular joint. Salt Lake City (UT): Elsevier; 2016; with permission.)

by a thicker layer of undifferentiated mesenchymal cells in the fibrocartilage cap of the condyle.

Imaging findings The condylar neck may be elongated and there may be regional overgrowth of the ipsilateral half of the mandible. The mandibular ramus may be bowed laterally and the inferior border of the mandible may be convex (it is usually fairly concave). An occlusal cant (tilt) in the coronal plane is noted, caused by this asymmetry, with the teeth on the affected side being more depressed (**Fig. 24**). The growth can continue until the third decade. If the condition is bilateral and in an older individual, acromegaly should be suspected.[2,4]

Imaging of Miscellaneous Conditions

Synovial chondromatosis
Definition Synovial chondromatosis can be primary (unrelated to DJD) or secondary to DJD. In the primary form, there is development of cartilaginous nodules within subsynovial connective

tissue that subsequently detach, ossify, and form loose articular bodies in the joint space.

Imaging findings Synovial chondromatosis is not a neoplastic process but can widen the joint space through mass effect on the condyle (displacement and remodeling) or remodeling of the fossa. Intracranial extension has been reported. On bone CT, multiple calcified nodules can be seen surrounding the condyle, and the joint space can be widened. It most commonly occurs in the superior compartment (**Fig. 25**). On T1WI, the tissue planes between the mass and the surrounding soft tissues can be defined, and the mass can be differentiated from a parotid gland tumor. Multiple hypointense nodules (loose articular bodies) may be observed. On T2WI, there is superior joint compartment effusion and there may be expansion. Contrast-enhanced T1WI reveals an enhancing synovium. In the form secondary to DJD, there is production of 1 or more cartilaginous or osseous fragments along with irritation and metaplasia of the synovial

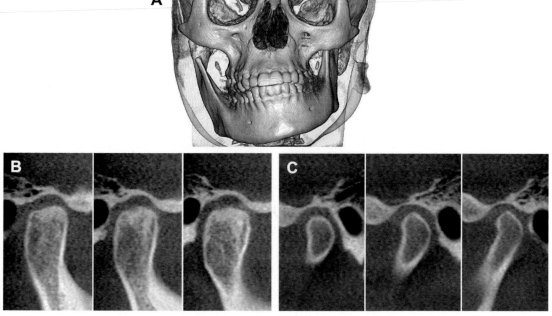

Fig. 24. (*A*) CBCT 3D frontal reformation shows mandibular asymmetry, deviation of the mandibular osseous midline to the left, and lateral bowing of the right ramus, indicating a large right condyle. (*B*) Sagittal oblique cross sections show a right condyle that appears to be too large for the fossa and overall larger than the left side (*C*). (*From* Tamimi D, Hatcher DC. Specialty imaging: temporomandibular joint. Salt Lake City (UT): Elsevier; 2016; with permission.)

membrane following unrelated breakdown of the articular surfaces caused by DJD. There are signs of advanced DJD (congruent articulation, osteophyte formation, joint space narrowing, and possible subchondral bone cyst formation). This form of synovial chondromatosis does not widen the joint space or displace the condyle (no mass effect).[2]

Calcium pyrophosphate dihydrate deposition disease

Definition Calcium pyrophosphate dihydrate deposition (CPPDD) is a metabolic disease in which calcium pyrophosphate crystals are deposited in the synovial fluid, resulting in calcification of the articular cartilage and leading to acute arthritis in some patients. Tumoral CPPDD disease is the

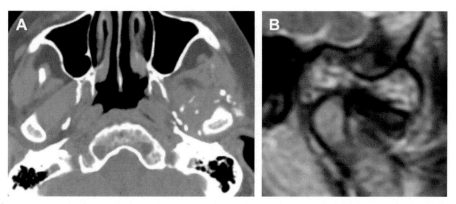

Fig. 25. (*A*) Noncontrast enhanced CT in a patient with synovial chondromatosis shows multiple small loose calcified articular bodies surrounding the left condyle. (*B*) Sagittal oblique T2WI MR shows a high-signal mass with small low-density bodies within. (*From* Tamimi D, Hatcher DC. Specialty imaging: temporomandibular joint. Salt Lake City (UT): Elsevier; 2016; with permission.)

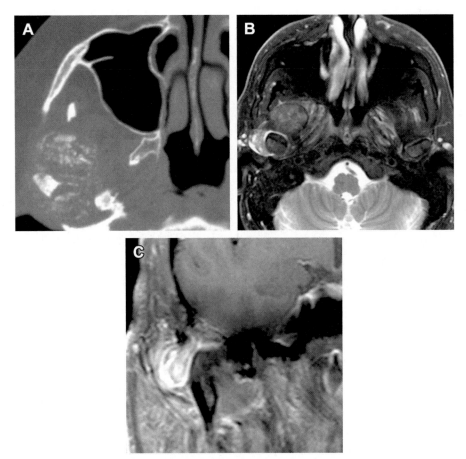

Fig. 26. (*A*) Axial bone CT of a patient with CPPDD disease shows a large erosive defect in the medial aspect of the condyle and fine granular soft tissue calcifications surrounding the condyle. (*B*) Axial MR T2WI with fat suppression (FS) shows a heterogeneous but predominantly low-signal-intensity lesion anterior to the condyle. Joint effusion is noted. (*C*) Coronal contrast-enhanced T1WI FS in the same patient shows enhancement of the inferolateral mass. (*From* Tamimi D, Hatcher DC. Specialty imaging: temporomandibular joint. Salt Lake City (UT): Elsevier; 2016; with permission.)

most prevalent type in the TMJs. It differs from gout, in which uric acid crystals are precipitated, therefore it is called pseudogout.

Imaging findings On bone CT, early CPPDD disease presents as fine, cloudlike calcifications with even distribution in the joint space, often encircling the condyle. Late CPPDD disease presents as a chunky, diffusely calcified mass that may have a ground-glass appearance. There can be associated bone remodeling and mass effect that may mimic malignancy because of extensive bone destruction, which makes it difficult to differentiate from chondrosarcoma. On MR imaging, T1WI shows a low-signal to intermediate-signal lesion because of the soft tissue mass in the joint space. Expansion of the joint capsule and joint space with or without joint effusion can be seen. Contrast enhancement yields a heterogeneously enhancing mass[2] (**Fig. 26**).

SUMMARY

The TMJ is a complex structure that is developmentally and functionally linked to the rest of the craniomandibular complex. The key to correct interpretation of TMJ imaging findings lies in a thorough knowledge of the anatomy of the TMJ and an understanding of the function and dysfunction of the TMJs in relation to the jaws, the teeth, and the cranial base.

REFERENCES

1. Kahn J, Tallents RH, Katzberg RW, et al. Prevalence of dental occlusal variables and intraarticular temporomandibular disorders: molar relationship, lateral guidance, and nonworking side contacts. J Prosthet Dent 1999;82:410–5.
2. Tamimi D, Hatcher DC. Specialty imaging: temporomandibular joint. Salt Lake City (UT): Elsevier; 2016.

3. Singh M, Detamore MS. Biomechanical properties of the mandibular condylar cartilage and their relevance to the TMJ disc. J Biomech 2009;42:405–17.

4. Westesson PL, Tallents RH, Katzberg RW, et al. Radiographic assessment of asymmetry of the mandible. AJNR Am J Neuroradiol 1994;15: 991–9.

5. Power A, Carter L. Osteochondroma of the mandibular condyle: an unusual case of dentofacial asymmetry. Dent Update 2015;42(4):369–70, 372. [Erratum appears in Dent Update 2015; 42(5):496].

6. Bonilla-Aragon H, Tallents RH, Katzberg RW, et al. Condyle position as a predictor of temporomandibular joint internal derangement. J Prosthet Dent 1999;82:205–8.

7. Larheim TA, Katzberg RW, Westesson PL, et al. MR evidence of temporomandibular joint fluid and condyle marrow alterations: occurrence in asymptomatic volunteers and symptomatic patients. Int J Oral Maxillofac Surg 2001;30:113–7.

8. Katzberg RW, Tallents RH. Normal and abnormal temporomandibular joint disc and posterior attachment as depicted by magnetic resonance imaging in symptomatic and asymptomatic subjects. J Oral Maxillofac Surg 2005;63:1155–61.

9. Hatcher DC, Blom RJ, Baker CG. Temporomandibular joint spatial relationships: osseous and soft tissues. J Prosthet Dent 1986;56:344–53.

10. Tallents RH, Katzberg RW, Murphy W, et al. Magnetic resonance imaging findings in asymptomatic volunteers and symptomatic patients with temporomandibular disorders. J Prosthet Dent 1996;75: 529–33.

11. Ahmad M, Schiffman EL. Temporomandibular joint disorders and orofacial pain. Dent Clin North Am 2016;60(1):105–24.

12. Look JO, Schiffman EL, Truelove EL, et al. Reliability and validity of axis I of the research diagnostic criteria for temporomandibular disorders (RDC/TMD) with proposed revisions. J Oral Rehabil 2010;37:744–59.

13. Ahmad M, Hollender L, Anderson Q, et al. Research diagnostic criteria for temporomandibular disorders (RDC/TMD): development of image analysis criteria and examiner reliability for image analysis. Oral Surg Oral Med Oral Pathol Oral Radiol Endod 2009;107:844–60.

14. Palconet G, Ludlow JB, Tyndall DA, et al. Correlating cone beam CT results with temporomandibular joint pain of osteoarthritic origin. Dentomaxillofac Radiol 2012;41:126–30.

15. Perrini F, Tallents RH, Katzberg RW, et al. Generalized joint laxity and temporomandibular disorders. J Orofac Pain 1997;11:215–21.

16. Al-Shwaikh H, Urtane I, Pirttiniemi P, et al. Radiologic features of temporomandibular joint osseous structures in children with juvenile idiopathic arthritis. Cone beam computed tomography study. Stomatologija 2016;18:51–60.

17. Damodar D, Chan N, Kokot N. Pigmented villonodular synovitis of the temporomandibular joint: case report and review of the literature. Head Neck 2015;37:E194–9.

18. Sawada K, Schulze D, Matsumoto K, et al. Osteochondroma of the coronoid process of the mandible. J Oral Sci 2015;57:389–92.

19. Mehra P, Arya V, Henry C. Temporomandibular joint condylar osteochondroma: complete condylectomy and joint replacement versus low condylectomy and joint preservation. J Oral Maxillofac Surg 2016; 74(5):911–25.

20. Wang Y, Li L, Chen M, et al. Osteochondroma with secondary synovial chondromatosis in the temporomandibular joint. Br J Oral Maxillofac Surg 2016;54: 454–6.

21. Giorgione C, Passali FM, Varakliotis T, et al. Temporo-mandibular joint chondrosarcoma: case report and review of the literature. Acta Otorhinolaryngol Ital 2015;35:208–11.

Radiographic Evaluation of Sleep-Disordered Breathing

Douglas D. Steffy, DDS, MS*, Clarence S. Tang, DDS, MD

KEYWORDS

- CBCT • Airway • Obstructive sleep apnea • Sleep-disordered breathing

KEY POINTS

- Anatomy and anatomic variations of the pediatric and adult airway, extending from the nasopharynx to the hypopharynx, are described.
- Airway anatomy and pathologies that relate to sleep-disordered breathing are discussed.
- Protocols for 3-dimensional radiographic interpretation of the airway are reviewed.

INTRODUCTION

In the litany of diseases afflicting modern civilizations, sleep-disordered breathing (SDB) is rapidly increasing in prevalence and financial impact on Western societies.[1] Comorbidities include hypertension, myocardial infarction, stroke, memory loss, diabetes, depression, insomnia, and daytime drowsiness. With a range of medical and surgical treatments each targeting a different aspect of the disease, it behooves providers to have an understanding of the anatomic, hereditary, environmental, and lifestyle considerations that play a role. This discussion focuses on the anatomic features pertinent to obstructive SDB.

In the current era, 3-dimensional imaging of the upper respiratory tract—specifically, cone beam computed tomography (CBCT) scans—aid in the prediction and diagnosis of patients who suffer from obstructive SDB. CBCTs are increasingly being used routinely for their value in providing general dental care, and as such can be an invaluable screening tool for identifying patients with potential obstructive SDB. For practitioners regularly acquiring such scans, it is imperative to become well-versed in the radiographic anatomy of the upper respiratory tract, including normal appearance, common abnormalities, incidental findings, and common pathologies that might increase the risk for SDB.[1]

CLINICAL ANATOMY OF THE UPPER RESPIRATORY TRACT

The upper respiratory tract extends from the nares to the larynx, encompassing the nasal and oral airways (**Fig. 1**). The nasal cavity extends from the nares to the posterior choanae, comprising the external nasal valves, internal nasal valves, nasal septum, and turbinates. The external nasal valve involves the lower lateral cartilages, the nasal septum, and floor. The internal nasal valve is found at the junction between the upper lateral cartilages and the septum, and should form an angle between 10° and 15°. The nasal septum, at the midline, is composed of the vomer, the perpendicular plate, and septal cartilage. The septum should be relatively straight with no significant deviations. The lateral walls of the nasal cavity should be either straight or slightly concave, upon which sit the 3 paired turbinates. The inferior and middle nasal turbinates should be relatively symmetric

United States Navy, James A. Lovell Federal Health Care Center, 3001 Green Bay Road, North Chicago, IL 60064, USA
* Corresponding author.
E-mail address: Dr.Steffy@beamreaders.com

Radiol Clin N Am 56 (2018) 177–185
http://dx.doi.org/10.1016/j.rcl.2017.08.012
0033-8389/18/Published by Elsevier Inc.

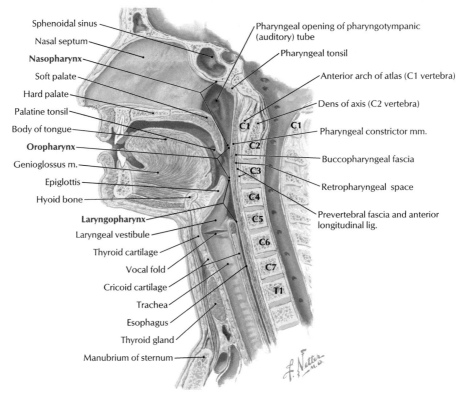

Sphenoidal sinus
Nasal septum
Nasopharynx
Soft palate
Hard palate
Palatine tonsil
Body of tongue
Oropharynx
Genioglossus m.
Epiglottis
Hyoid bone
Laryngopharynx
Laryngeal vestibule
Thyroid cartilage
Vocal fold
Cricoid cartilage
Trachea
Esophagus
Thyroid gland
Manubrium of sternum

Pharyngeal opening of pharyngotympanic (auditory) tube
Pharyngeal tonsil
Anterior arch of atlas (C1 vertebra)
Dens of axis (C2 vertebra)
Pharyngeal constrictor mm.
Buccopharyngeal fascia
Retropharyngeal space
Prevertebral fascia and anterior longitudinal lig.

C1 C1
C2
C3
C4
C5
C6
C7
T1

Fig. 1. Graphic from Netter's Anatomy shows the sagittal midline anatomy of the upper respiratory tract. (*Courtesy of* www.netterimages.com; with permission of Elsevier.)

and inferolaterally curved, with the concave surface facing toward lateral wall of the nasal cavity (**Fig. 2**).[2]

The nasopharynx begins at the posterior choanae and extends to the level of the hard palate. It is lined in the upper aspect with adenoidal tissue of varying thickness (**Fig. 3**). This tissue is sometimes referred to as the pharyngeal tonsils. The oropharynx begins at the level of the hard palate and includes the soft palate and uvula. Inferior to the uvula, along the lateral walls of the oropharynx posterior to the base of the tongue, paired palatine tonsils are present, as well as tonsils at the base of the tongue. Along with the pharyngeal tonsils, this collective of lymphoid tissue is often referred to as Waldeyer's ring. The hypopharynx begins at the base of the tongue, includes the epiglottis, and extends to the paired vocal cords.[2]

ANATOMIC VARIATIONS OF CLINICAL SIGNIFICANCE

Many normal variations of the upper respiratory tract can cause restricted airflow. Although these findings are not considered pathologic, they are

important to recognize and identify as possible contributors to SDB.

Nasal Cavity

The external and internal nasal valves have the smallest cross-sectional area (and therefore the highest resistance) of the passageways in the upper respiratory tract. Constricted nasal valves

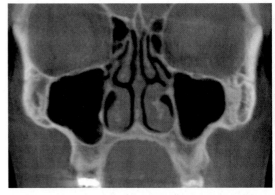

Fig. 2. Coronal cone beam computed tomography at the level of the nasal fossa and maxillary sinuses shows normal sinus, turbinate, and septal anatomy.

Medial view
Median (sagittal) section

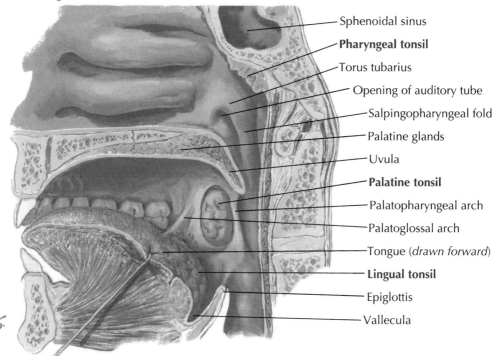

- Sphenoidal sinus
- **Pharyngeal tonsil**
- Torus tubarius
- Opening of auditory tube
- Salpingopharyngeal fold
- Palatine glands
- Uvula
- **Palatine tonsil**
- Palatopharyngeal arch
- Palatoglossal arch
- Tongue (*drawn forward*)
- **Lingual tonsil**
- Epiglottis
- Vallecula

Fig. 3. Graphic from Netter's Anatomy shows the sagittal anatomy, demonstrating key anatomic features of the oral cavity, nasal cavity, nasopharynx, and oropharynx areas. (*Courtesy of* www.netterimages.com; with permission of Elsevier.)

can be the result of malpositioned nasal cartilages, surgery, or trauma, and, although not considered strictly pathologic, is often an important cause of obstructed airflow.[3] The nasal septum is commonly deviated – by some estimates up to 80% of the time. The severity of this deviation varies greatly (**Fig. 4**).[3] Septal spurs are common and usually occur with deviation.

The middle and inferior nasal turbinates are highly variable in size and shape. Additionally, the turbinates are lined with mucosa, which can be enlarged. Together these 2 variables can cause significant obstruction of the nasal airway. Of note, turbinate size can be affected by the natural nasal cycle, an alternating pattern of partial congestion and decongestion of the nasal cavities that occurs every 2 to 3 hours. This occurs in the mucosa, predominantly surrounding the inferior turbinates, and results from the mucosa on 1 side becoming engorged with blood, while the contralateral side decongests by shunting away blood. This may result in the feeling of unilateral nasal congestion. It is important to understand this normal

physiologic process so as to avoid a radiographic misdiagnosis (**Fig. 5**).[4]

Another common incidental finding is pneumatization of the turbinates, referred to as concha bullosa (**Fig. 6**). Pneumatized turbinates, representing air-filled cavities within a turbinate or turbinates,

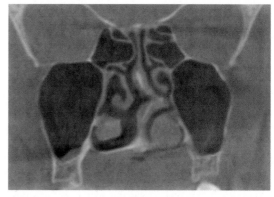

Fig. 4. Coronal cone beam computed tomography shows a deviated nasal septum with septal spur formation. This in narrowing the left nasal cavity and may increase upper airway resistance.

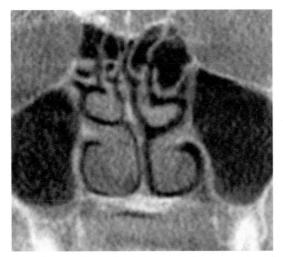

Fig. 5. Coronal cone beam computed tomography of the nasal fossa shows the natural nasal cycle. The mucosa on the right turbinates is enlarged when compared with the contralateral side.

can be enlarged enough to contribute to nasal airway constriction, either through physical occlusion of the airway or via displacement of adjacent structures, such as the nasal septum or infundibulum.[4]

Nasopharynx and Oropharynx

In the posterior nasopharynx and oropharynx, Waldeyer's ring may be the cause of significant partial or complete obstruction of the airway. This finding is more likely in a child or adolescent. Although the exact dimensions of this ring of

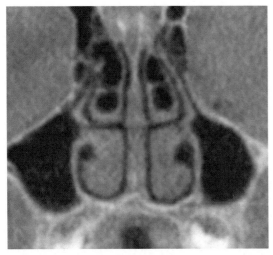

Fig. 6. Coronal cone beam computed tomography of the nasal fossa with pneumatized and enlarged middle nasal turbinates (concha bullosa).

tissue vary greatly, in general it is greatest in size around age 4, and begin to involute around age 10. By age 16, its dimensions are expected to be clinically insignificant. In an adult, the tonsillar tissues are not expected to be hypertrophic, and enlargement of these tissues may contribute not only to airway obstruction, but may be indicators of more insidious processes, such as chronic infection or neoplasm.

CERVICAL SPINE AND HEAD POSITION

When acquiring the CBCT scan in the seated position, the patient will most likely be positioned and stabilized using positioning devices to prevent motion artifact on the scan. These positioning devices may alter the natural head posture of the patient; thus, the position of the head on the scan should be correlated with the patient's clinical presentation. Patient head posture can affect the dimensions of the oropharynx, and if volumetric and cross-sectional analysis of the airway is produced, these measurements can change as the patient brings his or her head forward or back. Oropharyngeal patency is increased when the head is postured forward, and patients with small oropharyngeal dimensions can habitually adopt this mechanism to enable them to increase their airway patency. Patients with kyphotic or lordotic postures also have anterior head posture to make up for the excessive flexion of the thoracic spine.

Other conditions of the cervical spine that may decrease oropharyngeal and hypopharyngeal dimensions are the sequela of degenerative joint disease of the cervical spine. The development of osteophytes on the anterior aspect of the vertebral bodies and anterolisthesis can displace the prevertebral soft tissues into the lumen of the respiratory tract, thereby reducing the volume of respiratory tract (Fig. 7), but the significance of this condition for SDB is unknown.

CLINICAL PATHOLOGY OF THE UPPER RESPIRATORY TRACT

There are numerous upper respiratory tract pathologies that may contribute to airway obstruction. These range from congenital abnormalities, malformations, to acquired and pathologic entities. In the nasal cavity and nasopharynx areas, several pathologic conditions can cause partial or complete obstruction of the airway. Choanal atresia, which is a congenital condition that results in complete obstruction of the posterior nasal aperture, is the most common congenital

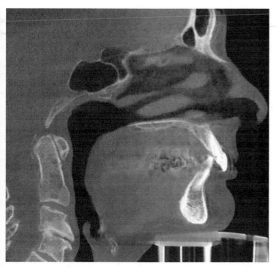

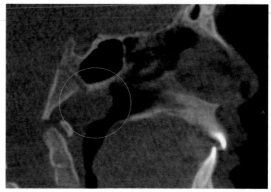

Fig. 8. Sagittal cone beam computed tomography (CBCT) shows enlarged adenoids (*yellow circle*) in the posterior wall of the nasopharynx.

Fig. 7. Sagittal cone beam computed tomography shows spondylolisthesis, or anterior positioning of the C4 vertebrae, with anterior osteophytes on C3 and C4, which are protruding into the airway space.

abnormality of the nasal cavity. This area should be examined for patency.[5]

The nasal cavity is also susceptible for sinus pathology, which, if left undetected or untreated, may invade into the nasal cavity, causing obstruction. A deviated septum not only can cause airway obstruction of the affected side, but also can interfere with sinus drainage, resulting in frequent sinonasal infections, which may contribute to breathing difficulties through the nose. Other lesions, such as fungal sinusitis, sinonasal polyposis, polyps, sinonasal ossifying fibromas, and inverted papilloma, can originate in the sinus and then expand into the nasal cavity. Sometimes, nasal obstruction is the first symptom the patient experiences.

As mentioned, in the posterior nasopharynx the adenoids can be quite enlarged in children (**Fig. 8**). Although this is a normal finding, if identified as the cause of significant breathing difficulties, surgical intervention may be warranted.

ADVANTAGES AND LIMITATIONS OF CONE BEAM COMPUTED TOMOGRAPHY FOR ANALYSIS OF THE UPPER RESPIRATORY TRACT

On a conventional large-volume CBCT scan, the airway is visible from the tip of the nose to the epiglottis. The hyoid bone is typically visible as well. A large-volume scan also includes the jaws, cranial base, and spine. The thyroid cartilage, and soft tissue components, such as the thyrohyoid ligament and triticeous

cartilage are not visible, unless they are secondarily calcified.

The advent of CBCT has brought many advantages for airway analysis. The small size and affordability of the machines enables many individual practices and practitioners to take CBCTs in their private offices. These practitioners are able to more precisely view and evaluate areas that previously were unable to be visualized on 2-dimensional radiography, including the paranasal sinuses, nasal cavity, the nasopharynx, the oropharynx, and the trachea, and are well-positioned to be able to identify common anatomic abnormalities contributing to obstructive SDB.

Another advantage of CBCT over other modalities, such as multidetector computed tomography, or MR imaging, is their time of acquisition. Children and some adolescents often require sedation for advanced imaging. Many CBCT manufacturers have created fast scan protocols for CBCT scans on young children, which lower the radiation dose and can be acquired in as little as 4.8 to 15.0 seconds, allowing high-quality images with minimal motion artifact. Although unnecessary radiographic examinations are never suggested, CBCT is a highly useful tool to evaluate children at risk for obstructive SDB.

One of the main limitations of CBCT is the lack of soft tissue contrast.[6,7] This limitation causes the soft tissues of the oropharynx and laryngopharynx, including the tonsils, lymph nodes, muscles, ligaments, blood vessels, salivary glands, and connective tissue, to appear isodense and therefore indistinguishable from each other. However, the soft tissue airway boundaries are easily identifiable.[6,7] As a screening tool, the airway can be examined for symmetry and smooth contours. If soft tissue pathology is visualized or suspected, appropriate further advanced imaging modalities, such as multidetector computed tomography or MR imaging, and a referral to the appropriate specialist should be recommended.[8]

An additional limitation of CBCT specific to evaluation of the airway for obstructive SDB is that patients are scanned upright and awake and are captured at a particular moment in time, which may or may not correlate with the dynamic airway at sleep in a supine position. The significance of capturing the image in natural head posture was discussed previously, thus, the importance of realizing that the volumetric and cross-sectional measurements may not correlate with the patient's actual oropharyngeal dimensions unless the head position on the scan and clinically are identical. The patient's tongue position during CBCT scan acquisition can also change the oropharyngeal dimensions on the scan. A neutral tongue position is encouraged.

CURRENT POSTPROCESSING PROTOCOLS FOR UPPER RESPIRATORY TRACT ANALYSIS

Airway analysis should be methodical, reliable, and repeatable. A suggested systematic method is to start at the beginning of the airway, which is the nasal cavity. The nasal valves should be analyzed for patency and symmetry. Any deviations in the nasal septum should be noted, because this can contribute to altered or restricted airflow. The nasal turbinates must be analyzed for normal size and shape. Pneumatized, enlarged, or paradoxic turbinates are important and significant findings, because they can all restrict airflow, or contribute to a clinical sensation of nasal obstruction (Fig. 9). The middle nasal turbinates are particularly susceptible to pneumatization and can become quite enlarged, partially or completely occluding the superior nasal compartment. Finally, the posterior nasopharynx should be analyzed for any significant soft tissue in the adenoid area, especially for occlusion of the posterior choanae. This finding will be very common in children, and although not pathologic, can be symptomatic.

The next area for analysis is the oropharynx. Two of the most useful measurements are minimum cross-sectional dimension and airway volume, and can be measured reliably and repeatedly using any of several software packages.[4]

The CBCT scan should be aligned in all 3 dimensions by identifying and orienting certain

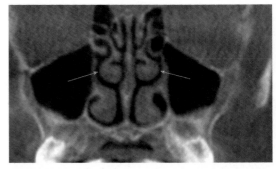

Fig. 9. Coronal cone beam computed tomography (CBCT) shows paradoxic middle nasal turbinates. Note the curvature of the middle turbinates medially (*yellow arrows*).

anatomic landmarks. An established method for doing this in the axial and coronal planes is by using the ossicles. The ossicles of the inner ear are an easily identifiable landmark and can be oriented parallel to each other in the axial and coronal planes (Figs. 10 and 11). In the sagittal plane, a line can be drawn from the posterior nasal spine to the basion (the most anterior point of the foramen magnum), and a second line at the superiormost level of the body of the C4 vertebrae (Fig. 12).[4,9] This second line should be oriented parallel to the first line. When the software airway dimension tool is set between these 2 parallel lines, it will automatically generate the minimum cross-sectional dimension, the anatomic location of greatest airway constriction, and the airway volume (Fig. 13).

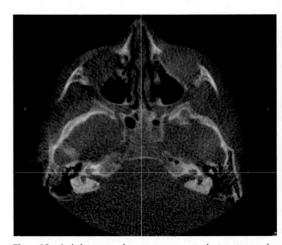

Fig. 10. Axial cone beam computed tomography (CBCT) demonstrates the orientation of the CBCT volume in the axial plane before airway evaluation. The coronal cross-hairs in the CBCT viewing software can be aligned with the middle ear ossicles.

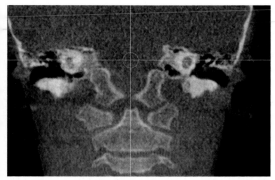

Fig. 11. Coronal cone beam computed tomography (CBCT) demonstrates the orientation of the CBCT volume in the coronal plane before airway evaluation. The axial cross-hairs in the CBCT viewing software can be aligned with the middle ear ossicles.

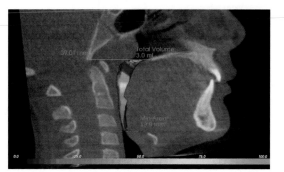

Fig. 13. Sagittal cone beam computed tomography (CBCT) with volumetric airway dimension, showing the minimum cross-sectional dimension. The measurement also indicates the level of greatest constriction in the respiratory tract. In this case, the greatest constriction is at the level of the epiglottis.

Several studies have been published that relate certain cross-sectional area dimensions thresholds to risk levels for obstructive breathing disorders. One such study relates the following values to risk level[8]:

- Minimum airway cross-sectional value:
  - Less than 52 mm^2 → high risk for obstructive sleep apnea;
  - From 52 to 100 mm^2 → intermediate risk for obstructive sleep apnea; and
  - Greater than 110 mm^2 → low risk for obstructive sleep apnea.

An additional useful measurement is the basion to hard palate linear dimension. Although it does not directly correlate with obstructive SDB risk level, this measurement can be particularly useful in children and adolescents undergoing

orthodontic growth modification, and can be used to compare the effects of intervention before, during, and after treatment. The total volume measurement can also be used to compare the airway volume in these patients. For example, if an adolescent is undergoing palatal expansion with orthodontic treatment, or an adult is having orthognathic surgery for jaw realignment, this tool can provide useful information on the effects of the intervention on the airway.

In addition to airway analysis and dimensions, there are several other developmental features that should also be analyzed,[1] specifically:

- Maxillary constriction and shallow palate;
- Mandibular retrognathia;
- A small mandible in the transverse dimension;
- Mandibular and palatal tori, which can crowd the tongue;
- Tooth crowding;
- Retroclination of the anterior teeth; and
- Posterior cross-bite.

Maxillary constriction is a common craniofacial abnormality that can contribute to abnormal positioning of the tongue, and can be seen in obligate mouth breathers, such as posterior posturing of the tongue, which can constrict the airway. Several measurements can easily be acquired on a CBCT to evaluate the palatal dimensions. In an adult, a palatal height index, as described by Korkhaus, is a simple formula that can be used to help determine if the palatal vault is too shallow, or the maxilla too constricted. The palatal height index is:

Palatal height index = palatal height × 100/ Posterior arch width.

This dimension is measured in the coronal plane at the level of the first molars. The posterior

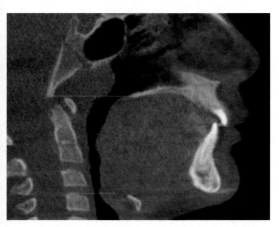

Fig. 12. Sagittal cone beam computed tomography with parallel lines drawn from the basion point to posterior nasal spine, and the level of C4, used for airway measurement boundaries.

arch width is the dimension between the midsagittal plane of the permanent maxillary first molars. The deepest part of the tooth's occlusal surface central groove can be used as a reference point for the midsagittal plane of the molars, because it can be reliably detected and used as a measurement point before and after palatal expansion. The palatal height measurement is a perpendicular line that connects the posterior arch width line to the deepest point of the hard palate, at the midline of the palate (**Fig. 14**). The formula is a percentage, and normal is considered 42%. If this dimension is significantly greater than 42%, the maxillary arch is inferred to be constricted. If the dimension is significantly less than 42%, the palate is inferred to be shallow (**Fig. 15**). Either a shallow or a constricted palatal vault can contribute to posterior posturing of the tongue.

The position of the mandible and maxilla must be evaluated for growth disturbances and altered position, which may cause constriction of the airway, such as in mandibular retrognathia.[10] This can be done by evaluating the relationship of the jaws to the skull base, using cephalometric measurements (**Fig. 16**).[11–13]

TREATMENT MODALITIES

Practitioners who use CBCT technology are in a unique position to evaluate their patients for obstructive SDB. In the pediatric population, pedodontists and orthodontists have the unique advantage of working with populations whose breathing disorders have not yet been diagnosed, and who are at a stage of development at which growth patterns are still easily modifiable for

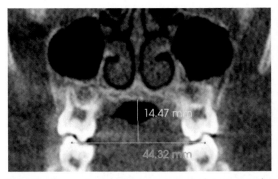

Fig. 15. Coronal cone beam computed tomography shows the anatomic landmarks of a subnormal palatal height index measurement (shallow palate).

treatment of obstructive SDB. Palatal expansion can be used to increase the transverse dimension of the palate, reducing palatal and nasal cavity constriction.

For adults, common medical treatments for obstructive SDB include medications, oral appliances, weight loss, and the use of continuous positive airway pressure devices. Surgical interventions include turbinectomy, septorhinoplasty, uvulopharyngopalatoplasty, genioglossus advancement, hyoid suspension, maxillomandibular advancement, and adjunctive procedures like bariatric surgery.

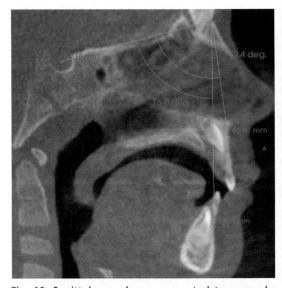

Fig. 16. Sagittal cone beam computed tomography with cephalometric analysis for evaluating anterior–posterior skeletal discrepancies of the maxilla and mandible in relation to the skull base. The Sella–Nasion A point and Sella–Nasion B point angle measurements are used to determine the position of the jaws in relation to the skull base. Smaller jaws predispose to narrowing of the oropharyngeal airway.

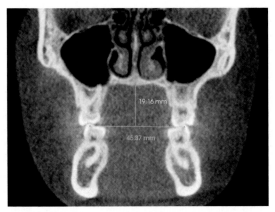

Fig. 14. Coronal cone beam computed tomography demonstrates the anatomic landmarks that are used for palatal height index measurement. This is an example of a normal palatal height index.

WHAT THE REFERRING PHYSICIAN NEEDS TO KNOW

An increased awareness and understanding of malocclusion and craniofacial anatomic structures should be viewed as more of a symptom than a distinct disease, and a better understanding of the interrelatedness between malocclusion and SDB and obstructive sleep apnea can improve diagnosis and treatment outcomes. The ability to identify known dentofacial anatomic risk indicators can help dentists and physicians to collaborate in providing coordinated care for patients with and at risk for obstructive sleep apnea and SDB.

SUMMARY

CBCT can be a readily available, inexpensive, noninvasive imaging modality that can identify obstructions and constrictions through the nasopharynx, oropharynx, and laryngopharynx. It can provide detailed dimensions and anatomic information that can identify risk levels and risk predictors for patients diagnosed with, or suspected to be at risk for obstructive sleep apnea and SDB. CBCT can also identify certain anatomic relationships, which can lead to properly identifying those at risk for obstructive sleep apnea and SDB. A thorough understanding of the anatomy, disease risks, at-risk populations, and how to perform a radiographic upper airway analysis are all critical skills and knowledge sets for successful treatment of a complicated and multifactorial medical condition.

REFERENCES

1. Boyd KL, Sheldon SH. Childhood sleep-disorder breathing: a dental perspective. In: Sheldon, Kryger, Ferber, et al, editors. Principles and practice of pediatric sleep medicine. 2nd edition. Philadelphia: WB Saunders; 2013. p. 273–9.
2. Koenig LJ, Harnsberger HR. Anatomy—oral cavity. In: Diagnostic imaging oral and maxillofacial. 1st edition. Amirsys; 2012. p. I-1-2–2-20.
3. Macari A, Bitar M, Ghafari J. New insights on age-related association between nasopharyngeal airway clearance on facial orphology. Orthod Craniofac Res 2012;15:188–97.
4. Vig K. Nasal obstruction and facial growth: the strength of evidence for clinical assumptions. Am J Orthod Dentofacial Orthop 1998;113:603–11.
5. Denolf P, Vanderveken O, Marklund M, et al. The status of cephalometry in the prediction of non-CPAP treatment outcome in obstructive sleep apnea patients. Sleep Med Rev 2016;27:56–73.
6. Ludlow J, Ivanovic M. Comparative dosimetry of dental CBCT devices and 64-slice CT for oral and maxillofacial radiology. Oral Surg Oral Med Oral Pathol Oral Radiol Endod 2008;106:106–14.
7. Pauwels R, Beinsberger J, Collaert B, et al. Effective dose range for dental cone beam computed tomography scanners. Eur J Radiol 2012;81:267–71.
8. Schendel S, Jacobson R, Khalessi S. Airway growth and development: a computerized 3-dimensional analysis. J Oral Maxillofac Surg 2012;70:2174–83.
9. Chiang C, Jeffres M, Miller A, et al. Three-dimensional airway evaluation in 387 subjects from one university orthodontic clinic using cone-beam computed tomography. Angle Orthod 2012;82(6):985–92.
10. Bitar M, Macari A, Ghafari J. Correspondence between subjective and linear measurements of the palatal airway on lateral cephalometric radiographs. Arch Otolaryngol Head Neck Surg 2010;1:43–7.
11. Celikoglu M, Bayram M, Sekerci A, et al. Comparison of pharyngeal airway volume among different vertical skeletal patterns: a cone-beam computed tomography study. Angle Orthod 2014;84(5):782–7.
12. Abramson Z, Susarla S, Troulis M, et al. Age-related changes of the upper airway assessed by 3-dimensional computed tomography. J Craniofac Surg 2009;20:657–63.
13. Chang Y, Koenig L, Pruszynski JE, et al. Dimensional changes of upper airway after rapid maxillary expansion: a prospective cone-beam computed tomographic study. Am J Orthod Dentofacial Orthop 2013;143:462–70.

Moving?

Make sure your subscription moves with you!

To notify us of your new address, find your **Clinics Account Number** (located on your mailing label above your name), and contact customer service at:

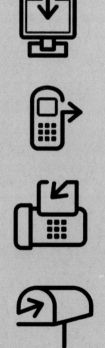

Email: journalscustomerservice-usa@elsevier.com

800-654-2452 (subscribers in the U.S. & Canada)
314-447-8871 (subscribers outside of the U.S. & Canada)

Fax number: 314-447-8029

Elsevier Health Sciences Division
Subscription Customer Service
3251 Riverport Lane
Maryland Heights, MO 63043

*To ensure uninterrupted delivery of your subscription, please notify us at least 4 weeks in advance of move.